Appalachian Whitewater

The Southern States

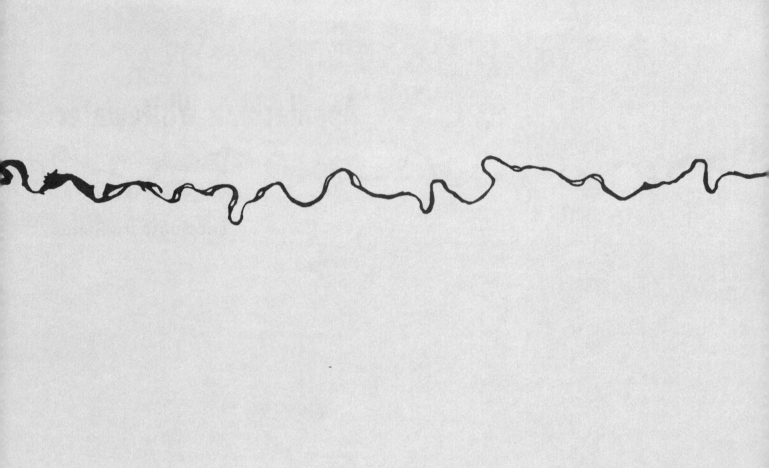

Appalachian Whitewater

The Southern States

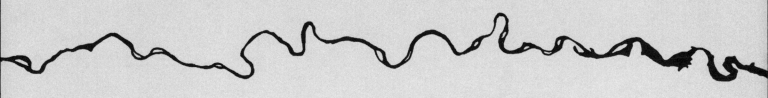

THIRD EDITION

The Premier Canoeing

and Kayaking Streams

of Alabama, Georgia,

Kentucky, Maryland,

North Carolina, South Carolina,

Tennessee, Virginia, and

West Virginia

Bob Sehlinger
Don Otey
Bob Benner
William Nealy
Ed Grove
Charlie Walbridge
and Bob Lantz

Menasha Ridge Press
Birmingham, Alabama

Copyright © 1988, 1998 by Bob Sehlinger, Don Otey,
Bob Benner, William Nealy, Ed Grove, Charlie Walbridge,
and Bob Lantz

Third edition, first printing
Printed in the United States of America

Library of Congress Cataloging-in-Publication Data:
Appalachian whitewater
Compiled by Bob Sehlinger and others.
Contents: v. 1. The Southern states
1. White-water canoeing—Appalachian region—Guide books.
2. Kayak touring—Appalachian region—Guide books.
3. Appalachian region—description and travel—Guide books.
I. Sehlinger, Bob, 1945-
GV776A55A67   1986   917.5   85-29762
ISBN 0-89732-242-8

Cover photo © Brian Gomsak
Cover design by Grant Tatum
Book design and river ornaments by B. Williams & Associates
Typeset by Bud Zehmer and Grant Tatum

Menasha Ridge Press
700 South 28th Street, Suite 206
Birmingham, Alabama 35233-3417
(800) 247-9437
www.menasharidge.com

Contents

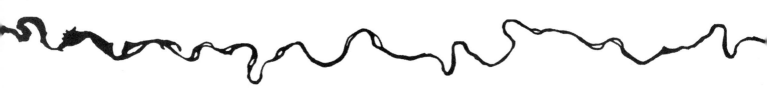

The Appalachian Mountain System

To appreciate the variety of whitewater opportunities described in this guidebook, it is good to begin with a brief discussion of Appalachian geography. The Appalachian Mountain system extends from the Gaspé Peninsula in Quebec, Canada, southwestward 1,500 miles to northern Georgia and Alabama. Only 80 miles wide in its northernmost reaches, the mountain range broadens to a considerable 350 miles in the south. Elevations vary from 300 feet above sea level at the far eastern edge of the range to lofty peaks exceeding 6,000 feet. New Hampshire and North Carolina have many of the highest mountains, and the highest peak in the range is Mount Mitchell in North Carolina with an elevation of 6,684 feet.

The Appalachian Mountains are seldom considered in their entirety. Explored, settled, and named by people from different nationalities over more than a hundred years, the Appalachians are more familiar to most of us when discussed in terms of component subranges. Extending southwest from Quebec and Maine are the White Mountains with their Presidential Range containing Mount Washington, the highest peak in the northeastern Appalachians at 6,288 feet, well above treeline at this latitude. Just west of the White Mountains are the Green Mountains, which become the Berkshires in Massachusetts. Covering parts of Vermont, Massachusetts, and Connecticut, the Green Mountains attain their highest elevations in Vermont, where summits range from 2,000 to 4,000 feet. Both the Green and the White Mountains are beautifully forested and embellished by spectacular highland lakes, a legacy of their history of glaciation.

Northwest of the Hudson River in New York are the Adirondacks, and to the west, the Catskills. A long plateau carved by many rivers runs southwest from the Catskills. This feature is known as the Allegheny Plateau in the north and as the Cumberland Plateau in the south. The Allegheny Plateau runs from the Mohawk Valley in New York to southeastern Kentucky. The Cumberland Plateau encompasses much of southeastern Kentucky,

east-central Tennessee, and northeastern Alabama. For the most part the Allegheny Plateau, which contains the Catskills and the Pocono and Allegheny Mountains of Pennsylvania and northern West Virginia, is more rugged and mountainlike than the sandstone ridges of the Cumberland Plateau.

The Blue Ridge Mountains begin in southeastern Pennsylvania and extend south to northeastern Georgia and northwestern South Carolina. To the immediate west of the Blue Ridge are the Cumberland Mountains of western Virginia, the Pisgah, Bald, and Black Mountains of North Carolina, and the Unicois, containing the Great Smoky Mountains, in North Carolina and Tennessee. These ranges boast some of the highest summits in the Appalachian system, as well as some of the greatest diversity of plant and animal life. Trees that are typical of northern states, such as spruce, birch, hemlock, and fir, grow on many of these southern mountaintops.

The Blue Ridge and its adjacent ranges are separated from the Allegheny and Cumberland Plateaus to the west by a series of river valleys known collectively as the Great Appalachian Valley. Beginning in the north with the St. Lawrence River valley and moving southwest, the Hudson River valley in New York, the Kittatinny valley in New Jersey, the Lebanon and Cumberland valleys in Pennsylvania and Maryland, the Shenandoah valley in Virginia, the Tennessee valley in Tennessee, and the Coosa valley in Georgia and Alabama all combine to form the Great Valley. While some sections of the Great Valley are broad and verdant, much consists of long, narrow, steep parallel ridges.

Born of powerful upheavals within the earth's crust and forged by the relentless force of moving water on the surface of the continent, the Appalachians are among the oldest mountains on earth. Yet, old as the mountains are, some of the rivers within the Appalachian system are older. Northeast of the New River in Virginia, the major Appalachian rivers flow into the Atlantic Ocean, sometimes through dramatic passages called water gaps.

Southwest of the New, however, the rivers (with only a couple of exceptions) flow to the Ohio River. During the faulting and folding which thrust the mountains up, these ancient west-flowing rivers were blocked in their course to the prehistoric sea which once covered mid-America. During the ensuing millennia, these rivers sculpted the landscape of the eastern United States, carving new routes to the sea and in the process creating the spectacular canyons and gorges which make the Appalachians a joy to the whitewater boater.

Water is, of course, the cutting agent, and the Appalachians generally have an abundance of this resource. Owing in part to its elevation, the Appalachian system receives an abundance of rainfall, exceeded in the United States only along the northwest Pacific coast.

Much of the annual rainfall, averaging 69 inches a year over most of the system, comes in great downpours. The brevity of these downpours, coupled with the steep gradient of many streams, accounts for water levels changing radically in very little time.

There is enough whitewater in the Appalachians to last the most avid paddler a lifetime. Many smaller streams are only occasionally runnable, but the larger ones, as well as those which are dam-controlled, are runnable year-round. Level of difficulty ranges from the splashy and scenic Class I to the virtually unrunnable. Throughout, the scenery is often spectacular, and river travel is frequently the only means of enjoying a true wilderness environment in the heavily populated eastern United States.

Stream Dynamics

Understanding hydrology—how rivers are formed and how they affect our activities—is at the very heart of paddling. To aid the paddler, we discuss the effects on paddling of seasonal variations of rainfall, water temperature, and volume, velocity, gradient, and stream morphology.

The most basic concept about water that all paddlers must understand is, of course, the hydrologic or water cycle, which moves water from the earth to the atmosphere and back again. Several things happen to water that falls to the earth: it becomes surface runoff that drains directly into rivers or their tributaries, or it is retained by the soil and used by plants, or it may be returned directly to the atmosphere through evaporation, or else it becomes groundwater by filtering down through subsoil and layers of rock. About 40 percent of each year's rainfall runs either directly into the streams or through the ground and then into the streams, and seasonal variations in the flow levels of watercourses are based on fluctuations in rainfall.

Local soil conditions have a great deal to do with stream flow, as do plant life, terrain slope, ground cover, and air temperature. In summer, during the peak growing season, water is used more readily by plants, and higher air temperatures encourage increased evaporation. The fall and winter low-water periods are caused by decreased precipitation, although since the ground may be frozen and plant use of water is for the most part halted, abnormally high amounts of rain, or water from melting snow, can cause flash floods because surface runoff is high—there's no place for the water to go but into creeks and rivers. Though surface runoff is first to reach the river, it is groundwater that keeps many larger streams flowing during rainless periods. Drought can lower the water table drastically. Soil erosion is related to the surface runoff—hilly land in intensive agricultural use is a prime target for loss of topsoil and flash flooding, as are areas where road building, other construction, or intensive logging is taking place.

The Water Cycle

The earth's water moves in a never-ending cycle from the atmosphere to the land and back to the atmosphere again. Although approximately 97 percent of the earth's water is contained in the oceans, with most of the remainder in ice caps, glaciers, and groundwater, atmospheric water and water in streams is what most concerns us. Atmospheric moisture flows constantly over the Appalachians, and the amount that falls on the region now is much the same as it was when only the Indians worried about dried-up springs and floods.

Beginning the cycle with the oceans, which cover some 75 percent of the earth's surface, the movement of the water follows these steps (see Figure 1):

1. Water from the surface of the oceans (and from the lands between) evaporates into the atmosphere as vapor. This water vapor rises and moves with the winds.
2. Eventually, either over the ocean or over the land, this moisture is condensed by various processes and falls back to the earth as precipitation. Some falls on the ocean; some falls on the land, where it becomes of particular concern to people.
3. Of the rain, snow, sleet, or hail that falls on the land, some runs off over the land, some soaks down into the ground to replenish the great groundwater reservoir, some is taken up by the roots of plants and is transpired as water vapor, and some is again evaporated directly into the atmosphere.
4. The water that flows over the land or soaks down to become groundwater feeds the streams that eventually flow back into the oceans, completing the cycle.

The key steps in this great circulation of the earth's moisture are evaporation, precipitation, transpiration, and stream flow. All occur constantly and simultaneously over the earth. Over the Appalachian river basins, the quantities in any part of the cycle vary widely from day to day or from season to season. Precipitation may be excessive or may stop entirely for days or even weeks.

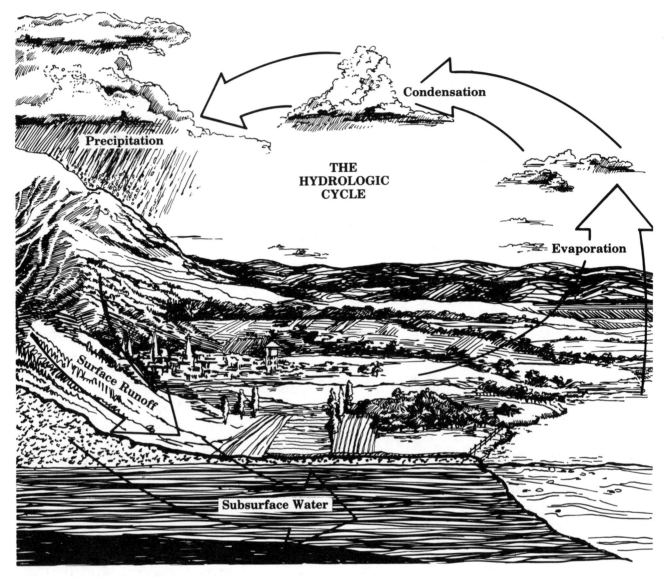

Figure 1. The Hydrologic Cycle

Evaporation and transpiration demands are low in winter but high in July and August. Stream flow depends on the interrelation of these processes.

Climate in the Appalachians

The mountains generally have cooler and wetter climates than neighboring low-lying elevations, with mean temperature dropping approximately three degrees Fahrenheit per 1,000 foot rise in elevation. The effects of mountains on air flow make the relation between elevation and precipitation a variable one. The dependence of temperature and precipitation on elevation plays an important role in determining the plant and animal life found in the area.

Water Temperature

Water temperature is another important factor to be considered by paddlers because of the obvious dangers of encountering cold water when they aren't prepared for it.

Surface water temperatures tend to follow air temperatures. Generally, the shallower the stream or reservoir, the closer the water temperature will be to the air temperature. Streams in the Appalachians show a wide variation in temperature throughout the year, ranging from a low of 32°F in winter to a high of about 88°F on some days in July, August, and early September. Streams also show a daily variation: the smaller the stream, the greater the variation, with the least variation occurring in large rivers. The Tennessee River may change only one or two degrees in a day, while changes in a small stream can be almost equal to the range in the day's air temperature.

Coal-burning steam plants, other non-hydroelectric power generation plants, and industrial users may influence the water temperature in some rivers through thermal discharges. Usually, the added heat is lost within 20 miles downstream from the discharge point, but this heat loss depends on the amount of water used, the temperature of the wastewater, the size of the discharge stream, the air temperature, and other factors.

Stream Evolution and Morphology

Often, someone new to boating will fix an inquisitive stare at a large boulder in midstream and ask, "How in blazes did that thing get in the middle of the river?" The frequency of being asked this and similar questions about the river has prompted us to include in this book a brief look at river dynamics, which is basically the relationship between geology and hydraulics, or, expressed differently, what effect flowing water has on the land surface and, conversely, how the land surface modifies the flow of water.

We all know that water flows downhill, moving from a higher elevation to a lower elevation and ultimately flowing into the sea, but contrary to what many people believe, the water on its downhill journey does not flow as smoothly as we might imagine the water in our home plumbing flows. Instead, to varying degrees, depending on the geology, it has to pound and fight every inch of the way, squeezing around obstructions, ricocheting from rock to rock, and funneling from side to side. Almost any river's course is tortuous at best, because the land was there first and is very reluctant to surrender to the moving water. Therefore it does so very slowly and grudgingly. In other words, the water must literally carve out a place in the land through which to flow. It accomplishes this work through erosion.

There are three types of moving water erosion: downward erosion, lateral erosion, and headward erosion. All three represent the wearing away of the land by the water. Downward erosion is at work continuously on all rivers and can be loosely defined as the moving water's wearing away the bottom of the river, eroding the rocks of the river bottom, allowing the river to descend deeper and deeper into the ground. A graphic example of downward erosion in its purest form is a river that runs through a vertical-walled canyon or gorge. Here the resistance of the rock forming the canyon walls has limited erosion to the sides. Down and down the river cuts without proportional expansion of its width. A gorge or canyon is formed this way.

Most of the time, however, two and usually three kinds of erosion are working simultaneously. When the water, through downward erosion, for example, cuts into the bottom of the river, it encounters geological substrata of varying resistance and composition. A layer of clay might overlay a shelf of sandstone, under which may be limestone or even granite. Since the water is moving downhill at an angle, the flowing water at the top of a mountain might be working against a completely different type of geological substratum than the water halfway down or at the foot of the mountain. Thus, to carve its channel, the water has to work harder in some spots than in others.

Where current crosses a seam marking the boundary between geological substrata of differing resistance to erosion, an interesting phenomenon occurs. Imagine that upstream of this seam the water has been flowing over sandstone, which is worn away by the erosive action of the current at a rather slow rate. As the current crosses the seam, it encounters limestone, which erodes much faster. Downward erosion wears through the limestone relatively quickly while the sandstone on top remains little changed over the same period. The result is a waterfall (see Figure 2). It may be only a foot high, or it may be 100 feet high, depending on the thickness of the layer eaten away. The process is complete when the less resistant substratum is eroded and the water again encounters sandstone or another equally resistant formation. The evolution of a waterfall by downward erosion is similar to covering your wooden porch stairs with snow so that from top to bottom the stairs resemble a nice snowy hill in the park, with the normal shape of the stairs being hidden. Wood (the stairs) and snow can both be eaten away by water. Obviously though, the water will melt the snow much faster than it will rot the wood. Thus, if a tiny stream of water is launched downhill from the top of

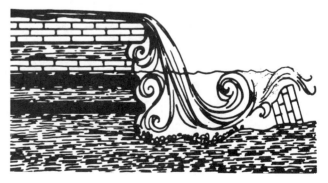

Figure 2. Downward Erosion: Waterfalls

the stairs, it will melt through the snow quickly, not stopping until it reaches the more resistant wood on the next stair down. Through a similar process, erosion forms a waterfall in nature.

Once a waterfall has formed, regardless of its size, headward erosion comes into play. Headward erosion is the wearing away of the base of the waterfall. This action erodes the substrata in an upstream direction toward the headwaters or source of the stream, thus it is called headward erosion. Water falling over the edge of the waterfall lands below with substantial force. As it hits the surface of the water under the falls, it causes a depression in the surface that water from downstream rushes to fill in. This is a hydraulic or hole. Continuing through the surface water, the falling current hits the bottom of the stream. Some of the water is disbursed in an explosive manner, some deflected downstream, and some drawn back to the top where it is recirculated to refill the depression made by yet more falling current. A great deal of energy is expended in this process, and the ensuing cyclical turbulence, which combines with bits of rock to make an abrasive mixture, carves slowly away at the rock base of the falls. If the falls are small, the turbulence may simply serve to smooth out the drop, turning a vertical drop into a slanting drop. If the falls are large, the base of the falls may be eroded, leaving the top of the falls substantially intact but precariously unsupported. After a time, the overhang thus created will surrender to gravity and fall into the river. Thus we see one way that huge

boulders happen to arrive in the middle of the river. Naturally the process is ongoing, and the altered facade of the waterfall is immediately attacked by the currents.

Lateral erosion is the wearing away of the sides of the river by the moving current. While occurring continuously on most rivers to a limited degree, lateral erosion is much more a function of volume and velocity (collectively known as discharge and expressed in cubic feet per second, cfs) than either downward or headward erosion. In other words, as more water is added to a river (beyond that simply required to cover its bottom), the increase in the volume and the speed of the current causes significant additional lateral erosion, while headward and downward erosion remain comparatively constant. Thus, as a river swells with spring rain, the amount of water in the river increases. Since water is noncompressible, the current rises on the banks and through erosion tries to enlarge the riverbed laterally to accommodate the extra volume. Effects of this activity can be observed every year following seasonal rains. Even small streams can widen their beds substantially by eroding large chunks of the banks and carrying them downstream. Boulders and trees in the river are often the result of lateral erosion undercutting the bank.

Through a combination of downward erosion, lateral erosion, and meandering, running water can carve broad valleys between mountains and deep canyons through solid rock. Downward and lateral erosion act on the terrain to determine the morphology (depth, width, shape,

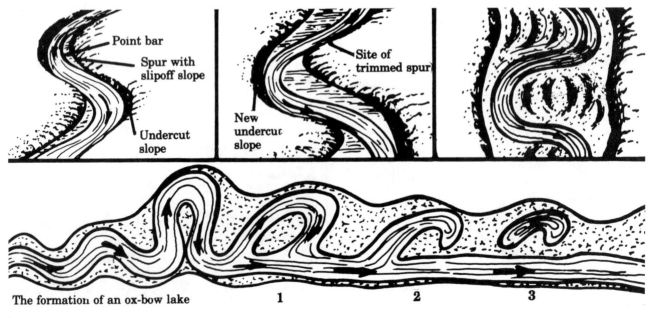

The formation of an ox-bow lake   1   2   3

Figure 3. Floodplain Features

and course) of a river. Headward erosion serves to smooth out the rough spots that remain.

Curves in a river are formed much as waterfalls are formed: as the water follows the path of least resistance, its path twists and turns as it is diverted by resistant substrata. Rivers constantly change and do not continue indefinitely in their courses once they are formed. Water is continuously seeking to decrease the energy required to move from the source of the river to the mouth. Understanding this fact is essential to understanding erosion.

Moving water erodes the outside of river bends and deposits much of the eroded matter on the inside of the turn, thereby forming a sand or gravel bar. Jagged turns are changed to sweeping bends. The result in more mature streams is a meander, or the formation of a series of horseshoe-shaped and geometrically predictable loops in the river (see Figure 3). A series of such undulating loops markedly widens the valley floor. Often, as time passes, the current erodes the neck of a loop, creating an island in midstream and eliminating a curve in the river.

As we have observed, headward erosion works upstream to smooth out the waterfalls and rapids. Lateral erosion works to make more room for increased volume, and downward erosion deepens the bed and levels obstructions and irregularities. When a river is young (in the geological sense), it cuts downward and is diverted into sharp turns by differing resistance from underlying rock layers. As a stream matures, it carves a valley, sinking even deeper relative to sea level and leaving behind, in many instances, a succession of terraces marking previous valley floors.

In the theoretically mature stream, the bottom is smooth and undisturbed by obstructing boulders, rapids, or falls. Straight stretches in the river give way to serpentine meanders, and the river has a low gradient from the source to the sea. Of course, there are no perfect examples of a mature stream, although rivers such as the Ohio and the Mississippi tend to approach the mature end of the spectrum. In contrast, a stream exhibiting a high gradient and frequent rapids and sharp turns is described as a young stream in the evolutional sense of the word (stream maturity having more to do with the evolutional development of a stream than with actual age; see Figure 4).

All streams carry a load that consists of all the particles, large and small, that are a result of the multiple forms of erosion we have discussed. The load, then, is solid matter transported by the current. Rocky streams at high altitudes carry the smallest loads. Their banks and bottoms are more resistant to erosion, and their tributary drainages are usually small. Scarcity of load is evident in

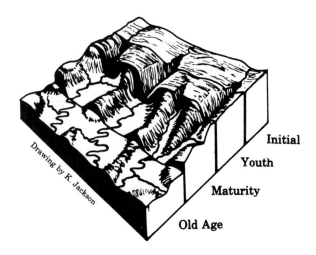

Figure 4. Stream Dissection Cycle: Evolution of a Landscape

the clarity of the water. Rivers such as the Mississippi and Ohio carry enormous loads collected from numerous tributaries as well as from their own banks and bottoms. Water in these and in similarly large rivers is almost always dark and murky with sediment. Since it takes a lot of energy to move a load, many rivers transport conspicuous (readily visible) loads only during rainy periods when they are high, fast, and powerful. When the high waters abate, there is insufficient energy to continue to transport the large load that then, for the most part, settles as silt or alluvium on the bottom of the stream.

Understanding stream dynamics gives any boater an added advantage in working successfully with the river. Knowledge of stream evolution and morphology tells a paddler where to find the strongest current and deepest channel, where rapids and falls are most likely to occur, and what to expect from a given river if the discharge increases or decreases. But more, understanding the river's evolution and continuing development contributes immeasurably to the paddler's aesthetic experience and allows for a communion and harmony with the river that otherwise might be superficial.

Components of Stream Flow

Being able to recognize potential river hazards depends on a practical knowledge of river hydrology—why the water flows the way it does. Since river channels vary greatly in depth and width and the composition of streambeds and their gradients also enter into the river's character, the major components of stream flow bear explanation.

Discharge is the volume of water moving past a given point of the river at any one time. The river current, or velocity, is commonly expressed as the speed of water movement in feet per second (fps), and stage is the river's height in feet based on an arbitrary measurement gauge. These terms are interrelated; higher water levels mean increased volume and velocity.

Another factor in assessing stream difficulty is gradient, which is expressed in feet per mile. As gradient increases, so does velocity. The streams profiled in this book have gradients that range from about 1 foot per mile to an astounding 200 feet per mile. The gradient in any stream or section of a stream changes with the landforms, the geology of the basin. If a river flows over rock or soil with varying resistance to erosion, ledges, waterfalls, and rapids sometimes form and dramatically affect gradient.

Velocity is also affected by the width and depth of the streams. Rapids form where streams are shallow and swift. Large obstructions in shallow streams of high velocity cause severe rapids. Within a given channel, there are likely to be rapids with different levels of difficulty. The current on straight sections of river is usually fastest in the middle. The depth of water in river bends is determined by flow rates and soil types. Water tends to cut away the land and form deep holes on the outsides of bends where the current is the swiftest.

Paddler Information

Rating the River

For years concerned paddlers have sought to rate rivers objectively, and central among their tools has been the International Scale of River Difficulty. While certainly useful, the International Scale (provided in part V of the Safety Code of the American Whitewater Affiliation found later in this chapter) lacks precision and invites subjective, judgmental error. A more objective yardstick is the River Rating Chart, which allows boaters to assign points to a stream based on various aspects of river difficulty (see Table 2). While more complex, it does succeed in describing a river more or less as it really is. Gone is the common confusion of a single rapid's being described as Class II by the veteran while the novice perceives a roaring Class IV. Also eliminated is the double standard by which a river is rated Class III for open canoes but only Class II for decked boats. Additionally, this system helps eliminate regional classification discrepancies. Points are awarded as prescribed for conditions observed on the day the river is to be run. The total number of points describes the general level of difficulty.

Once the basic difficulty rating is calculated for a river, however, how is it to be matched against the skill level of a prospective paddler? The American Whitewater Affiliation relates the River Rating Chart back to the International Scale of River Difficulty and to traditional paddler classifications (see Table 1).

Making the foregoing comparisons helps, but only to the extent that the individual paddler understands the definitions of "Practiced Beginner," "Intermediate," "Experienced," and so on. Most paddlers find these traditional titles ambiguous and hard to differentiate and probably classify themselves according to self-image. When this occurs, we are back to where we started.

Rating the Paddler

Correctly observing the need for increased objectivity in rating paddlers as well as in rating rivers, several paddling clubs have developed self-evaluation systems where paddlers are awarded points that correspond to the point scale of the River Rating Chart (Table 2). Thus an individual can determine a point total through self-evaluation and compare his or her skill, in quantified terms, to any river rated through use of the chart. The individual paddler, for instance, may compile 18 points through self-evaluation and note that this rating compares favorably with a river difficulty rating of 17 points and unfavorably with a difficulty rating of 23 points. It should be emphasized here, however, that river ratings via the river difficulty chart pertain to a river only on a given day and at a specific water level.

Table 1. A Comparison of Ratings

International Scale	Approximate Difficulty	River Ratings (from Table 2)	Approximate Paddler Skill Required
I	Easy	0-7	Practiced Beginner
II	Requires Care	8-14	Intermediate
III	Difficult	15-21	Experienced
IV	Very Difficult	22-28	Highly Skilled (Several years with organized group)
V	Exceedingly Difficult	29-35	Team of Experts
VI	Utmost Difficulty- Near Limit of Navigability	36-42	Team of Experts with every precaution

Table 2. River Rating Chart*

Points	Obstacles, Rocks, and Trees	Waves	Turbulence	Bends	Length (feet)	Gradient (ft/mile)	Resting or Rescue Spots	Water Velocity (mph)	Width and Depth	Temp (°F)	Accessibility
0	None	Few inches high, avoidable	None	Few, very gradual	<100	<5, regular slope	Almost anywhere	<3	Narrow (≤75 ft) and shallow (≤3 ft)	>65	Road along river
1	Few; passage almost straight through	Low (up to 1 ft), regular, avoidable	Minor eddies	Many, gradual	100–700	5–15, regular slope		3–6	Wide (>75 ft) and shallow (≤3 ft)	55–65	<1 hour travel by foot or water
2	Courses easily recognizable	Low to med. (up to 3 ft), regular, avoidable	Medium eddies	Few, sharp, blind; scouting necessary	701–5,000	16–40, ledges or steep drops		7–10	Narrow (≤75 ft) and deep (>3 ft)	45–54	1 hour to 1 day travel by foot or water
3	Maneuvering course not easily recognizable	Med. to large (up to 5 ft), mostly regular, avoidable	Strong eddies and cross-currents		>5,000	>40, steep drops, small falls	A good one below every danger spot	>10 or flood	Wide (>75ft) and deep (>3 ft)	<45	>1 day travel by foot or water
4	Intricate maneuvering; course hard to recognize	Large, irregular, avoidable; or med. to large, unavoidable	Very strong eddies, strong cross-currents								
5	Course tortuous, frequent scouting needed	Large, irregular, avoidable; or med. to large, unavoidable	Large-scale eddies and cross-currents, some up and down								
6	Very tortuous; always scout from shore	Very large (>5 ft), irregular, unavoidable; special equipment required					Almost none				

Source: Prepared by Guidebook Committee—AWA (from "American White Water," Winter 1957).

*To rate a river, match the characteristics of the river with descriptions in *each* column. Add the points from each column for a total river rating.

Some paddler self-evaluation systems seem to emphasize strength and individual fitness at the expense of river skills, perhaps encouraging fit but inexperienced individuals onto rivers too difficult for them. To shift the focus towards river skills, author Bob Sehlinger has redefined the paddler rating system, creating a more complex, exhaustive, and objective paddler self-evaluation. Heavy emphasis is placed on paddling skills, with descriptions adopted from several different evaluation formats, including a nonnumerical system proposed by Dick Schwind ("Rating System for Boating Difficulty," *American Whitewater Journal*, vol. 20, num. 3, May/June 1975).

The paddler rating system that follows will provide a numerical point summary. The paddler can then use this information to gauge whether a river of a given ranking is within his or her capabilities.

Paddler Rating System

Instructions: All items, except the first, carry points that are added to obtain an overall rating. All items except "Rolling Ability" apply to both open and decked boats. Rate open and decked boat skills separately.

1. Prerequisite Skills. Before paddling on moving current, the paddler should:

a. Have some swimming ability
b. Be able to paddle instinctively on nonmoving water (on lakes). (This presumes knowledge of basic strokes.)
c. Be able to guide and control the canoe from either side without changing paddling sides
d. Be able to guide and control the canoe (or kayak) while paddling backwards
e. Be able to move the canoe (or kayak) laterally
f. Understand the limitations of the boat
g. Be practiced in "wet exit" if in a decked boat

2. Equipment. Award points on the suitability of your equipment to whitewater. Whether you own, borrow, or rent the equipment makes no difference. Award points for either Open Canoe or Decked Boat, not both.

Open Canoe

0 Points: Any canoe used for tandem with seats mounted too low to safely place the paddler's feet under while kneeling; any canoe used for solo that offers no mid-area braced kneeling position
1 Point: Canoe with moderate rocker and full depth; should be at least 14 feet long for tandem and at least 13 feet for solo and have bow and stern painters

2 Points: Whitewater canoe with strong rocker design, full bow, full depth amidships, no keel; meets or exceeds minimum length requirements as described under "1 Point"; made of hand-laid fiberglass, Kevlar, Marlex, or ABS Royalex; has bow and stern painters. Or a canoe as described under "1 Point" but with extra flotation.
3 Points: A whitewater canoe as described under "2 Points" but with extra flotation

Decked Boat (K1 or 2, C1 or 2)

0 Points: Any decked boat lacking full flotation, spray skirt, or foot braces
1 Point: Any fully equipped, decked boat with a wooden frame
2 Points: Decked boat with full flotation, spray skirt and foot braces; has grab loops; made of hand-laid fiberglass, Marlex, or Kevlar
3 Points: Decked boat with foam wall reinforcement and split flotation; Neoprene spray skirt; has knee braces, foot braces, and grab loops; made of hand-laid fiberglass or Kevlar only

3. Experience. Compute the following to determine preliminary points, then convert the preliminary points to final points according to the conversion table. This is the only evaluation item where it is possible to accrue more than 3 points.

Number of days spent paddling each year:

Class I rivers	x 1 =	____
Class II rivers	x 2 =	____
Class III rivers	x 3 =	____
Class IV rivers	x 4 =	____
Class V–VI rivers	x 5 =	____
Preliminary subtotal	=	____
Number of years of paddling experience	x	____
Total preliminary points		____

Conversion Table

Preliminary Points	Final Points
0–20	0
21–60	1
61–100	2
101–200	3
201–300	4
301–up	5

4. Swimming

0   Points: Cannot swim
1   Point: Weak swimmer
2   Points: Average swimmer
3   Points: Strong swimmer (competition level or skin diver)

5. Stamina

0   Points: Cannot run a mile in 10 minutes or less
1   Point: Can run a mile in 7 to 10 minutes
2   Points: Can run a mile in less than 7 minutes

6. Upper Body Strength

0   Points: Cannot do 15 push-ups
1   Point: Can do 15 to 25 push-ups
2   Points: Can do more than 25 push-ups

7. Boat Control

0   Points: Can keep boat fairly straight
1   Point: Can maneuver in moving water; can avoid big obstacles
2   Points: Can maneuver in heavy water; knows how to work with the current
3   Points: Finesse in boat placement in all types of water; uses current to maximum advantage

8. Aggressiveness

0   Points: Does not play or work river at all
1   Point: Timid; plays a little on familiar streams
2   Points: Plays a lot; works most rivers hard
3   Points: Plays in heavy water with grace and confidence

9. Eddy Turns

0   Points: Has difficulty making eddy turns from moderate current
1   Point: Can made eddy turns in either direction from moderate current; can enter moderate current from eddy
2   Points: Can catch medium eddies in either direction from heavy current; can enter very swift current from eddy
3   Points: Can catch small eddies in heavy current

10. Ferrying

0   Points: Cannot ferry
1   Point: Can ferry upstream and downstream in moderate current
2   Points: Can ferry upstream in heavy current; can ferry downstream in moderate current
3   Points: Can ferry upstream and downstream in heavy current

11. Water Reading

0   Points: Often in error
1   Point: Can plan route in short rapid with several well spaced obstacles
2   Points: Can confidently run lead through continuous Class 2; can predict the effects of waves and holes on boat
3   Points: Can confidently run lead in continuous Class 3; has knowledge to predict and handle the effects of reversals, side currents, and turning drops

12. Judgment

0   Points: Often in error
1   Point: Has average ability to analyze difficulty of rapids
2   Points: Has good ability to analyze difficulty of rapids and make independent judgments as to which should not be run
3   Points: Has the ability to assist fellow paddlers in evaluating the difficulty of rapids; can explain subtleties to paddlers with less experience

13. Bracing

0   Points: Has difficulty bracing in Class 2 water
1   Point: Can correctly execute bracing strokes in Class 2 water
2   Points: Can correctly brace in intermittent whitewater with medium waves and vertical drops of 3 feet or less
3   Points: Can brace effectively in continuous whitewater with large waves and large vertical drops (4 feet and up)

14. Rescue Ability

0   Points: Self-rescue in flatwater
1   Point: Self-rescue in mild whitewater
2   Points: Self-rescue in Class 3; can assist others in mild whitewater
3   Points: Can assist others in heavy whitewater

15. Rolling Ability

0   Points: Can only roll in pool
1   Point: Can roll 3 out of 4 times in moving current

2 Points: Can roll 3 out of 4 times in Class 2 whitewater

3 Points: Can roll 4 out of 5 times in Class 3 and 4
whitewater

Add your points from items 2 through 15. To see what types of rivers might be appropriate for your skill level, compare your skill level rating to the river difficulty rating in Table 2. While these systems provide a better way to choose what rivers are appropriate for you than the International Scale of River Difficulty alone, there is no guarantee of a smooth trip.

Hazards and Safety

Hazardous situations likely to be encountered on the river must be identified and understood for safe paddling. The American Whitewater Affiliation's safety code is perhaps the most useful overall safety guideline available. (The much-discussed International Scale of River Difficulty is included in Part V of the code.)

Safety Code of the American Whitewater Affiliation

This code has been prepared using the best available information and has been reviewed by a broad cross section of whitewater experts. The code, however, is only a collection of guidelines. Attempts to minimize risks should be flexible—not constrained by a rigid set of rules. Varying conditions and group goals may combine with unpredictable circumstances to require alternate procedures.

I. Personal Preparedness and Responsibility

1. Be a competent swimmer, with the ability to handle yourself underwater.
2. Wear a life jacket. A snugly-fitting vest-type life preserver offers back and shoulder protection as well as the flotation needed to swim safely in whitewater.
3. Wear a solid, correctly-fitted helmet when upsets are likely. This is essential in kayaks or covered canoes and recommended for open canoeists using thigh straps and rafters running steep drops.
4. Do not boat out of control. Your skills should be sufficient to stop or reach shore before reaching danger. Do not enter a rapid unless you are reasonably sure that you can run it safely or swim it without injury.
5. Whitewater rivers contain many hazards that are not always easily recognized. The following are the most frequent killers:

A. High water. The river's speed and power increase tremendously as the flow increases, raising the difficulty of most rapids. Rescue becomes progressively harder as the water rises, adding to the danger. Floating debris and strainers make even an easy rapid quite hazardous. It is often misleading to judge the river level at the put-in, since a small rise in a wide, shallow place will be multiplied many times where the river narrows. Use reliable gauge information whenever possible, and be aware that sun on snowpack, hard rain, and upstream dam releases may greatly increase the flow.

B. Cold. Cold drains your strength and robs you of the ability to make sound decisions on matters affecting your survival. Cold water immersion, because of the initial shock and the rapid heat loss which follows, is especially dangerous. Dress appropriately for bad weather or sudden immersion in the water. When the water temperature is less than 50°F, a wetsuit or drysuit is essential for protection if you swim. Next best is wool or pile clothing under a waterproof shell. In this case, you should also carry waterproof matches and a change of clothing in a waterproof bag. If, after prolonged exposure, a person experiences uncontrollable shaking, loss of coordination, or difficulty speaking, he or she is hypothermic and needs your assistance.

C. Strainers. Brush, fallen trees, bridge pilings, undercut rocks, or anything else which allows river current to sweep through can pin boats and boaters against the obstacle. Water pressure on anything trapped this way can be overwhelming. Rescue is often extremely difficult. Pinning may occur in fast current, with little or no whitewater to warn of the danger.

D. Dams, weirs, ledges, reversals, holes, and hydraulics. When water drops over an obstacle, it curls back on itself, forming a strong upstream current which may be capable of holding a boat or a swimmer. Some holes make for excellent sport; others are proven killers. Paddlers who cannot recognize the differences should avoid all but the smallest holes. Hydraulics around man-made dams must be treated with utmost respect regardless of their height or the level of the river. Despite their seemingly benign appearance, they can create an almost escape-proof trap. The swimmer's only exit from the "drowning machine" is to dive below the surface where the downstream current is flowing beneath the reversal.

    E. Broaching. When a boat is pushed sideways against a rock by strong current, it may collapse and wrap. This is especially dangerous to kayak and decked canoe paddlers; these boats will collapse and the combination of indestructible hulls and tight outfitting may create a deadly trap. Even without entrapment, releasing pinned boats can be extremely time-consuming and dangerous. To avoid pinning, throw your weight downstream toward the rock. This allows the current to slide harmlessly underneath the hull.

6. Boating alone is discouraged. The minimum party is three people or two craft.

7. Have a frank knowledge of your boating ability, and don't attempt rivers or rapids that lie beyond your ability.

    A. Develop the paddling skills and teamwork required to match the river you plan to boat. Most good paddlers develop skills gradually, and attempts to advance too quickly will compromise your safety and enjoyment.

    B. Be in good physical and mental condition, consistent with the difficulties which may be expected. Make adjustments for loss of skills due to age, health, or fitness. Any health limitation must be explained to your fellow paddlers prior to starting the trip.

8. Be practiced in self-rescue, including escape from an overturned craft. The eskimo roll is strongly recommended for decked boaters who run rapids of Class IV or greater, or who paddle in cold environmental conditions.

9. Be trained in rescue skills, CPR, and first aid with special emphasis on recognizing and treating hypothermia. It may save your friend's life.

10. Carry equipment needed for unexpected emergencies, including footwear that will protect your feet when walking out, a throw rope, a knife, a whistle, and waterproof matches. If you wear eyeglasses, tie them on and carry a spare pair on long trips. Bring cloth repair tape on short runs, and a full repair kit on isolated rivers. Do not wear bulky jackets, ponchos, heavy boots, or anything else which could reduce your ability to survive a swim.

11. Despite the mutually supportive group structure described in this code, individual paddlers are ultimately responsible for their own safety, and must assume sole responsibility for the following decisions:

    A. The decision to participate on any trip. This includes an evaluation of the expected difficulty of the rapids under the conditions existing at the time of the put-in.

    B. The selection of appropriate equipment, including a boat design suited to their skills and the appropriate rescue and survival gear.

    C. The decision to scout any rapid, and to run or portage according to their best judgment. Other members of the group may offer advice, but paddlers should resist pressure from anyone to paddle beyond their skills. It is also their responsibility to decide whether to pass up any walk-out or take-out opportunity.

    D. All trip participants should constantly evaluate their own and their group's safety, voicing their concerns when appropriate and following what they believe to be the best course of action. Paddlers are encouraged to speak with anyone whose action on the water is dangerous, whether they are a part of your group or not.

II. Boat and Equipment Preparedness

1. Test new and different equipment under familiar conditions before relying on it for difficult runs. This is especially true when adopting a new boat design or outfitting system. Low-volume craft may present additional hazards to inexperienced or poorly conditioned paddlers.

2. Be sure your boat and gear are in good repair before starting a trip. The more isolated and difficult a run, the more rigorous this inspection should be.

3. Install flotation bags in non-inflatable craft, securely fixed in each end, designed to displace as much water as possible. Inflatable boats should have multiple air chambers and be test inflated before launching.

4. Have strong, properly sized paddles or oars for controlling your craft. Carry sufficient spares for the length and difficulty of the trip.

5. Outfit your boat safely. The ability to exit your boat quickly is an essential component of safety in rapids. It is your responsibility to see that there is absolutely nothing to cause entrapment when coming free of an upset craft. This includes:

    A. Spray covers that won't release reliably or that release prematurely.

B. Boat outfitting too tight to allow a fast exit, especially in low-volume kayaks or decked canoes. This includes low hung thwarts in canoes lacking adequate clearance for your feet and kayak footbraces which fail or allow your feet to become wedged under them.

C. Inadequately supported decks which collapse on a paddler's legs when a decked boat is pinned by water pressure. Inadequate clearance with the deck because of your size or build.

D. Loose ropes which cause entanglement. Beware of any length of loose line attached to a white-water boat. All items must be tied tightly and excess line eliminated; painters, throw lines, and safety rope systems must be completely and effectively stored. Do not knot the end of a rope, as it can get caught in cracks between rocks.

6. Provide ropes that permit you to hold on to your craft so that it may be rescued. The following methods are recommended:

A. Kayaks and covered canoes should have grab loops of 1/4"+ rope or equivalent webbing sized to admit a normal sized hand. Stern painters are permissible if properly secured.

B. Open canoes should have securely anchored bow and stern painters consisting of 8–10 feet of 1/4" line. These must be secured in such a way that they are readily accessible, but cannot come loose accidentally. Grab loops are acceptable, but are more difficult to reach after an upset.

C. Many rafts and dories have taut perimeter lines threaded through the loops provided. Footholds should be designed so that a paddler's feet cannot be forced through them, causing entrapment. Flip lines should be carefully and reliably stowed.

7. Know your craft's carrying capacity and how added loads affect boat handling in whitewater. Most rafts have a minimum crew size which can be added to on day trips or in easy rapids. Carrying more than two paddlers in an open canoe when running rapids is not recommended.

8. Car top racks must be strong and attach positively to the vehicle. Lash your boat to each crossbar, then tie the ends of the boat directly to the bumpers for added security. This arrangement should survive all but the most violent vehicle accident.

III. Group Preparedness and Responsibility

1. Organization. A river trip should be regarded as a common adventure by all participants, except on instructional or commercially guided trips as defined below. Participants share the responsibility for the conduct of the trip, and each participant is individually responsible for judging his or her own capabilities and for his or her own safety as the trip progresses. Participants are encouraged (but are not obligated) to offer advice and guidance for the independent consideration and judgment of others.

2. River Conditions. The group should have a reasonable knowledge of the difficulty of the run. Participants should evaluate this information and adjust their plans accordingly. If the run is exploratory or no one is familiar with the river, maps and guidebooks, if available, should be examined. The group should secure accurate flow information; the more difficult the run, the more important this will be. Be aware of possible changes in river level and how this will affect the difficulty of the run. If the trip involves tidal stretches, secure appropriate information on tides.

3. Group equipment should be suited to the difficulty of the river. The group should always have a throw line available, and one line per boat is recommended on difficult runs. The list may include: carabiners, prussick loops, first aid kit, flashlight, folding saw, fire starter, guidebooks, maps, food, extra clothing, and any other rescue or survival items suggested by conditions. Each item is not required on every run, and this list is not meant to be a substitute for good judgment.

4. Keep the group compact, but maintain sufficient spacing to avoid collisions. If the group is large, consider dividing into smaller groups or using the "buddy system" as an additional safeguard. Space yourselves closely enough to permit good communication, but not so close as to interfere with one another in rapids.

A. The lead paddler sets the pace. When in front, do not get in over your head. Never run drops when you cannot see a clear route to the bottom or, for advanced paddlers, a sure route to the next eddy. When in doubt, stop and scout.

B. Keep track of all group members. Each boat keeps the one behind it in sight, stopping if necessary. Know how many people are in your group and take head counts regularly. No one should paddle ahead or walk out without first informing the group. Weak paddlers should stay at the center of a group, and not allow themselves to lag behind. If the group is large and contains a wide range of abilities, a designated "sweep boat" should bring up the rear.

C. Courtesy. On heavily used rivers, do not cut in front of a boater running a drop. Always look upstream before leaving eddies to run or play. Never enter a crowded drop or eddy when no room for you exists. Passing other groups in a rapid may be hazardous: it's often safer to wait upstream until the group has passed.

5. Float plan. If the trip is into a wilderness area or for an extended period, plans should be filed with a responsible person who will contact the authorities if you are overdue. It may be wise to establish checkpoints along the way where civilization could be contacted if necessary. Knowing the location of possible help and preplanning escape routes can speed rescue.

6. Drugs. The use of alcohol or mind-altering drugs before or during river trips is not recommended. It dulls reflexes, reduces decision-making ability, and may interfere with important survival reflexes.

7. Instructional or Commercially Guided Trips. In contrast to the common adventure trip format, in these trip formats, a boating instructor or commercial guide assumes some of the responsibilities normally exercised by the group as a whole, as appropriate under the circumstances. These formats recognize that instructional or commercially guided trips may involve participants who lack significant experience in whitewater. However, as a participant acquires experience in whitewater, he or she takes on increasing responsibility for his or her own safety, in accordance with what he or she knows or should know as a result of that increased experience. Also, as in all trip formats, every participant must realize and assume the risks associated with the serious hazards of whitewater rivers. It is advisable for instructors and commercial guides to acquire trip or personal liability insurance.

A. An "instructional trip" is characterized by a clear teacher/pupil relationship, where the primary purpose of the trip is to teach boating skills, and sometimes is conducted for a fee.

B. A "commercially guided trip" is characterized by a licensed, professional guide conducting trips for a fee.

IV. Guidelines for River Rescue

1. Recover from an upset with an eskimo roll whenever possible. Evacuate your boat immediately if there is imminent danger of being trapped against rocks, brush, or any other kind of strainer.

2. If you swim, hold on to your boat. It has much flotation and is easy for rescuers to spot. Get to the upstream end so that you cannot be crushed between a rock and your boat by the force of the current. Persons with good balance may be able to climb on top of a swamped kayak or flipped raft and paddle to shore.

3. Release your craft if this will improve your chances, especially if the water is cold or dangerous rapids lie ahead. Actively attempt self-rescue whenever possible by swimming for safety. Be prepared to assist others who may come to your aid.

A. When swimming in shallow or obstructed rapids, lie on your back with feet held high and pointed downstream. Do not attempt to stand in fast moving water; if your foot wedges on the bottom, fast water will push you under and keep you there. Get to slow or very shallow water before attempting to stand or walk. Look ahead! Avoid possible pinning situations including undercut rocks, strainers, downed trees, holes, and other dangers by swimming away from them.

B. If the rapids are deep and powerful, roll over onto your stomach and swim aggressively for shore. Watch for eddies and slackwater and use them to get out of the current. Strong swimmers can effect a powerful upstream ferry and get to shore fast. If the shores are obstructed with strainers or undercut rocks, however, it is safer to "ride the rapid out" until a less hazardous escape can be found.

4. If others spill and swim, go after the boaters first. Rescue boats and equipment only if this can be done safely. While participants are encouraged (but not obligated) to assist one another to the best of their ability, they should do so only if they can, in their judgment, do so safely. The first duty of a rescuer is not to compound the problem by becoming another victim.

5. The use of rescue lines requires training; uninformed use may cause injury. Never tie yourself into either end of a line without a quick-release system. Have a knife handy to deal with unexpected entanglement. Learn to place set lines

effectively, to throw accurately, to belay effectively, and to properly handle a rope thrown to you.

6. When reviving a drowning victim, be aware that cold water may greatly extend survival time underwater. Victims of hypothermia may have depressed vital signs, so they look and feel dead. Don't give up; continue CPR for as long as possible without compromising safety.

V. International Scale of River Difficulty

This is the American version of a rating system used to compare river difficulty throughout the world. This system is not exact; rivers do not always fit easily into one category, and regional or individual interpretations may cause misunderstandings. It is no substitute for a guidebook or accurate firsthand descriptions of a run.

Paddlers attempting difficult runs in an unfamiliar area should act cautiously until they get a feel for the way the scale is interpreted locally. River difficulty may change each year due to fluctuations in water level, downed trees, geological disturbances, or bad weather. Stay alert for unexpected problems!

As river difficulty increases, the danger to swimming paddlers becomes more severe. As rapids become longer and more continuous, the challenge increases. There is a difference between running an occasional Class IV rapids and dealing with an entire river of this category. Allow an extra margin of safety between skills and river ratings when the water is cold or if the river itself is remote and inaccessible.

The Six Difficulty Classes

Class I: Easy. Fast-moving water with riffles and small waves. Few obstructions, all obvious and easily missed with little training. Risk to swimmers is slight; self-rescue is easy.

Class II: Novice. Straightforward rapids with wide, clear channels that are evident without scouting. Occasional maneuvering may be required, but rocks and medium-sized waves are easily missed by trained paddlers. Swimmers are seldom injured and group assistance, while helpful, is seldom needed.

Class III: Intermediate. Rapids with moderate, irregular waves which may be difficult to avoid and which can swamp an open canoe. Complex maneuvers in fast current and good boat control in tight passages or around ledges are often required; large waves or strain-

ers may be present but are easily avoided. Strong eddies and powerful current effects can be found, particularly on large-volume rivers. Scouting is advisable for inexperienced parties. Injuries while swimming are rare; self-rescue is usually easy but group assistance may be required to avoid long swims.

Class IV: Advanced. Intense, powerful but predictable rapids requiring precise boat handling in turbulent water. Depending on the character of the river, it may feature large, unavoidable waves and holes or constricted passages demanding fast maneuvers under pressure. A fast, reliable eddy turn may be needed to navigate dangerous hazards. Scouting is necessary the first time down. Risk of injury to swimmers is moderate to high, and water conditions may make self-rescue difficult. Group assistance for rescue is often essential but requires practiced skills. A strong eskimo roll is highly recommended.

Class V: Expert. Extremely long, obstructed, or very violent rapids which expose a paddler to above average endangerment. Drops may contain large, unavoidable waves and holes or steep, congested chutes with complex, demanding routes. Rapids may continue for long distances between pools, demanding a high level of fitness. What eddies exist may be small, turbulent, or difficult to reach. At the high end of the scale, several of these factors may be combined. Scouting is mandatory, but often difficult. Swims are dangerous, and rescue is difficult, even for experts. A very reliable eskimo roll, proper equipment, extensive experience, and practiced rescue skills are essential for survival.

Class VI: Extreme. One grade more difficult than Class V. These runs often exemplify the extremes of difficulty, unpredictability, and danger. The consequences of errors are very severe and rescue may be impossible. For teams of experts only, at favorable water levels, after close personal inspection, and taking all precautions. This class does not represent drops thought to be unrunnable, but may include rapids that are only occasionally run.
Adopted 1959; Revised 1989

Injuries and Evacuations

Even allowing for careful preparation and attention to the rules of river safety, it remains a fact that people and boats are somewhat more fragile than rivers and rocks. Accidents occur on paddling trips, and all boaters should understand that accidents can happen to them. Although virtually any disaster is possible on a river, including drowning, there are specific traumas and illnesses that occur more frequently than others. These include the following:

1. Hypothermia
2. Dislocated shoulder (especially common in decked boating)
3. Sprained or broken ankles (usually sustained while scouting or getting into or out of the boat)
4. Head injuries (sustained in falls on shore or during capsize)
5. Hypersensitivity to insect bite (anaphylactic shock)
6. Heat trauma (sunburn, heat stroke, heat prostration, dehydration, etc.)
7. Food poisoning (often resulting from sun spoilage of lunch foods on a hot day)
8. Badly strained muscles (particularly of the lower back, upper arm, and the trapezius)
9. Hand and wrist injuries
10. Lacerations

Many paddlers are well prepared to handle the first aid requirements when one of the above injuries occurs on the river, but they are ill prepared to handle continued care and evacuation.

You and your paddling partners should have up-to-date CPR and first aid training and should improve your rescue skills by taking the courses in river rescue offered by many river outfitters. In addition, study works about river rescue such as *The American Canoe Association's River Safety Anthology*, edited by Charlie Walbridge and Jody Tinsley; *River Rescue*, by Les Bechtel; *The American Canoe Association's 1992–1995 River Safety Report*, edited by Charlie Walbridge; and *The American Canoe Association's River Safety Flashcards*. These can help prepare you for continued care and evacuation of the injured or ill.

Be prepared for such contingencies. Carry topographic maps and know where you are in relation to roads. If an emergency occurs, don't panic. If possible, send two people out to find help, carrying written instructions about the nature of the injury or illness and the specific location of the victim or a rendezvous point if the remainder of the party is beginning an evacuation. Because helicopter rescues are available only near military bases or high-use areas and because helicopters need more room to land and hover than Appalachian river valleys typically allow, don't expect a dramatic helicopter rescue. If you have the manpower and know-how, you may decide to carry out the victim, being sure to keep him or her safe, calm, and warm during the evacuation. Otherwise, once help is sent for, psychologically prepare yourself for a long wait.

Hypothermia

Although this guide is by no means a first aid manual, hypothermia, the lowering of the body's core temperature, is so common and so deadly that it deserves special attention here. Hypothermia can occur in a matter of minutes in water just a few degrees above freezing, but even 50°F water is unbearably cold. To make things worse, panic can set in when the paddler is faced with a long swim through rapids. Heat loss occurs much more quickly than believed. When the body's temperature drops appreciably below the normal 98.6°F, sluggishness sets in, breathing is difficult, coordination is lost to even the most athletic person, pupils dilate, speech becomes slurred, and thinking becomes irrational. Cold water robs the victim of the ability and desire to save him- or herself. Finally unconsciousness sets in, and then, death. A drop in body temperature to 96°F makes swimming and pulling yourself to safety almost impossible, and tragically, the harder you struggle, the more heat your body loses. Body temperatures below 90°F lead to unconsciousness, and a further drop to about 77°F usually results in death. (But this same lowering of the body temperature slows metabolism and delays brain death in cases of drowning; therefore, rescue efforts have a higher chance of success.)

Paddlers subjected to spray and wetting from waves splashing into an open boat are in almost as much danger of hypothermia as a paddler completely immersed after a swim. The combination of cold air and water drains the body of precious heat at an alarming rate, although it is the wetness that causes the major losses, since water conducts heat away from the body 20 times faster than air. Clothes lose their insulating properties quickly when immersed, and skin temperatures will rapidly drop to within a few degrees of the water temperature. The body, hard-pressed to conserve heat, will then reduce blood circulation to the extremities. This reduction in blood flowing to arms and legs makes movement and heavy work next to impossible. Muscular activity increases heat loss because blood forced to the extremities is quickly cooled by the cold water. It's a vicious, deadly cycle.

The best safeguards against cold-weather hazards are recognizing the symptoms of hypothermia, preventing exposure to cold by wearing proper clothing (wool or synthetic fabrics, waterproof outerwear, wet suits, or dry suits), understanding and respecting cold weather and water, and knowing how to treat hypothermia when it is detected. Actually, cold weather deaths may be attributed to a number of factors: physical exhaustion, inadequate food intake, dehydration, and psychological elements such as fear, panic, and despair. Factors such as body fat, the metabolic rate of an individual, and skin thickness are variables in a particular person's reaction and endurance when immersed in cold water.

Exercise may warm a mildly hypothermic person, and shivering is involuntary exercise. But the key to bringing victims out of serious hypothermia is heating their bodies from an external source. In a field situation, strip off all wet clothes and get the victim into a sleeping bag with another person. Skin-to-skin transfer of body heat is by far the best method of getting the body's temperature up. By all means, don't let the victim go to sleep, and give him or her warm liquids. Build a campfire if possible. Mouth-to-mouth resuscitation or CPR may be necessary in extreme cases when breathing and pulse have stopped, but remember that a person in the grips of hypothermia has a significantly reduced metabolic rate, so check carefully before administering this treatment.

Paddlers' Rights and Responsibilities

While it is essential to have knowledge of first aid and rescue techniques, it is also very important to know your legal rights and responsibilities while on the river. A paddler's legal right to run a river is based on the concept of navigability. This situation is somewhat unfortunate since navigability as a legal concept has proven both obscure and somewhat confused over the years. The common law test of navigability specifies that only those streams affected by the ebb and flow of the sea tides are navigable. Obviously, if this were the only criterion, none of the streams in the Appalachians would be navigable. Fortunately, most states expressly repudiate the common law test and favor instead the so-called civil law test—thus a stream is considered navigable if it is capable of being navigated in the ordinary sense of that term, which relates essentially to commerce and transportation. But even if a stream is not navigable from a legal perspective according to the civil law test, it may still be navigable in fact, meaning that its navigability does not depend on any legislative act but is based rather on the objective capability of the stream to support boating. Thus, a creek swollen by high waters may become navigable for a time.

If a stream is navigable according to the civil law test, ownership of the streambed is public. In this case, the public possesses all navigation rights as well as incidental rights to fish, swim, and wade. Property rights to those who own land along a navigable stream extend only to the ordinary low water mark. If the water later recedes or islands form in the bed of the stream, the property remains that of the state.

On the other hand, if a stream is only navigable sometimes (as in the case of a seasonal stream), the title of the land under the water belongs to the property owners over whose land the stream passes. However, the ownership is subject to a public easement for such navigation as the condition of the stream will permit.

Regardless of the question of navigability, the right of landowners to prohibit trespassing on their land along streams (if they so desire) is guaranteed. Therefore, access to rivers must be secured at highway rights-of-way or on publicly-owned lands if permission to cross privately owned land cannot be secured. Legally, paddlers are trespassing when they camp, portage, or even stop for a lunch break if they disembark from their boats onto the land. If approached by a landowner while trespassing, by all means be cordial and explain your reason for being on the property. Never knowingly camp on private land without permission. If you do encounter a perturbed landowner, be respectful and keep tempers under control.

Landowners, in granting access to a river, are extending a privilege that should be appreciated and respected. Do not betray a landowner's trust if you are extended the privilege of putting in, taking out, or camping. Do not litter or drive on grass or planted fields. Leave gates the way you find them (typically, closed). In some cases, property owners may resent outsiders arriving to float through what the landowner may consider private domain. Indeed, it is not unusual for landowners firmly to believe that they own the river that passes through their land.

Landowners certainly have the right to keep you off their land, and the law will side with them unless they inflict harm on you; in that case, they may be both civilly and criminally liable. If you threaten a landowner verbally and physically move with apparent will to do harm, the landowner has all the rights of self-defense and self-protection in accordance with the perceived danger that you impose. Likewise, if the landowner points a firearm at you, fires warning shots, assaults, injures, or wounds you or a boater in your group, you are certainly in the right to protect yourself.

Although the chance of such a meeting may be rare, paddlers nonetheless should know their rights, and the rights of the landowners. Without question, confrontations between belligerent paddlers and cantankerous landowners are to be avoided. On the other hand, good manners, appreciation, and consideration go a long way when approaching a landowner for permission to camp or launch. The property owner may be interested in paddling and flattered that the paddler is excited about the countryside and so may be quite friendly and approachable. Cultivate and value this friendship and avoid giving landowners cause to deny paddlers access to the river at some time in the future.

Courtesy and respect should be extended to the river environment as well as to landowners. Many of the streams listed in this guide flow through national parks and forests, state-owned forests and wildlife management areas, and privately owned lands that in some cases are superior in quality and aesthetics to lands under public ownership. It is the paddling community's responsibility to uphold the integrity of these lands and their rivers by using these waterways in an ecologically sound way. Litter, fire scars, pollution from human excrement, and the cutting of live trees are unsightly and affect the land in a way that threatens to ruin the outdoor experience for everyone.

Paddlers should pack out everything they pack in: all paper litter and such nonbiodegradable items as cartons, foil, plastic jugs, and cans. Help keep our waterways clean for those who follow. If you are canoe camping, leave your campsite in better shape than you found it. If you must build a fire, build it at an established site, and when you leave, dismantle rock fireplaces, thoroughly drown all flames and hot coals, and scatter the ashes. Never cut live trees for firewood (in addition to destroying a part of the environment, they don't burn well). Dump all dishwater and bathwater in the woods away from watercourses, and emulate the cat—bury all excrement. Let's all show these rivers the respect they deserve.

How to Use this Guide

This series of guidebooks on the whitewater of the Appalachian Mountains is divided into two volumes. *Appalachian Whitewater: The Southern Mountains* covers the Appalachian streams of Alabama, Georgia, Kentucky, Maryland, North Carolina, South Carolina, Tennessee, Virginia, and West Virginia. *Appalachian Whitewater: The Northern Mountains* covers Maine, Vermont, New Hampshire, Connecticut, Massachusetts, New York, Pennsylvania, Delaware, Maryland, and West Virginia. The emphasis in each volume is on the classic whitewater streams, though a number of lesser known but no less spectacular streams are also included. No attempt is made to review a river from source to mouth. Rather, only the better whitewater sections of each stream are detailed.

For each stream in this guide you will find a stream description and at least one stream data list and map. For our purposes, we are defining a stream as flowing water; this may be a river, a creek, or a branch or fork of a river.

Stream Descriptions

Stream descriptions are intended to give you a feel for the streams and their surroundings and are presented in general, nontechnical terms.

Stream Data

Each stream data list provides technical and quantitative information, as well as some additional descriptive information. For added emphasis, certain facts will occasionally be covered in both the stream description and in the data list. Each list begins with the specific stream section to which the data apply and the counties in which the stream is located. Fuller explanations of many of the categories on the data lists are as follows:

Difficulty. The level of difficulty of a stream is given according to the International Scale of River Difficulty, provided in the previous chapter. Such ratings are relative and pertain to the stream described under more or less ideal water levels and weather conditions. For streams with two International Scale ratings, the first represents the average level of difficulty of the entire run and the second (expressed parenthetically) represents the level of difficulty of the most difficult section or rapids on the run. Paddlers are cautioned that changes in water levels or weather conditions can alter the stated average difficulty rating appreciably. We strongly recommend that paddlers also assess the difficulty of a stream on a given day by using the River Difficulty Rating Chart (Table 2 in the previous chapter).

Gradient. Gradient is expressed in feet per miles and refers to the steepness of the streambed over a certain distance. It is important to remember that gradient, or drop, as paddlers refer to it, is an average figure and does not tell the paddler when or how the drop occurs. A stream that has a listed gradient of 25 feet per mile may drop gradually in one- or two-inch increments (like a long, rocky slide) for the course of a mile, or it may drop only slightly over the first nine-tenths of a mile and then suddenly drop 24 feet at one waterfall. As a general rule, gradient can be used as a rough indicator of level of difficulty for a given stream: the greater the gradient, the more difficult the stream. In practice, gradient is almost always considered in conjunction with other information.

Average Width. Rivers tend to start small and enlarge as they go toward their confluence with another river. The average width is an approximate measure. Pools form in some places, and in other places the channel may constrict, accelerating the current. It should be remembered that wide rivers create special problems for rescuers.

Velocity. Velocity represents the speed of the current, on the average, in nonflood conditions and can vary incredibly from section to section on a given stream, depending on the stream's width, volume, and gradient at any point along its length. Velocity is a partial indicator of how much reaction time you might have on a certain river. Paddlers should remember that a high velocity stream does not allow them much time for decision and action.

Rivers are described here as slack, slow, moderate, and fast. Slack rivers have current velocities of less than a half mile per hour; slow rivers have velocities over a half mile per hour but less than two miles per hour. Moderate velocities range between two and four miles per hour, and fast rivers are those that exceed four miles per hour.

Rescue Index. Many of the streams in this book run through wild areas. A sudden serious illness or injury could become an urgent problem if you can't get medical attention quickly. To give you an idea of how far you may be from help, a brief description is given of what might be expected. Accessible means that you might need up to an hour to secure assistance, but evacuation is not difficult. Accessible but difficult means that it might take up to three hours to get help, and evacuation may be difficult. Remote indicates it might take three to six hours to get help, and extremely remote means that you might be six hours from help and would need expert assistance to get a victim out.

Hazards. Hazards are dangers to navigation. Because of the nature of rivers and ongoing human activity, many existing hazards may change, and new ones might appear. Low-hanging trees, which can be a nuisance, may become deadfalls, blowdowns, and strainers. Human intervention creates hazards such as dams, low bridges, powerboat traffic, and fences (an especially dangerous strainer). Some watersheds have soils that cannot retain much water, and the streams in that watershed may have a flash flood potential. Additionally, geologically young rivers, usually whitewater rivers, may have undercut rocks, keeper hydraulics, difficult rapids, and a scarcity of eddies.

Scouting. This guidebook attempts to list specific spots on rivers where scouting is required, that is, recommended for the continuation of life and good health. Because hazards may change quickly, this guidebook also strongly recommends that you scout anytime you cannot see what is ahead (on whitewater or flatwater and even on familiar rivers). That small, turning drop that you have run a thousand times may have a big log wedged across it today.

Portages. Dams should be portaged. Additionally, portages are recommended for certain rapids and other dangers. The fact, however, that a portage is not specified in

this guidebook at a certain spot or rapid does not necessarily mean that you should not portage. It is the mark of good paddlers to be able to make safe and independent decisions about their own abilities for a given river or rapid.

Scenery. Taste is relative, and our preference is that you form your own conclusions about the beauty of these streams. Knowing, however, that it takes a long time to run all of the Appalachians' major drainages, we include a comparative scenery rating based on our own perceptions. The ratings run from unattractive, through uninspiring, through gradations of pretty and beautiful, to spectacular. To give you some examples, here are our ratings of some popular canoeing streams:

> Little Miami River (Ohio): Pretty in spots to pretty
> Whitewater River (Indiana): Pretty in spots to pretty
> Nantahala River (North Carolina): Pretty to beautiful in spots
> Current River (Missouri): Beautiful in spots to beautiful
> Elkhorn River (Kentucky): Beautiful in spots to beautiful
> New River (West Virginia): Beautiful in spots to beautiful
> Red River (Kentucky): Exceptionally beautiful to spectacular
> Chattooga III, IV (Georgia): Exceptionally beautiful to spectacular

Highlights. This category includes special scenery, wildlife, whitewater, local culture and industry, history, and unusual geology.

Gauge. Where possible, we give the most direct number to find information about current water levels. If there are other phone numbers to call, we list them under Additional Information. You may also want to check the World Wide Web (see appendixes).

Runnable Water Level (Minimum). The lowest water level at which a given stream is navigable is referred to as the minimum runnable water level. Where possible, water levels are expressed in terms of volume as cubic feet per second (cfs). The use of cfs is doubly informative in that knowledge of volume at a gauge on one stream is often a prime indicator of the water levels of ungauged runnable streams in the same watershed, or for other sections of the gauged stream, either up- or downstream.

Runnable Water Level (Maximum). In this book, "runnable" does not mean the same thing as "possible."

The maximum runnable water level refers to the highest water level at which the stream can be run with reasonable safety. This level may vary for open and decked boats. With the exception of the few streams that can be run only during times of extremely high water, this categorically excludes rivers in flood.

Sources of Additional Information. Various sources of additional information on water conditions are listed. Professional outfitters can provide both technical and descriptive information and relate the two to paddling. Tennessee Valley Authority (TVA) and the various hydraulics branches of the respective district Corps of Engineers offices can provide flow data in cfs but will not be able to interpret the data for you in terms of paddling. Other sources listed (forest rangers, police departments, etc.) will normally provide only descriptive information,

for example, "The creek's up pretty good today," or, "The river doesn't have enough water in it for boating."

Maps

The maps in this guide are not intended to replace topographic quadrangles for terrain features. Rather, they are intended to illustrate the general configuration of the stream, its access points, and surrounding shuttle roads. Some of the maps are congested to the point that access letters may not be exactly where they should be. A county map to the area may help in finding the put-in and take-out points. Keep in mind that you may have to scout the area before launching. Letters on the map correspond to letters found in the text. A brief explanation of the different symbols can be found below.

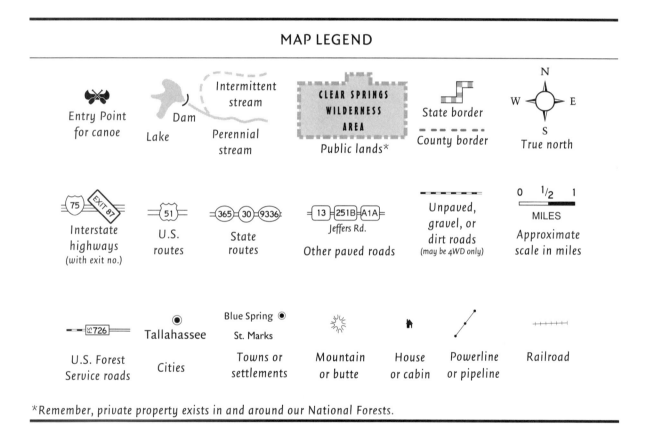

MAP LEGEND

Entry Point for canoe	Dam — Lake — Perennial stream / Intermittent stream	CLEAR SPRINGS WILDERNESS AREA — Public lands*	State border — County border	N W E S True north
Interstate highways (with exit no.)	U.S. routes	State routes	Other paved roads — Jeffers Rd.	Unpaved, gravel, or dirt roads (may be 4WD only)	Approximate scale in miles — 0 ½ 1 MILES
U.S. Forest Service roads	Tallahassee Cities	Blue Spring — St. Marks — Towns or settlements	Mountain or butte	House or cabin	Powerline or pipeline	Railroad

Remember, private property exists in and around our National Forests.

ALABAMA

Little River Canyon

To one unfamiliar with the infinite variety of landscapes in the southeastern United States, the term "Alabama whitewater" may seem to present a ludicrous contradiction. Laughter may begin in earnest when Alabama canyons are mentioned. Laugh no more, for it is all there in the Little River Canyon in northeastern Alabama.

Located approximately nine miles east of Fort Payne in northeast Alabama, the Little River Canyon is an impressive cleft in the sandstone-granite countryside with a sparkling clear stream running through it. The Little River has deep mirror-surfaced pools, gentle ripples, and boulder-smashing, highly technical whitewater.

Because of the extreme seasonal water level fluctuations, the difficulty of an emergency exit from the bottom of the canyon, and the boating skills required to successfully complete the run, the first stop before any trip begins at the river gauge at Little River Canyon Mouth Park. The USGS gauge is just downstream of the beach area in the park. Acceptable levels are a minimum of four feet and a maximum of six feet. It is possible to run the river at higher levels, but the mutilated carcasses of canoes, kayaks, and rafts scattered throughout the canyon offer the mute testimonies of those who tried and failed. Boaters should have advanced skill levels before attempting the Upper Two Mile section of Little River Canyon (the section starting approximately two miles above the old chairlift at Eberharts Point), and intermediate to advanced skills when entering the canyon at Eberharts Point.

The put-in is one of the more memorable parts of the trip. One descends approximately 600 feet straight down from the rim of the canyon to its floor. For the Upper Two Mile put-in (A), park at the pull-off approximately three miles from AL 35 on the Canyon Rim Parkway (AL 176). This is where the road takes a sharp right turn to travel around the first major side canyon. Carry your boat straight down the point. No marked trail exists at this put-in. For the lower section, begin at the sight of the old chairlift at Eberharts Point on the parkway. This put-in

has a wide, clearly marked trail to the left of the chairlift. Both put-ins are arduous carries to the river, but do not succumb to the urge to weep and toss your boat into the abyss. The river is well worth the struggle.

Scenery ranges from delightful to magnificent. The water is usually clear, with deep, shimmering, turquoise pools. Cedars, pines, hardwoods, and, in spring, a profusion of wildflowers adorn the cliffs on either side of the river. Small tributaries plummet to merge with the primary flow, creating many intimate coves with excellent photographic potential.

Do not become too enthralled with the scenic vistas, for the river demands your full attention at times. Rapids are numerous and good boat control is essential. If dependable eddy turns, ferrying skills, and good judgment calls are not part of your paddling program, then do not venture here.

Section: Upper Two Miles to Eberharts Point
Counties: De Kalb, Cherokee
USGS Quads: Jamestown, Little River, Fort Payne
Highlights: Scenery, wildlife, whitewater, geology
Scenery: Spectacular
Difficulty: Class IV–V
Gradient: 80 feet per mile
Average Width: 30–50 feet
Velocity: Fast
Rescue Index: Remote to extremely remote
Hazards: Strainers, undercut rocks, flash flooding
Scouting: At rapids and blind curves
Portages: As needed according to water level and skill level
Gauge: Alabama Power, (800) LAKES11

Runnable Water Level	Minimum	Maximum
Gauge at River		
Canyon Mouth Park	4.0 feet	6.0 feet

Additional Information: DeSoto State Park, (205) 845-0051; Canyon Mouth Park Campground, (205) 845-9605; Alabama Outdoors (205) 870-1919

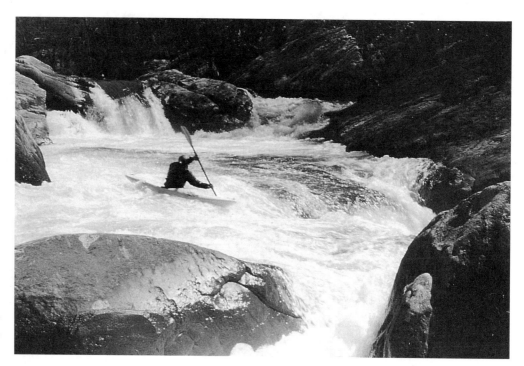

Richard Vest paddling through Cable Falls. Photo courtesy Matthew Vest.

Little River Canyon • Alabama

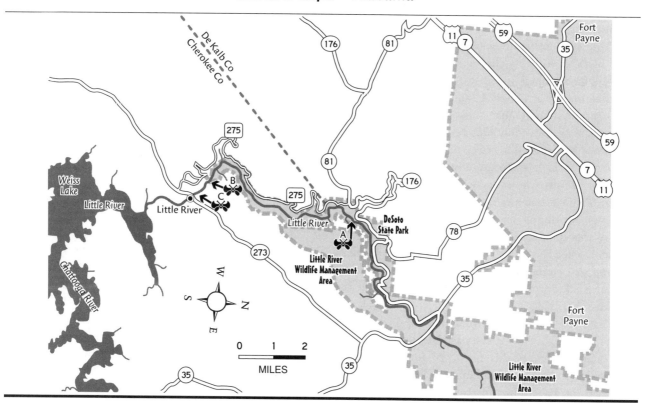

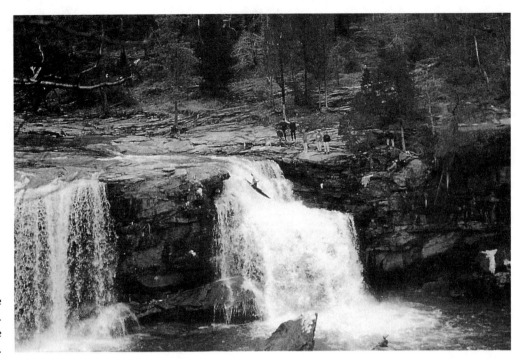

Brad Hinds going over the edge at Little River Falls. Photo by Jason Lawrence (courtesy of Brad Hinds).

Most rapids are not described in detail here. Scout anything that is not clearly visible. Often there is more than one possible route and at least one impossible one. Huge boulders will often obscure the downstream view. The heaviest rapids (Class IV–V) are found in the Upper Two Mile section, while below the chairlift the water (Class III–IV) is still very challenging.

While many rapids in Little River Canyon are both technical and treacherous, Humpty Dumpty deserves this description more than most. After running Road Block (Class IV, a five-foot drop off the side of a boulder and into a V-shaped slot), eddy on the right bank and walk a few yards downstream to scout Humpty Dumpty (Class V). A series of holes and waves form the Class II–III entrance. Run this down the middle and eddy right to take your bearing on the six-foot ledge that forms the maw of this monster. Take the ledge directly over the middle. Do not be tempted to eddy right at the brink of the drop. A cavernous abyss located between the boulders can suck down boat and boater. Be upright at the bottom of the ledge or prepared for a very quick roll because the eddy behind the hydraulic is all the time you have to move right and avoid a nasty slot straight ahead. Once you succeed at this move, go for the boulder-choked alley on the right, running towards the center of the river. You have now run Humpty Dumpty without

scrambling your eggs! Take a deep breath and prepare for the many thrills to come.

Below the chairlift there is one rapid of special merit. Bottleneck (Class IV), is recognized by the tight succession of three technical drops, the last of which is reminiscent of Crack in the Rock on Section IV of the Chattooga River. After choosing one of the three slots in this drop, eddy out and scout the fourth and final drop from the right. Huge boulders dam the river completely on the left and form a tight sluice on the right. The top of the sluice chokes the river down to a width of about 10–12 feet. Enter as far right as possible to avoid the hole on the left, and ride the water as it cushions off the slanted boulders on the right. Move left across the middle of the sluice and catch the tongue at the bottom to avoid the deep hole on the right.

The canyon ends abruptly and with it goes the whitewater. Drift gently into Canyon Mouth Park (B). Carry your boat the short distance across the sandy beach to the parking area, take a hot shower in the conveniently located bathhouse, and congratulate yourself and your companions on another good day on the river.

If Canyon Mouth Park is closed, an alternative takeout is approximately one mile further downstream at the AL 273 bridge (C).

Locust Fork of the Black Warrior River

The Locust Fork of Alabama's Black Warrior River is the Deep South's top cruising river. Each year "the Fork" is enjoyed by boaters from Mississippi, Louisiana, Tennessee, and Florida in addition to a multitude of Alabama boaters. A piedmont river bracketed by high shale bluffs and rolling hills, the Fork drops a respectable 23 feet per mile in the five and a half miles from the AL 79/US 231 bridge to the AL 160 bridge. This section is usually runnable from midwinter to late spring with frequent "thunderstorm runs" throughout the summer and fall. In terms of technical difficulty, at optimal water flows the Fork ranks between the Nantahala River and Section III of the Chattooga (minus Bull Sluice). The majority of the Locust Fork rapids are of the funneling ledge-shoal variety. Two rapids require bank scouting: The first, Double Trouble (at mile 2), is preceded by a long pool and a distinct horizon line. Take out top left to scout and set up throw ropes. At optimal to high levels a nasty boulder sieve forms at the bottom of this long rapid to the right of the last drop. The second blind rapid, Powell Falls (mile 4.5), is safely runnable from low to optimal levels to the right of the midstream scouting rock. At high levels this eight-foot slanting ledge creates a riverwide hydraulic followed by a one-acre strainer where an island used to be.

The USGS gauge is located just upstream of the AL 79/US 231 bridge on river left. Read the gauge before running the Fork! Absolute minimum running level (read "too *?#@?! low!") is 1.8 feet. "Low" is 2.2 feet; at this

Locust Fork of the Black Warrior River • Alabama

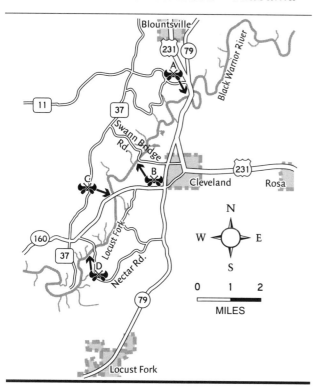

Section: AL 79/US 231 bridge to Nectar Covered Bridge
County: Blount
USGS Quad: Blount
Highlights: Covered bridges, wildlife, whitewater, geology
Scenery: Very good to excellent
Difficulty: Class II–IV
Gradient: 23 feet per mile
Average Width: 25–60 feet
Velocity: Slow to fast
Rescue Index: Accessible to accessible but difficult
Hazards: Strainers, undercut rocks, Powell Falls, logjams, Skirum Bluff Pool (at flood stage)
Scouting: Double Trouble, Powell Falls
Portages: None
Gauge: Alabama Power, (800) LAKES11

Runnable Water Levels	Minimum	Maximum
	1.8 feet	8.0 feet

Additional Information: Pardue Grocery, (205) 274-2586; Locust Fork Racing Organization, (205) 442-1345

level you'll have a fun technical Class II run. "Medium" is 2.4 to 3.2 feet (Class II to III+). Optimal running level is 3.6 to 4.2 feet (Class III to IV-). "High" is 4.4 feet and up; rapids begin washing out at 5.0 feet, and the river leaves its banks at around 6.0 feet. Above 8.0 feet (flood stage), you get your basic big-water, acid-trip experience: standing waves in the trees, monster holes, whirlpools, etc. Both banks become a continuous mega-strainer from put-in to take-out. If you must run this stretch at high water levels, take out at or before Swann Covered Bridge; farther downstream Powell Falls creates a riverwide hydraulic followed half a mile later by a potentially deadly whirlpool consuming the first two-thirds of the river at Skirum Bluff. Every major accident (including several fatalities) that has occurred on the Fork in the past has been caused by a combination of extremely high water, inexperience, inadequate equipment, and lack of skill.

Relations between boaters and locals have improved greatly over the past several years. Treat those you meet with respect and they should respond accordingly. Presently boater/local relations are good and hopefully will remain so. In general, however, when in Blount County, Alabama, be discreet and considerate when dealing with the locals. Public nudity, profanity, consumption of alcohol and/or controlled substances, partying, trespassing, and other aspects of normal boater behavior are not tolerated here.

Call Pardue's Grocery and Texaco Station at (205) 274-2586 for water levels and conditions. When you get off the river be sure to stop by Pardue's, located on AL 79 a quarter of a mile on the right before you reach the river, for the best barbecue in Blount County.

GEORGIA

Chattooga River

The Chattooga River is now and will remain one of the nationÕs most popular rivers. It has something for everyone: easy water suitable for beginners to raging Class V rapids for the whitewater crazies. The scenery is nothing short of spectacular for almost the entire length of the river. Its excellence rivals any river in this country.

The river ßows from North Carolina to form the border between South Carolina and Georgia for approximately 40 miles, until it ßows into Tugaloo Lake. Fortunately, the Chattooga is protected under the National Wild and Scenic Rivers Act and is managed by the U.S. Forest Service, Sumter National Forest, South Carolina. The Forest Service divides the river into four sections according to the major access points. Section I is from Burrells Ford near the North Carolina border to the GA 28 bridge. The Forest Service regulations state that Òall boating is prohibited above Highway 28,Ó although it is open for hiking and Þshing. We will not discuss Section I in this book.

Chattooga Section II

Section II of the Chattooga begins at the GA 28 bridge (A), with easy access and parking on the Georgia side of the bridge, and continues downriver to Earls Ford. This section is approximately seven miles long and is a good day trip for beginning boaters. Initially the stream is shallow and rocky with only a slight gradient. Considerable volume is added when the West Fork of the Chattooga ßows in from the right, approximately 100 yards below the GA 28 bridge.

For the Þrst few miles of Section II the Chattooga is a meandering, gentle valley stream, ßowing through an area with a rich history. It was once the site of one of the largest Native American settlements in the southeast, Chattooga Old Town. Inhabited by the Cherokee, Chattooga Old Town became a major trading center after Europeans came to the area. The valley was ideally suited

for agriculture, and Europeans with a lust for land soon appropriated it as their own. It remained in agricultural use until recently. Just off the river on the South Carolina side are the remains of a large farmhouse owned by the Russell family. The main building was burned in 1988, but eight other structures still stand as evidence of the early agricultural period. This area was also visited by colonial naturalist William Bartram and was described in his travels. The Bartram Trail, named in his honor, parallels the river down to Earls Ford.

Through the valley the river remains close to SC 28, and several seasonal private homes are scattered along the South Carolina shore. Near the end of the valley is Long Bottom Ford, reached from SC 28. This is an alternate put-in for Section II (B) and a take-out for a trip down the West Fork. There is a paved parking area, boat launching ramp, and chemical toilets at the Long Bottom access point. After reaching the end of the valley, the terrain begins to revert to its wilderness character and the river quickens its pace. Large hemlocks and white pines thrust from the rocky banks and small islands. In the spring, youÕll Þnd a profusion of wildßowers and ßowering shrubs, including wild azaleas in ßaming orange and white.

After passing several large islands in the stream, you will reach the long deep pool that precedes Turn Hole Rapid, the Þrst rapid that most paddlers deem worthy of naming. The rapid is not very difÞcult, but it can trick the unwary. The approach is through a shallow shoal area that has several possible routes. The main drop is usually entered near the left side. It calls for a quick turn to the right, which is necessary to avoid being pushed into the rocky bank. At average water levels, you can run near the center of the stream, straight across the main ledge, if you desire. The drop is about three feet.

Continuing downstream through another half mile or so of mild Class I and II rapids, you will come around the bend to see a group of large boulders and rock slabs

Section: GA 28 to Earls Ford

Counties: Rabun (GA), Oconee (SC)

USGS Quads: Satolah, Whetstone, Rainy Mountain

Highlights: Scenery, wildlife, whitewater, local culture and industry, history, geology

Scenery: Exceptionally beautiful

Difficulty: Class I–II (III)

Gradient: 11.5 feet per mile

Average Width: 20–65 feet

Velocity: Slow to moderate

Rescue Index: Accessible but difficult

Hazards: Strainers, deadfalls

Scouting: Big Shoals Rapid

Portages: As conditions and skill level require

Gauge: Chattooga Whitewater Shop, (864) 647-9083

Runnable Water Levels	Minimum	Maximum
US 76 bridge	0.8 feet	3.5 feet

Additional Information: Nantahala Outdoor Center, (864) 647-9014; Wildwater, Ltd., (864) 647-9587; Southeastern Expeditions, (404) 329-0433

extending almost completely across the river. This is Big Shoals and it should be scouted. The approach to the rapid is blind because of the large rocks; occasionally logs or entire trees have become lodged in the main chutes. Scout from the boulders to the right of center.

Big Shoals, rated a Class III by the Forest Service, is a veritable whitewater gymnasium—an excellent place for beginners to play and train. There are several routes to run, a large pool at the bottom for easy recovery, and a relatively simple portage back up and over the rocks if you wish to try again. The easiest and most popular route at Big Shoals is next to the right bank, which offers a nice tongue dropping swiftly into a small reversal wave at the head of the pool below. Other possible routes are over the curler in the right center and, at most water levels, the chute on the far left side.

Down to Earls Ford the river has many long, slow pools and a sprinkling of Class I and II whitewater. Look for wildlife in this section—many hawks nest near the stream and deer are frequently seen early and late in the day. You will easily recognize Earls Ford where Warwoman Creek, a fairly large stream, enters the river on the right. There is a well-used sand-and-gravel beach on the left. If you are getting out here, you are about to begin the worst part of your trip—the quarter-mile carry uphill to the parking lot.

Chattooga Section III

Earls Ford (C) marks the beginning of Section III, described by many as ideal for open canoeists (it is quite attractive to decked boaters as well). The scenery is nothing short of spectacular and rapids range in difficulty from Class I to Class V. We have been running this section for years, as both private boaters and professional outfitters, and we have never become tired of it.

By the time it reaches Earls Ford, the flow volume in the river has increased significantly and the average gradient to US 76 is much steeper than that of Section II. The first rapid encountered is a fairly straight drop over a three-foot ledge. Drop over to the right of center. From the large eddy and pool below this drop, look downstream and to the left for the entrance to Warwoman Rapid. This tricky Class III rapid should be entered on the left, heading toward the right. After the small initial drop, make a quick turn to the left and back downstream. There is a pillowed rock in the center of the chute; if you don't make your turn quickly, it can pin your boat or capsize it.

The next noteworthy stretch of river is through the Rock Garden. This run is noted more for its scenic value than for the difficulty of its rapids. You'll weave between huge boulders and fingerlike slabs of granite that often overshadow the stream. The rapids are mild, but stay on your toes.

Three Rooster Tails Rapid is the next challenge. After a sharp bend in the river, the course narrows and spills over a series of funneling rocky ledges under overhanging rocks. Three pluming waves (the rooster tails) can be seen in the center of the channel. The easiest run is just to the right of these pluming waves.

Just below this rapid, the river widens and slows to relative tranquillity. As you look far downstream you will see Dicks Creek (Five Finger) Falls coming into the river on the right. This is a picturesque waterfall where Dicks Creek cascades over a 50- to 60-foot drop into the river. Slightly upstream of these falls on the Chattooga is a low shelf of rock that forms part of a definite river horizon line. At low water, you can stop on this shelf or you can stop 300 yards upstream on the right to scout from the bank. Dicks Creek Ledge is given a Class IV rating in Forest Service literature. There are several possible routes—one of them is a portage over the rocks in the center. Most who run the rapid try to make the S turn over the two drops. Start the first drop heading toward the right and be prepared to make an extreme cut back to

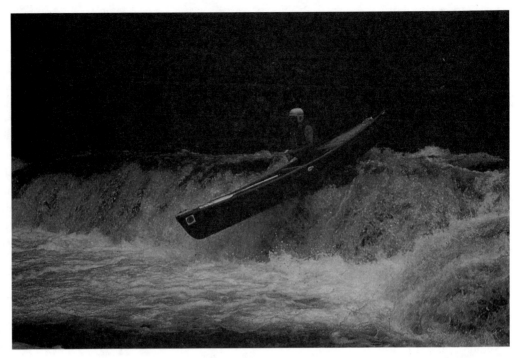

Second Ledge on Section III
of the Chattooga River.
Photo by Ed Grove.

the left at the bottom of the second drop. The **S** turn maneuver becomes increasingly difficult at higher water levels.

A short distance beyond Dicks Creek Ledge you'll observe a large rocky island. Down the right side of this island is a series of Class III drops called Stairsteps Rapid. This is not one of the major rapids on Section III. If you are doing well at this point, selecting an appropriate course through the Stairsteps should not be difficult.

Just below Stairsteps is another island, which announces Sandy Ford Rapid. The favored route in the past was to the right of this island also, but because this is a narrow channel, downed trees are always a possibility. Most paddlers now go to the left of the island. Sandy Ford (D) is recognizable by the sand beaches on both sides of a pooled area. Gravel road access is on both sides of the river, but Sandy Ford Road on the South Carolina side is recommended.

The fabled Narrows of the Chattooga River is the next major rapid. As you round the bend below Sandy Ford you'll come into a large pooled area. Get out on the lower left end of this pool to scout the entrance to the Narrows. The river drops over a series of ledges, decreasing in width as it drops. The biggest holes are just to the left of center; the least turbulent path is to the far right. Take your pick.

It should be noted that the area immediately below this series of drops has highly irregular boiling currents, an extremely fast-moving current and strong eddy lines, and numerous undercut rocks. For these reasons, the Forest Service has given the Narrows a Class IV rating. If you should find yourself swimming in the Narrows, avoid all contact with rocks, except from the downstream side. We highly recommend that an experienced boater lead the

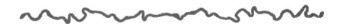

Section: Earls Ford to US 76 bridge

Counties: Rabun (GA), Oconee (SC)

USGS Quad: Rainy Mountain

Difficulty: Class I–IV (V)

Gradient: 30 feet per mile

Average Width: 30–65 feet

Velocity: Moderate to fast

Rescue Index: Remote to extremely remote

Hazards: Strainers, deadfalls, rapids, undercut rocks, keeper hydraulics

Scouting: Dicks Creek Ledge, Narrows, Keyhole (Painted Rock) Rapid, Bull Sluice

Portages: Bull Sluice and others as conditions require

Scenery: Spectacular

Highlights: Scenery, wildlife, whitewater, geology

Gauge: Chattooga Whitewater Shop, (864) 647-9083

Runnable Water Levels	Minimum	Maximum
US 76 bridge	0.8 foot	3.5 feet

Additional Information: Nantahala Outdoor Center, (864) 647-9014; Wildwater, Ltd., (864) 647-9587; Southeastern Expeditions, (404) 329-0433

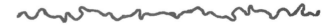

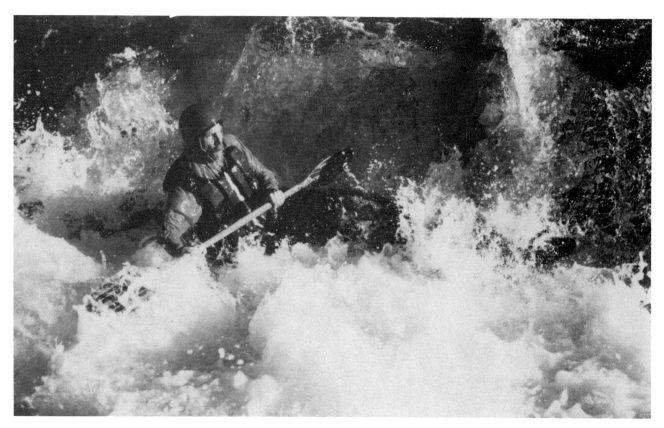

Surfing Bull Sluice on the Chattooga River. Photo by Butch Clay.

way, setting up a safety rope at strategic points through the Narrows.

Open canoes needing to bail and others needing a breather may eddy out on the left below the first series of drops. The river continues to narrow and drop until it's only a few feet wide, creating some strangely turbulent currents. The final drop in the Narrows is around the right side of an undercut rock. As you drop, make a hard left turn very quickly to avoid being forced into the rock face on the right. The Narrows' combination of whitewater, high rock faces, and drooping ferns has made this a favorite spot on the river. If you brought your camera, you should record this scenic spot on film.

One of the more dramatic rapids on Section III is not far downstream. Second Ledge is a breathtaking and heart-stopping six-foot vertical drop. It may be scouted from the left bank at any water level or from the rocks in the center of the stream at lower levels. Most paddlers run straight over the top of this one. Keep your boat parallel to the current and maintain brisk speed. Be ready to brace firmly when you hit the aerated water at the bottom. Second Ledge is not extremely difficult, but it will get your adrenaline pumping.

Less than two miles from Second Ledge is Eye of the Needle, a Class III plunge. Most of the current is pushed against the left bank, down a narrow chute that cuts slightly back to the right. The current does most of the work for you in this rapid. Beware of leaning too far to the right as you progress down the chute; you may need a strong brace to stay upright.

For approximately the next four miles the river alternates between long pools and Class I and II rapids. When Fall Creek Falls enters the river from about 25 feet up on the left bank, you'll know that Roller Coaster and Keyhole are just ahead. Roller Coaster is a fast, bucking ride down an extended series of large standing waves. Go for the center of the waves for the most excitement. A large pool at the base of Roller Coaster allows you to bail and recover if necessary.

Immediately around the bend is Keyhole, or Painted Rock, Rapid. Much of the current is pushing strongly toward a huge boulder at the bottom of the drop. To avoid this rock, begin to the right of center and continue to work right as you descend. You may also run down the extreme left, but a move to the right of the boulder is still essential. If the water level is extremely low, the far left or far right may be your only choices. Keyhole is rated a Class IV rapid by the Forest Service.

Chattooga River • Georgia

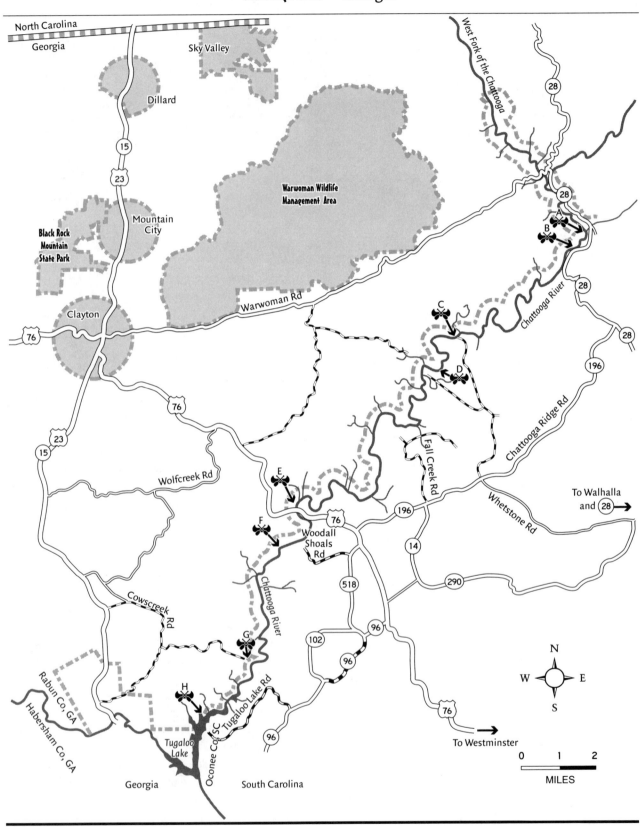

North Carolina

Georgia

Sky Valley

Dillard

15

23

Black Rock
Mountain
State Park

Mountain
City

Warwoman Wildlife
Management Area

Clayton

76

West Fork of the Chattooga

28

28

A

B

Warwoman Rd

C

Chattooga River

28

28

D

196

Chattooga Ridge Rd

Fall Creek Rd

76

23

15

Wolfcreek Rd

E

196

Whetstone Rd

To Walhalla
and 28

76

Woodall
Shoals
Rd

14

F

Cowscreek Rd

Chattooga River

518

290

G

102

96

96

H

Rabun Co, GA

Habersham Co, GA

Tugaloo Lake Rd

Oconee Co, SC

96

76

To Westminster

N

W ⊕ E

S

Tugaloo
Lake

Georgia

South Carolina

0   1   2

MILES

About three more miles of Class I and II water bring you to Bull Sluice. Even those who have run this rapid many times usually stop to scout it. Changing water levels alter the difficulty of Bull Sluice considerably and may also alter your plan of attack. It is often given a Class V rating and the total drop is over 10 feet.

You will know when you have arrived at Bull Sluice because of the extremely large boulders extending from the Georgia side of the river that seem to block the entire stream. Pull out well above these rocks on the Georgia (right) side and walk down to do your scouting. Inexperienced paddlers and those unfamiliar with the sluice have been known to enter the Class III rapids just above the Bull only to find themselves committed to running the thundering lower drops against their will.

Bull Sluice has been run in an infinite variety of watercraft by an infinite variety of people. On any given day you will see examples of the worst and best whitewater technique at Bull Sluice. Unfortunately, too many people have begun to take this rapid lightly. There have been fatalities here, and on several occasions people, both in and out of their boats, have been stuck in the upper hydraulic for uncomfortably long periods of time. The lower drop is much rockier beneath the surface than it appears. Look at it carefully before you decide to run it. The portage is on the right side over the boulders.

If you decide to run Bull Sluice, here is one of many possible routes: Follow the Class III entrance rapid down the South Carolina (left) side and hit the eddy on the left that is just above the major drop. If you are in an open canoe and have taken on a lot of water, this is the place to bail it out. It is a good spot for one to reconnoiter from river level what lies ahead. Peel out very high from this eddy and head straight over the first of the double drops just to the left of the center of the upper hole. The current will tend to push you to the left, so use it to your advantage to hit the second drop head on. Good luck!

A few hundred yards below Bull Sluice is the US 76 bridge (E). This marks the end of Section III and the beginning of Section IV. Boating access is from the large paved parking lot on the South Carolina side of the bridge. The US 76 bridge also provides a footpath to Bull Sluice for those who want to get a glimpse of the giant rapid without getting on the water.

Chattooga Section IV

In spite of the myriad attractions of Section III, the reputation of Section IV as an ultimate whitewater experience is probably what brings the throngs to the Chattooga. Skilled boaters from throughout the country try to

Section: US 76 bridge to Tugaloo Lake
Counties: Rabun (GA), Oconee (SC)
USGS Quad: Rainy Mountain
Difficulty: Class I–V (VI)
Gradient: 45 feet per mile
Average Width: 10–60 feet
Velocity: Moderate to fast
Rescue Index: Remote to extremely remote
Hazards: Strainers, deadfalls, rapids, undercut rocks, keeper hydraulics
Scouting: Woodall Shoals, Seven Foot Falls, Raven Rock, Five Falls
Portages: Woodall Shoals, Five Falls, others as conditions require
Scenery: Spectacular
Highlights: Scenery, wildlife, whitewater, geology
Gauge: Chattooga Whitewater Shop, (864) 647-9083

Runnable Water Level	Minimum	Maximum
US 76 Bridge gauge	0.8 foot	4.0 feet (expert)

Additional Information: Nantahala Outdoor Center, (864) 647-9014; Wildwater, Ltd., (864) 647-9587; Southeastern Expeditions, (404) 329-0433

make at least one pilgrimage to Section IV. Because of the greater difficulty and frequency of the rapids on this section, it should be attempted only by those with a high degree of competency. Because it is advisable that only advanced boaters attempt to paddle Section IV, this portion of the guidebook will give attention only to the more hazardous or unusual rapids.

Surfing Rapid, just around the first bend below the put-in at US 76 bridge (E), is exactly what it sounds like—an excellent spot for surfing or playing the river. The best wave is to the far right. Screaming Left Turn is located approximately 200 yards below Surfing Rapid. Large boulders direct the main stream to the far right (at higher levels, a run downriver to the left is possible, but it dumps you into a rather sticky hole). The river then flushes through an extremely sharp turn back to the left—almost all the way to the left bank. Head back across to the right for the best run of the lower part of this rapid. Screaming Left Turn is designated a Class IV by the Forest Service.

Approximately half a mile downstream you will reach a point where the river appears to be choked by large mounds of granite. This rapid is called Rock Jumble. Several routes are possible, but the best is probably to the left of center. Just below, the river calms into a pooled area known locally as Sutton's Hole, a popular swimming

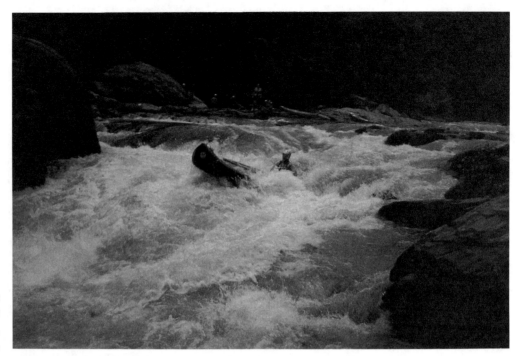

In the Five Falls at Corkscrew Rapid, Section IV of the Chattooga River. Photo by Ed Grove.

hole and a good rest stop. At this point, you are not far from what is probably the most dangerous spot on the river—Woodall Shoals, a Class VI rapid. When you see a granite shelf extending far into the river from the South Carolina (left) side, you are approaching Woodall. Stop on the rocks on the left side to scout. Do not be deceived by the way this rapid appears. The first drop creates a vicious recirculating hydraulic that has taken the lives of many people. The portage is over the rocks to the left and recenters well below the hydraulic.

One option for navigating this rapid is the Cheat Chute just off the far right bank. When this drop becomes too rocky to run (1.4 and lower) it is possible for expert paddlers to run the hydraulic on the left. If you attempt this drop, take all safety precautions. The rest of the river gives you enough thrills, so don't needlessly risk your neck here. Below the first drop, about 50 yards of Class III water takes you down into a large pool. Dirt-road access (USFS Road 757, Woodall Shoals Road) on the South Carolina side gives you a chance to enter or leave the river from here (F).

Beyond the pool the river begins to narrow and drop swiftly. When the river appears to drop out of sight on the left, stop on the right and scout the next rapid—Seven Foot Falls. A large granite outcropping splits the stream with a sheer seven-foot drop on the left and a more gradual descent to the right. If you choose the left route, run the drop sideways to avoid a rock just beneath the surface and be quick at the bottom or you will be literally smashed into the rock wall on the left. The right side is easier, but success is not guaranteed.

The next few miles provide many Class II–III rapids with the first sizable series marked by Stekoa Creek cascading in from the Georgia side. The larger sheer drop of Long Creek Falls entering from the South Carolina side is not too far beyond and is an excellent place to stop for a break.

As you continue downstream, Deliverance Rock (Class IV), a gargantuan boulder on the right, looms into view. Local lore suggests this rock was named after the crew from the movie *Deliverance* flipped their boats and lost some expensive gear here. Approach from the right side of the river above the rock. As you reach the rock, make a sharp right turn as you continue downstream.

Raven Rock Rapid (Class IV), also called Ravens Chute or Raven Cliff Rapid, is the next challenge and is easily recognized by the imposing cliffs below the rapid on the left side. Scouting should be done from the left shore. A good route starts on the left and follows the top of the long, curling diagonal wave to the right. Then head back to the left again to the base of the cliff.

A mile or so of more moderate water brings you to Camp Creek Road, which can be discerned by a sandy beach on the right. Camp Creek Road (G) is unpaved but it is the last opportunity for exit before the most formidable section of whitewater on the Chattooga—the Class III–V Five Falls. All of the Five Falls should be scouted from the shore.

The first rapid, First Fall, or Entrance Rapid, can be scouted from the right. Start on the left but immediately move toward the right, going over two small ledges. Slide down a narrow chute then head quickly across to the left bank to scout the second fall, Corkscrew. From the left bank you can get right on top of the drop and look into the chaos of Corkscrew. The bigger holes can be avoided by staying to the left in the first part of your descent. Eddy out on the right at the bottom. If you decide to portage, the right bank is slightly easier.

Scout Crack in the Rock from the right side. Cracked boulders split the river into three narrow falls, each of which drops about five feet. Run the far right or the center crack but avoid the left crack at all costs. Portage on the left. Below Crack in the Rock, ferry to the left bank for scouting Jawbone. Enter this rapid in the center, pushing hard to get back to the eddy on the left below the first drop. Peel out high on the big curler and head toward the right and the safety of the eddy on the right side of the river above the large boulder in the center of the stream. This is Hydroelectric Rock. A large hole in the rock with water flushing through it resembles a pipe that funnels water down to turbines in a dam. This hole is often lodged with debris and a swim into it could be your last. Ferry back to the left side of the stream below Hydroelectric Rock. The hazards in Jawbone are magnified greatly by its proximity to Sock-Em-Dog. Frequently, a swim in Jawbone becomes a continuing swim through Sock-Em-Dog.

Impressive at all water levels, Sock-Em-Dog is the last of the Five Falls. The Forest Service believes this one deserves a Class V rating. If you don't like the looks of Sock-Em-Dog, portage on the left. If you feel you must run the drop, start from the right as the current pushes strongly to the left. There is a smooth hump of water near the center of the top of the fall. This is sometimes referred to as the "launching pad." Keep up your speed and go over the top of the launching pad or just to the right of it. Crosscurrents are powerful. There is always the chance of landing at the bottom on rocks or in the hydraulic that can be a keeper at times. If you are unsuccessful, the large pool at the bottom gives ample time and space for recovery.

At the end of this calm area is Shoulder Bone Rapid. A jutting granite escarpment in the river is reminiscent of a shoulder bone, hence the name. Enter at the tip of the "bone" and head to the right. A few Class II to III rapids remain before the rollicking Chattooga becomes dispassionate Lake Tugaloo. The next two miles across the lake to the take-out are painfully slow, so you might as well enjoy the scenery to take your mind off the agony in your body. Take out on the left at Tugaloo Lake Road (H). Parking can be a problem here, especially on the weekends because this parking is shared with many local anglers.

A water-resistant map of the Chattooga is available from the U.S. Forest Service, Andrew Pickens Ranger District 112, Andrew Pickens Circle, Mt. Rest, SC 29664, (864) 638-9568.

Upper Chattahoochee River

The Chattahoochee River is one of the major rivers draining the state of Georgia, and its remarkable diversity is an accurate reflection of Georgia topography. It is navigable by canoe or kayak from the dramatic mountain headwaters to the Florida border, where it becomes the Apalachicola River, and remains navigable all the way to the Gulf of Mexico. There has been a metamorphosis of the river from an isolated crystalline mountain stream of a few decades ago to an overcrowded and abused stream today. Increased construction of riverbank homes and businesses, lumbering scars, hordes of weekend paddlers, and the gradually increasing turbidity of the water itself have begun to take their toll on the Chattahoochee. Please treat it with care.

In spite of the changes, however, the Chattahoochee remains a sparkling jewel in Georgia's mountain crown. At higher water levels the headwaters above Robertstown and Helen are navigable by skilled boaters. The uppermost access is via unpaved U.S. Forest Service roads. The river is extremely small here, but the scenery and gradient combine to make a run that borders on the spectacular when the water level is right. The lower sections of the river must approach flood levels before a run on this section is feasible.

From USFS Road 44 (A) to Robertstown (B) the river drops extremely quickly through a rocky, constricted channel bordered by hemlocks, mountain laurel, and rhododendron. There are many sections barely wide enough for a boat to pass through and occasional blind turns and drops. There is little margin for error. Scout as much of the river as possible from the road before putting in, and scout all major drops while on the water. This section is seldom traveled but is a real treat for advanced boaters. Those who catch it when the water is right won't forget it.

On reaching the valley floor, the river calms into steady Class I riffles and remains that way through Helen (C,D). There are no obstacles except for one low wooden bridge near Robertstown that may present problems at some water levels.

The town of Helen deserves some mention at this point. The economy here was once based on agriculture and logging. In the 1960s some residents decided that revitalization was needed and began remodeling the town as a Bavarian alpine village in an effort to boost tourism. They were successful. Helen is now a major north Georgia tourist attraction.

The Chattahoochee continues its gentle pace through Helen and down to Nora Mill, where a portage is necessary. Portage either through the woods on the left bank, or use the highway parallel to the river on the right bank. Begin your portage well away from the mill as the property owners don't seem to be overly fond of canoeists.

Below the mill the river takes a significant bend and crosses the highway twice. At the second crossing (GA 75, F) the river is adjacent to the Nacoochee Indian Mound. This mound and the surrounding valley have produced numerous Cherokee artifacts. Valley farmers still report uncovering arrowheads and bits of pottery during spring plowing. All of this land is private property and is definitely not open for public digging. Please respect landowners' rights.

The Nacoochee Valley is a pleasant pastoral float through mostly open farmland with some wooded areas. There are often many downed trees, however, that can cause problems. Near the end of the valley, Sautee Creek enters from the left. Many boaters put in to Sautee Creek on Lynch Mountain Road, an unpaved county road, next to the GA 17 bridge over the creek (G). The float down the creek is only 100 yards to the main stream of the Chattahoochee.

From the Sautee Creek junction down to GA 255 (H) is one of the longest undisturbed stretches of the river. The terrain is heavily forested with large white pines and frequent rock outcroppings. The evidence of intrusion by man is less obvious here than elsewhere, and a pleasant illusion of isolation settles in. This used to be a good section for camping, but increased development makes

Section: USFS Road 44 (52) to Lake Sidney Lanier

Counties: White, Habersham Hall

USGS Quads: Jacks Gap, Cowrock, Helen, Leaf Clarkesville, Lula

Difficulty: Class I–IV

Gradient: 3 to 95+ feet per mile

Average Width: 20–50 feet

Velocity: Moderate

Rescue Index: Accessible to accessible but difficult

Hazards: Strainers, deadfalls, difficult rapids, low bridges

Scouting: Entire section above Robertstown, Smith Island Rapid, Three Ledges, Horseshoe Rapid

Portages: Rapids as necessary, Nora Mill dam

Scenery: Pretty to exceptionally beautiful

Highlights: Scenery, wildlife, whitewater, local culture and industry (Helen), history

Gauge: Wildewood Outfitters, (706) 865-4451 or (800) 553-2715

Runnable Water Levels	Minimum	Maximum
GA 115 gauge	0.8 foot	6 feet

Additional Information: US Forest Service, Chattahoochee National Forest, (770) 536-0541

camping difficult these days. Rapids are fairly frequent but never go beyond a mild Class II.

Access at the GA 255 bridge is on the White County side of the river, upstream of the bridge. The property owner on the right side should not be disturbed. Use the public highway right-of-way.

This section begins with several Class I rapids and smooth pools. Then the river enters a long, slow area nicknamed "the Dead Sea" because its stillness offers a marked contrast to the rapids above and below. It is a beautiful area and should not be slighted. Large trees on either side form a cool green tunnel of vegetation that occasionally opens into rolling pastured vistas. The Dead Sea section is partially formed by the natural damming effect of Smith Island and is the first warning sign that the Smith Island rapid is near. The next indicator is a large, gently sloping granite face on the right bank.

The Smith Island rapid is the first of the significant rapids on the upper Chattahoochee. It should be scouted by first-time paddlers or by anyone running the river at extreme water levels; however, do not scout by landing on the island. The island and the left bank are private property and are protected by the courts after many years of land disputes. Scout cautiously by landing on the right bank and walking down below the island to look back upstream, but be aware of the local landowners' rights.

The left side of the island is the best route. It is a Class II rapid at almost any water level; at high water it becomes a solid Class III. Enter the rapid from the left side of the main stream at the tip of the island, and gradually work back to the right side (the left bank of the island) for the final plunging chute. This chute ends in a fairly deep pool next to a large rock face. Recover on the island if necessary.

The channel going to the right of the island may be scouted from the right bank of the river. It can be run at higher water levels (above three feet on the GA 115 gauge), but most of the time it is too shallow and rocky to be worthwhile. It does provide a nice view, however, if you look back upstream from below the island. Stay to the right of center for the best course below the island. Rapids are Class I down to the GA 115 bridge.

If you are putting in the river at the GA 115 bridge (I), enter on the Habersham County side at the Wildewood Shop Outpost. Parking, boat rentals, and shuttle services are available from the Duncan bridge access point to this location. Parking is now restricted in this area. Whitewater buffs will find the section from the GA 115 bridge to Duncan bridge the most pleasant. None of the rapids are intimidating at normal water levels, but altogether they are frequent enough and challenging enough to keep you occupied.

Just below the bridge you'll encounter a small, sloping drop into a long, wide, pooled area that disappears around the bend to the left. After rounding the bend, look downstream beyond the shallow shoals and you should be able to distinguish the tip of an island. The river has become quite wide here (over 100 feet) but is very shallow. The island you see marks the beginning of Buck Island Shoals, a fairly continuous quarter-mile section of Class II water. The best run is to the left of the first three small islands, then work back to the right center for the rest of the shoals. The gradient here is constant and fairly steep. This section has "eaten" experienced decked boaters at extremely high water levels when waves may exceed four feet in height. At low or average water levels one would encounter only minor technical problems.

After a series of Class I and pooling water, watch for a large granite outcropping on the right—this indicates the imminence of the Three Ledges. Many consider this to be the most fun or challenging series of rapids. Looking downstream to the left of center you will observe a large, low, flat rock protruding above water level. Run just to the left of this rock over the first ledge. Immediately ferry to the right of center for ledge number two, a more gradual slope that angles back to the left. You are now approaching the third ledge, a straight drop of about three

Upper Chattahoochee River • Georgia

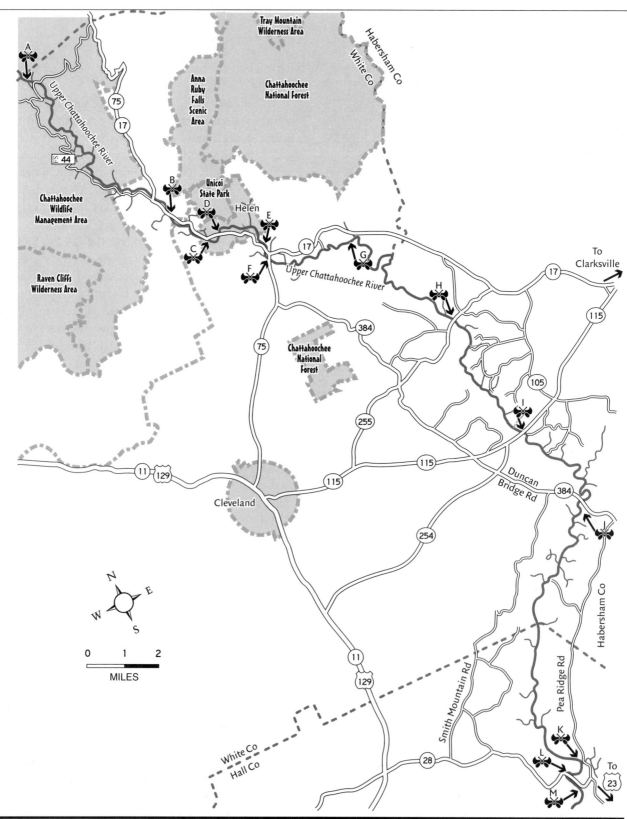

Upper Chattahoochee River • Georgia

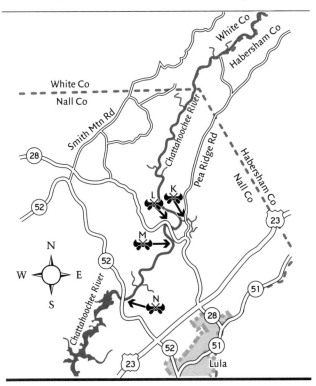

feet. Go straight over and you will do just fine. The hole at the base of this one is a great place to play.

The river then continues in a Class I and pool series, with the exception of one washboard series of small diagonal ledges that is interesting. After passing this, watch again for another long pool with granite outcroppings on the right. This denotes the approach to Horseshoe Rapid (Class II+). You can see a long, low ledge of rocks where the river hooks around, giving Horseshoe its name. Enter on the left, and be ready to cut hard back to the right. Just below Horseshoe Rapid the Soquee River enters on the left followed shortly by a small creek falls that also enters on the left. You are now almost to the Sandy Bottoms/Duncan bridge access point (J).

The next reasonable access point below Duncan bridge is Belton bridge on the backwaters of Lake Lanier. The scenery remains quite good, and there are a few Class I–II rapids; however, once you hit the backwater of the lake forward progress becomes painful. Plan at least another half a day to get to Belton bridge.

Amicalola Creek

The Amicalola Creek, which gets its name from the Cherokee phrase for "tumbling water," is called a creek on most maps, but this is something of a misnomer. The scenery is spectacular, the rapids are sometimes stupendous. It is hard to describe this stream without superlatives, so if it is only a creek, it is simply the best whitewater creek in the state.

Located entirely in Dawson County, its upper east fork, Little Amicalola Creek, contains the famous Amicalola Falls. Amicalola Falls State Park encompasses the southern end of the Appalachian Trail, which stretches from there to Mount Katahdin in Maine.

The stream does not become navigable until below the junction of the Little Amicalola with the main Amicalola. The small wooden bridges near Alton (A,B) mark the highest normal put-in point. These are small county roads surrounded by private property. Please be extremely courteous and respectful of the rights of landowners in this area.

Check the gauge for this section first. It is in the pool just upstream of the GA 53 bridge, toward the east bank. With 0.8 foot or more, the upper section has enough water to be a comfortable run. For the most part it provides easy floating and quiet beauty, but a few rapids require extra care. Early in the run, the stream turns east and comes to a shallow and rocky series of Class II ledges. In midrun, Cochrane Creek enters on the left and increases the water volume considerably. In the next half mile are three good rapids that may require scouting. The first is a wide, five-foot ledge. Look for a little chute into a pool just left of the downstream island. The next rapid is more complex; from a right-side approach several routes are possible. The third rapid is a three-and-a-half-foot ledge that can be sneaked through on the extreme right; the main route left of center can be a boat-buster. The remaining miles provide easy floating through forest recently damaged by a tornado.

By the time it reaches Devils Elbow (C), the Amicalola has a more respectable volume. A covered bridge here was burned by vandals in the mid-1970s, but some timbers are still visible along the banks and, unfortunately, in the streambed. The three and a half miles from the covered bridge ruins to the GA 53 bridge is an excellent afternoon trip. The mountain flora common in the first section continues, and there are more frequent rock outcroppings. Because it starts flat and builds gradually to several Class II rapids, this section has proved to be an excellent training course for beginners. The last Class II rapid, just a quarter of a mile from the bridge, has a feisty little hole at the bottom that creates a good surfing wave. There is a good recovery pool if upsets occur.

Below GA 53 (D) the Amicalola is for experienced boaters only. The rapids crescendo to Class IV+ ratings when the water is high and even at low water they rate a solid Class III. It is runnable from a level of 0.6 at the GA 53 gauge, but if the level is above 1.2, boaters should be confident. The first two miles below the highway average over 80 feet per mile drop. The first mile is almost continuous rapids, so be adept at self-rescue.

The Edge of the World is the name given the first set of rapids below the bridge. The boater will see a definite rocky horizon line all across the river. A large logjam in the center of the stream provides a good vantage point for scouting. The Edge is composed of two large drops of five to six feet each with several small drops interspersed. Begin on the left side for the first drop and work all the way across to the right side over the smaller ledges. The second large drop is a straight shot near the right bank.

The Class II–III action continues for another half mile of maneuvering before slowing to any sizable pool. Pools interspersed with Class II rapids continue for another half mile to Off the Wall Rapid. Off the Wall can be recognized by the steep, sloping granite face on the right bank. A large portion of the stream flow is diverted by boulders into a narrow channel on the right. The water rebounds off the granite face and makes a quick drop. Draw to the left of the protruding rock at the bottom of the chute.

Scenery surpasses the expectations of most travelers

Section: Goshen Road (Alton) to Etowah River
County: Dawson
USGS Quads: Amicalola, Nelson, Juno, Matt
Difficulty: Class I–IV (V)
Gradient: 5–80 feet per mile
Average Width: 30–40 feet
Velocity: Fast
Scenery: Exceptionally beautiful to spectacular
Highlights: Scenery, wildlife, whitewater
Rescue Index: Accessible to extremely remote
Hazards: Strainers, deadfalls, undercut rocks, difficult rapids
Scouting: At major rapids below GA 53
Portages: As required by water level
Gauge: Visual only. Gauge on river right above Highway 53
   Bridge.

Runnable Water Levels	Minimum	Maximum
Above GA 53	0.8 foot	3.5 feet
Below GA 53	0.6 foot	3.5 feet

Additional Information: Amicalola River Rafting, (706) 265-6892;
   Amicalola Falls State Park, (706) 265-8888

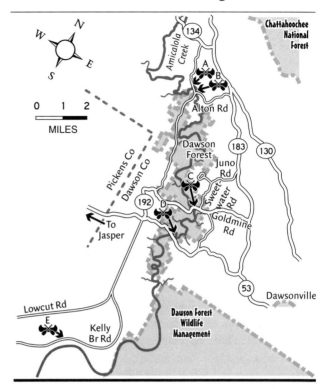

Amicalola Creek • Georgia

on their first descent. Lacy hemlocks and towering pines jut out from rocky precipices. Sheer walls occasionally rise several hundred feet above water level. Tributary streams cascade into the crystalline Amicalola and the influences of nearby civilization are seldom evident. Savor it.

Class I–II rapids are abundant and quickly bring you to Split Rock Rapid. Here the stream divides into three channels with the center channel seemingly splitting a large boulder. The left channel is blocked by large fallen trees, but the center and right channels are runnable; the center channel is preferable.

The action begins to moderate, but the streamside environment remains extraordinary. Just about the time you think the Amicalola has shown you all of its thrills,

you reach Roostertail Rapid. The stream drops steeply with good routes along the left (the roostertail) and the far right. The center is usually too shallow and rocky.

The intense whitewater is now done and the stream begins to change character altogether. Rapids become less frequent and the current is almost slack. The Etowah River merges from the left a few miles below Roostertail Rapid, increasing the volume but not the velocity of the flow. Relax and enjoy this section in contrast to the adrenaline rush of the upper section, or stroke hard if the day is waning. It always takes longer than you think it will. The take-out is on the right bank next to the new bridge and newly graveled road.

Cartecay River

The Cartecay was for years a sleeper hit among Georgia's many fine whitewater streams. It rolled along unnoticed near Ellijay, known only to a few area anglers and local boaters. However, this situation is gradually changing and the Cartecay is now attracting some well-deserved attention.

The navigable section of the river lies entirely within Gilmer County in northwestern Georgia. The Cartecay is a tributary of the once mighty but now dammed Coosawattee River. There are many launch and take-out spots providing a variety of trips for all skill levels. The upper section is two and a half miles of scenic Class I rapids from Holt Bridge Road (Highway 52, A) to Lower Cartecay Road (B). The trip from Lower Cartecay Road to Blackberry Mountain is full of fun. There is a public take-out at the covered bridge. The lower part of the river should be done only if you are prepared for eight miles of Class II–III whitewater with three miles of calm water.

The first few miles are slow and easy paddling through a scenic mountain valley. Thickets of mountain laurel, large pines, and various hardwoods will often suddenly part to expose rolling pastures and views of the surrounding mountains. The flow here is Class I. The only hazards are occasional downed trees that may block the narrow streambed.

As the valley ends the gradient gets steeper and easy Class II rapids begin to appear. Just below the first large island, the **S** turn is the first rapid of significant technical difficulty. Go to the left of the island and scout from the left shore. The terrain in this area is reminiscent of the third section of the Chattooga and has often been called a miniature version of the Narrows.

Seeing the covered bridge at Blackberry Mountain signals the first big drop on the river, called Stegall Mill. The drop can be scouted on the left and a small pool is all that separates it from several tight rapids below. Stegall Mill can be run straight down the center over the pluming wave in the main chute or in the chute on the left by cheating the wave to its left side. Eddy left in the pool

below or be ready to brace and recover for the technical turns that follow.

The Cartecay, like the Chattooga, is a drop-and-pool stream, with sudden bursts of rapids interrupted by long, nearly placid stretches. This pattern continues as the river meanders along until it reaches a series of small islands. At the bottom of the second island after the covered bridge, pull out on the left to scout the second major drop, the Narrows at Clear Creek. At normal water levels you should run near the left bank. At water levels over three feet, a potentially hazardous hydraulic reversal develops at the base of the falls. Portage is easiest on the right.

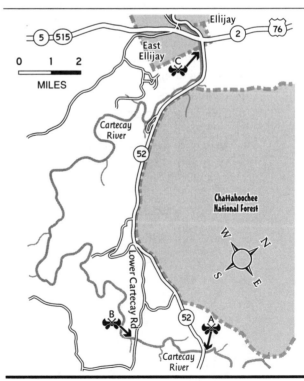

Cartecay River • Georgia

Section: GA 52 to East Ellijay
County: Gilmer
USGS Quads: Tickanetly, Ellijay
Difficulty: Class I–III
Gradient: 10 to 40+ feet per mile
Average Width: 20–40 feet
Velocity: Moderate
Rescue Index: Accessible to remote
Hazards: Strainers, deadfalls, difficult rapids
Scouting: First Fall, Clear Creek Falls
Portages: None required
Scenery: Pretty to exceptionally beautiful
Highlights: Scenery, wildlife, whitewater
Gauge: Beacon Sports Center, (706) 276-3600

Runnable Water Level	Minimum	Maximum
	1.0 foot	Up to flood stage

Additional Information: Mountain Outdoor Expeditions, (706) 635-2524; Beacon Sports Center, (706) 276-3600

The Narrows is the last drop on the river, but the pace remains brisk with some interesting Class II ripples before reaching the lower valley. Here the river slows almost to a halt and signs of civilization reappear in abundance. Highway noises filter through the woods. Riverside homes and pastures are again noticeable and a mobile-home park marks the end of all seclusion. A Class II rapid just above the river gauging station on the right bank denotes the end of the trip. Take out on the highway right-of-way on the right bank (C).

Talking Rock Creek

Talking Rock Creek is navigable from GA 5 in Pickens County to GA 136 (in some places marked GA 156) in Murray County. A few miles of the stream are in southwestern Gilmer County, but there is no road access to this portion. Approximately the last two miles of paddling prior to reaching the access at GA 136 (156) are across the Carters Lake reservoir. At this point Talking Rock Creek has merged with the Coosawattee River.

At the upper access at GA 5 (A), the stream is quite small and flows through a valley almost the entire distance to county road 198 (B), a distance of almost three miles. Although this section is scenic and pleasant to paddle when water is high, most boaters prefer to put in at (B) or where the river next crosses GA 136 (C). Below point B the streamside environment becomes much steeper and the flow volume is more conducive to easy floating because Town Creek has entered just above the bridge. Shoals become more frequent but are not extremely difficult.

GA 136 (C) provides easy access to a splendid canoeing experience. Talking Rock Creek enters a gorge environment of beauty and isolation. Terrain is extremely rugged and sheer walls often rise 100 feet or more above the stream. There are many rapids, some quite long but few rank above Class II difficulty. Numerous deep, quiet pools give ample opportunity for swimming, fishing, or just relaxing. This is an excellent area for camping and this section is long enough for two full, relaxed days. It may be traversed in one day, but the boater should allow maximum daylight time. There is no good access until reaching GA 136 again (D).

Of particular interest is the scenery along the entire route. At low water levels there are many small islands

Section: Blaine to Carters Lake Reservoir
Counties: Pickens, Gilmer, Gordon, Murray
USGS Quads: Talking Rock, Oakman
Difficulty: Class I–III
Gradient: 19 (30+) feet per mile
Velocity: Moderate
Average Width: 20–45 feet
Rescue Index: Accessible but difficult to remote
Hazards: Strainers, deadfalls, difficult rapids, powerboat trams
Scouting: Rapids as required by ability level
Portages: None required
Scenery: Beautiful to spectacular
Highlights: Scenery, wildlife, whitewater
Gauge: Visual only

Runnable Water Levels	Minimum	Maximum
GA 136 bridge	1.5 feet	6.0 feet

Additional Information: Beacon Sports Center, (706) 276-3600

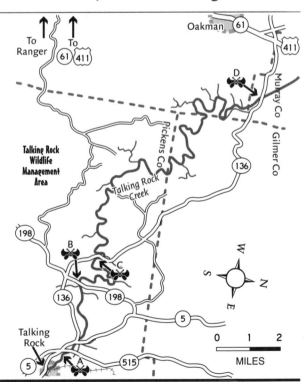

Talking Rock Creek • Georgia

of river grasses and flowers in midstream that create a maze for canoeists. Sheer rock walls often will be on the sides of the stream. The name Talking Rock Creek probably came from the echoes that reverberate from the cliffs when any loud noise is made. One imposing bluff on the right side about two-thirds of the way down this section contains what appears to be the entrance to a cave that is well above stream level. The gorge area also holds one of the last stands of virgin timber in the state of Georgia.

Talking Rock Creek is subject to rapid fluctuations in water level, and the difficulty of navigation is appreciably increased in extreme high water. Due to the lack of easy access and the incumbent difficulty of evacuation if problems arise, inexperienced boaters are advised to float this section only when the water is moderate to low.

KENTUCKY

Russell Fork of the Levisa Fork of the Big Sandy River

Flowing out of Virginia and joined by the Pound River, the Russell Fork cuts a 1,600-foot gorge in the lonely Pine Ridge Mountains, forming what is referred to as the "Great Breaks of the Pine Ridge." This incredible chasm with giant vertical walls and pounding whitewater defines the Kentucky-Virginia border for several miles before plunging out of the mountains near Elkhorn City, Kentucky.

There are three runnable sections of the Russell Fork. The put-in for the first section is in Dickenson County, Virginia, just below the John Flannagan Dam. It's a quick paddle in mostly Class I–II water. The traditional launching point is at the Bartlick Bridge off VA 611 (A), just below the confluence of the Pound and Russell Fork Rivers. From here, there is a 2.8-mile paddle in Class II (III) water to the Garden Hole access road (B). Anyone who feels the slightest bit overwhelmed should be aware that this is the last chance to stop before the bottom falls out. Soon the drop increases markedly, steep sandstone walls rise on both sides, and the Russell Fork pounds its way for 3.8 miles along a giant semicircular loop at the base of the mountain. Here, hidden by the shadows of the gorge, is a hellish continuum of thundering vertical Class IV–V+ drops and foam-blasted boulder gardens where the river gradient reaches an amazing 180 feet per mile.

The rapids in this section include the consecutive five-, eight-, and nine-foot vertical drops of Triple Drop, the awesome El Horendo with drops of 10 and 15 feet spaced only a boat length apart, the boulder-strewn S turn at Red Cliff, and the appropriately named Climax. These are rugged rapids that only the most confident of paddlers should attempt. Once seldom paddled, this section has recently become the standard against which all other eastern rivers are compared.

The numerous dangers of the Russell Fork should not be taken lightly. The pushy water, frequent undercuts, and intensely long and complex rapids make this a very unforgiving stream. The Russell Fork is a "river of inches," where boat placement becomes an exacting art and mis-

takes usually lead to more than a bruised ego. Commercial rafting was introduced to the river in 1988 and private paddlers must now compete for "must make" eddies with rafts, increasing the intensity of the run. First-time paddlers running the river without benefit of a knowledgeable guide will find it necessary to extensively scout most of the rapids—an extremely difficult proposition among the house-sized rocks lining the banks.

After this demanding section paddlers may take out at the access point a short distance from KY 80 (C), or continue the two miles through Class II rapids to Elkhorn City, Kentucky (D).

The efforts of local paddlers have swayed Elkhorn City officials and the U.S. Army Corps of Engineers to con-

Russell Fork of the Levisia Fork, Big Sandy River • KY/VA

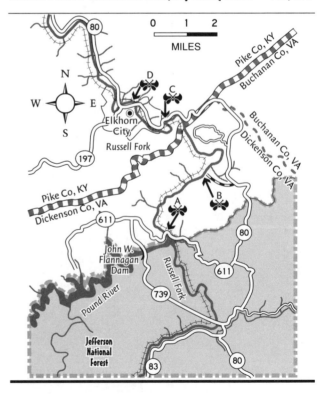

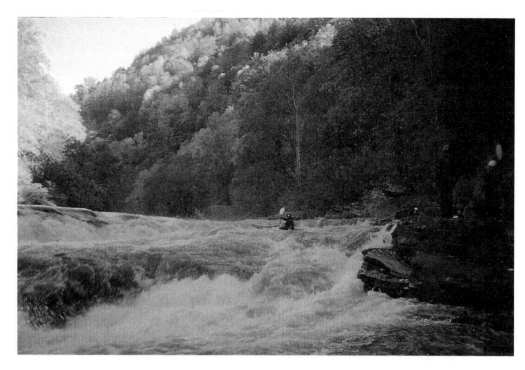

Richard Vest in El Horendo on
the Russell Fork.
Photo courtesy Matthew Vest.

Section: Pound River Dam to Elkhorn City
Counties: Dickenson (VA), Pike (KY)
USGS Quad: Elkhorn City
Difficulty: Class IV–V+
Gradient: 5–180+ feet per mile
Average Width: 35–60 feet
Velocity: Fast
Rescue Index: Accessible but difficult to remote
Hazards: Undercut rocks, keeper hydraulics, difficult rapids,
    scarcity of eddies
Scouting: Entire run on foot prior to running
Portages: Routes around most rapids are available at 1,300 cfs
Scenery: Spectacular to exceptionally beautiful
Highlights: Scenery, history, geology, whitewater
Gauge: John Flannagan Dam, (540) 835-1438
Runnable Water level   Minimum   Maximum
                         Open 900 cfs   2,000 cfs
Additional Information: U.S. Army Corps of Engineers, (540)
    635-9544; Break Center State Park, (540) 865-4413

duct special water releases from the John Flannagan Dam each October. Although the river can be run anytime throughout the year depending on rainfall, in October the Corps of Engineers will occasionally schedule weekend flows of 1,350 cfs, considered an optimal level. Elkhorn City, in an effort to boost tourism with whitewater, has also scheduled Fall Festival events to coincide with the water releases.

North Fork of the Cumberland River

The North Fork of the Cumberland River (locally referred to simply as the Cumberland) originates near Harlan at the confluence of the Poor Fork of the Cumberland and Catron Creek, and it flows west, draining the eastern Kentucky counties of Harlan, Bell, Knox, Whitley, McCreary, and Pulaski.

Between Harlan (A) and Pineville (D), the North Fork flows over a mud and gravel bed with infrequent small shoals and rapids (Class I+) and occasional large rocks in evidence in the stream and along the banks. From a width of approximately 50 feet at its origin, the Cumberland broadens quickly to 85 to 105 feet. Running west through the steep, rugged hills of the Cumberland Plateau, the river winds through forest and coal country, under hanging wooden footbridges, and past the cabins of miners and the ever-present coal tipples along the railroad tracks. As the Cumberland passes Pineville, it settles down into a mud bottom with steep banks, broadens a bit, and flows smoothly as it progresses through the deep valleys past Barbourville toward Williamsburg.

To canoe the Cumberland from Pineville (D) to Williamsburg (H) is to become intimately acquainted with the land and the people of eastern Kentucky, whose lifestyle and institutions are visible and alive all along the river. Although only steep wooded hillsides meet your searching eyes, you are never out of earshot of the rumbling coal trucks or the raspy barking of a dog defending an unseen cabin in some lonely hollow.

The Cumberland from Harlan to Pineville is frequently runnable from November through mid-May or whenever the Williamsburg gauge reads in excess of 1,300 cfs. Access is reasonably good, provided you are accustomed to steep banks. From Pineville to Williamsburg the river is usually runnable when the Williamsburg gauge reads in excess of 700 cfs. The section from Harlan to Williamsburg is best suited for one-day runs (pick your own) rather than canoe camping.

From Williamsburg (H) to Cumberland Falls (J), the river flows through the Daniel Boone National Forest. In this section the river continues to widen until in some places it is almost 200 feet across. The gradient increases here and some mild whitewater (Class II) is encountered, with boulders in the stream and some shoals spanning the entire width of the river. This section (beyond the mouth of Jellico Creek) is extremely remote and makes a good canoe-camping run at moderate water levels (500–1,100 cfs) and a fair whitewater run at higher levels (1,100–1,900 cfs). Rock replaces the mud bottom of the upper sections, and the current runs swiftly and continuously, with very few pools. Boulders line the banks in increasing numbers, and some flat, accessible terraces have been carved along the streamside. In the last three miles before reaching the KY 90 bridge, exposed rock palisades become visible on the right as the Cumberland begins to enter the deep gorge that will carry it over the falls and beyond to Lake Cumberland.

Section: Harlan to west of Pineville
Counties: Bell, Harlan
USGS Quads: Harlan, Wallins Creek, Balkan, Varilla, Middlesboro North, Pineville
Difficulty: Class I+
Gradient: 3 feet per mile
Average Width: 50–100 feet
Velocity: Fast
Rescue Index: Accessible to accessible but difficult
Hazards: Deadfalls
Scouting: None required
Portages: None required
Scenery: Pleasant to pretty in spots
Highlights: Scenery, local culture, history
Gauge: U.S. Army Corps of Engineers, (800) 261-5033

Runnable Water Levels	Minimum	Maximum
Williamsburg gauge	1300 cfs	Up to flood stage

Additional Information: U.S. Army Corps of Engineers, (309) 529-2604

North Fork of the Cumberland River • Kentucky

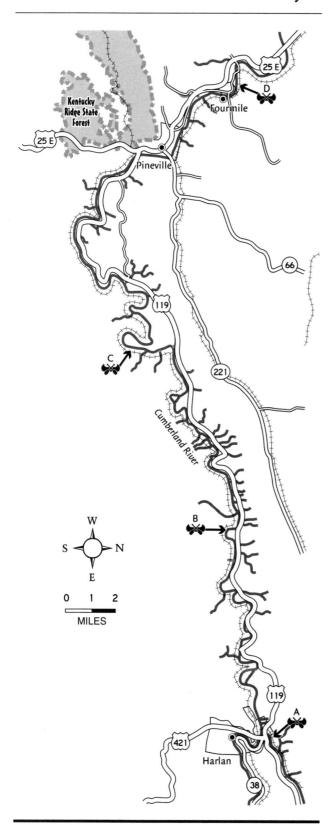

About one mile upstream of the falls, the river curves sharply to the left and the KY 90 bridge becomes visible downstream. Move to the right of the river for the take-out on the upstream side of the bridge (at the picnic ground and parking lot). Failure to move promptly to the right can have tragic consequences for the unlucky or inexperienced. One of the larger shoals (Class II) of this section is situated across the entire river just upstream of the take-out. If you run it on the left and fill or capsize, you will find yourself in the main current heading for the entrance rapids to Cumberland Falls several hundred yards downstream. If you run the shoals on the right and take water or turn over, you will be in much slower current and (except at excessive levels, i.e., 1,900+ cfs) you'll be washed into the bank as the river narrows near the bridge, or alternately swept downstream past the bridge into a huge eddy that forms along the bank near the visitors' parking lot.

Access for this section is not plentiful, but is good where it exists. The Cumberland from Williamsburg to Cumberland Falls is normally runnable from November to early June or whenever the Williamsburg gauge reads 400 cfs or higher.

The next section of the North Fork of the Cumberland is a Kentucky-protected Wild River and is one of the most popular whitewater runs in the state. Referred to as "The Cumberland Below the Falls" by local paddlers, the river here runs through a mammoth rock gorge with boulders lining the river marking the age-old erosion of the falls. This run should be attempted only by experienced boaters, and extra flotation is recommended for open boats.

The run begins with a long carry from the visitors' parking lot at Cumberland Falls to a beach a quarter mile away at the bottom of the falls (K). Scenery is spectacular right from the put-in, and most paddlers take the opportunity to paddle back upstream for a truly awe-inspiring view of the falls. Eighty yards from the falls is as close as you can safely paddle without fighting a fantastically strong reversal current trying to pull you into the falls.

Moving downstream, several easy Class II rapids that require no scouting are encountered before arriving at the Class III Center Rock Rapid. This rapid can be identified by the large boulders on each side that constrict the river to a channel of approximately 20 feet, and by the degree of drop that substantially exceeds that encountered previously. The rapid consists of a 25-foot-long, stairstep chute followed 50 feet later by a 3-foot vertical drop directly in front of a huge boulder that splits the current. This is Center Rock. The first drop is usually run straight

North Fork of the Cumberland River • Kentucky

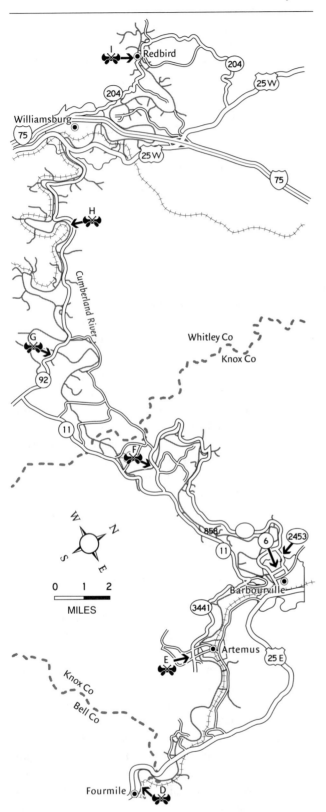

Section: West of Pineville to Williamsburg

Counties: Bell, Knox, Whitley

USGS Quads: Pineville, Artemus, Barbourville, Rockholds, Saxton, Williamsburg

Difficulty: Class I+

Gradient: 3 feet per mile

Average Width: 50–100 feet

Velocity: Fast

Rescue Index: Accessible to accessible but difficult

Hazards: Deadfalls, dams

Scouting: None required

Portages: Dam at power plant nine miles below Pineville

Scenery: Pleasant to pretty in spots

Highlights: Scenery, local culture, industry

Gauge: U.S. Army Corps of Engineers, (800) 261-5033

Runnable Water Levels	Minimum	Maximum
Williamsburg gauge	1300 cfs	Up to flood stage

Additional Information: U.S. Army Corps of Engineers, (309) 529-2604; Sheltowee Trace Outfitters, (606) 376-5567 or (800) 541-7238; Cumberland Falls State Resort Park, (606) 528-4121 or (800) 325-0063

down the center, while the strategy for the second is to angle the bow to the right and drop straight into the eddy on the right at the bottom of the drop. An alternative strategy for the second drop is to ride the pillow off the right side of Center Rock. We recommend that you scout this rapid.

Continuing downstream, the river lapses into a series of pools followed by rock gardens (at low to moderate water) and Class II rapids. The drops are small, but several of the rapids are quite technical. One of these, at about mile four, has an undercut boulder situated in mid-channel, splitting the flow. This should be run along the far right bank. Moving on, there are more long pools and small rapids. At mile five there is a slanting, two-and-a-half-foot drop with a playful hole at the bottom that spans the entire river. This is known as Surfing Rapid and is a delightful place to stop for lunch.

Beyond Surfing Rapid the run becomes more intense. At a half mile downstream of Surfing Rapid, the river disappears to the right around a house-sized rock and immediately cuts left again, crashing into a boulder on the right and down a 30-foot-long chute. This fast and furious, borderline Class III run serves up an exciting ride. Run right of center and play the pillow off the boulder.

The next rapid, a quarter mile distant, is a turning, four-foot drop known as Screaming Right Turn Rapid. At

North Fork of the Cumberland River • Kentucky

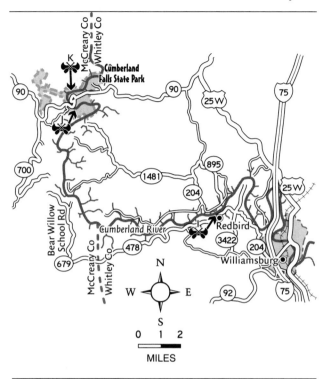

MILES

Section: Williamsburg to Cumberland Falls

Counties: Whitley, McCreary, Cumberland Falls

USGS Quads: Williamsburg, Wofford, Cumberland Falls

Difficulty: Class I–II

Gradient: 2.61 feet per mile

Average Width: 70–105 feet

Velocity: Fast

Rescue Index: Remote to extremely remote

Hazards: Falls at end of run

Scouting: None required

Portages: None required, but you must take out before the falls

Scenery: Pretty to beautiful in spots

Highlights: Scenery, wildlife

Gauge: U.S. Army Corps of Engineers, (800) 261-5033

Runnable Water Levels	Minimum	Maximum
	500 cfs	Up to flood stage

Additional Information: U.S. Army Corps of Engineers, (309) 529-2604; Sheltowee Trace Outfitters, (606) 376-5567 or (800) 541-7238; Cumberland Falls State Resort Park, (606) 528-4121 or (800) 325-0063

North Fork of the Cumberland River • Kentucky

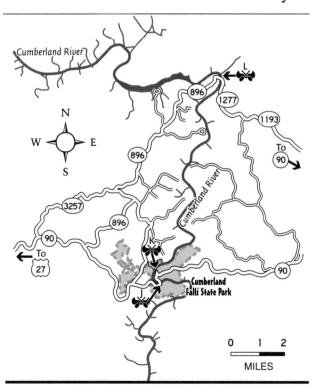

MILES

Section: Cumberland Falls to the mouth of the Laurel River

Counties: Whitley, McCreary

USGS Quads: Cumberland Falls, Sawyer

Difficulty: Class III

Gradient: 11.75 feet per mile

Average Width: 40–80 feet

Velocity: Fast

Rescue Index: Remote to extremely remote

Hazards: Undercut rocks, keeper hydraulics at certain water levels, difficult rapids

Scouting: At major or blind rapids

Portages: None required, but you should consider carrying at major rapids

Scenery: Beautiful to exceptionally beautiful

Highlights: Scenery, wildlife, geology

Gauge: U.S. Army Corps of Engineers, (800) 261-5033

Runnable Water Levels	Minimum	Maximum
	300 cfs	Up to flood stage

Additional Information: U.S. Army Corps of Engineers, (309) 529-2604; Sheltowee Trace Outfitters, (606) 376-5567 or (800) 541-7238; Cumberland Falls State Resort Park, (606) 528-4121 or (800) 325-0063

low to moderate water levels the main flow drops over a one-and-a-half-foot ledge and splashes almost immediately onto a rock that diverts the current sharply to the right over a three-foot, slanted drop. The most popular strategy here is to cut right after the first ledge, using the pillow to turn the boat. At higher water levels the river overflows the obstructing rock and a four-foot vertical drop (and a mean hydraulic) is created completely across the river. Scouting is definitely required in this situation.

The next large rapid, known as Stair Steps, is a long, delightful, borderline Class III stretch that looks much worse than it really is. It is easily recognized by the large hole at the top with a shark-fin–shaped rock just below it. Decked boaters may want to punch the hole. For open boaters, the best route is to run right of the hole and then hug the right bank all the way to the bottom. Scout on the right.

The last major rapid is appropriately named Last Drop. In this Class III area, the current winds to the right along the upstream side of a large boulder and then suddenly cuts left, dropping vertically three feet. Next the current is split by a building-sized boulder in the middle of the river. Run to the right at the top, staying to the inside of the turn and away from the upstream face of the boulder. Cut hard left, taking the vertical drop as close to the boulder as possible. Go around the building-sized boulder that splits

the current on the far right. At high water this rapid (like several others) changes drastically, forming a super-mean hole at the top. Scout (or portage) to the right. Last Drop marks the end of the whitewater section of the Cumberland (although several small shoals are encountered farther downstream due to the low level of the lake pool).

From here it is a scenic three-and-a-half-mile paddle through the lake to the take-out at the mouth of the Laurel River (L). Access is excellent at the take-out. The pool level of Lake Cumberland varies considerably throughout the year. When the lake is high, usually in late May, June, and part of July, all of the rapids below Screaming Right Turn Rapid are underwater. As the lake pool slowly drops toward the end of the summer, additional rapids are uncovered. During the fall through the spring, all of the rapids are uncovered. If you paddle when the lake is high, be prepared for a tedious seven miles of lake water to the take-out. An alternative to the long paddle out is to arrange for a tow from Sheltowee Trace Outfitters, (800) 541-7238. Other dangers include logs that occasionally become trapped in the more narrow chutes and strong headwinds while paddling off the lake. Off-the-river dangers include the possible vandalizing of vehicles (especially vans) left at the take-out. The Cumberland River below the falls is the only whitewater river in Kentucky that is normally runnable all year.

Rockcastle River

The Rockcastle River originates in Laurel County and drains portions of Jackson, Rockcastle, Laurel, and Pulaski counties. One of KentuckyÕs most popular rivers, the Rockcastle offers something for every type of canoeist.

The upper section from KY 490 (A) to KY 80 (C) ßows over a sand and rock bed through hilly woods and farmland in the heart of the Daniel Boone National Forest. Runnable from late fall to midsummer, this section is scenic and has banks of varying steepness and some very mild (Class I+) whitewater. A favorite run for canoe campers, the current is good and dangers of navigation are limited to deadfalls. Access to the upper section is good except for steep mud banks at the KY 80 bridge. Canoe rentals and shuttle services are available from a nearby professional outÞtter.

The lower Rockcastle, from KY 80 (C) to KY 192 (D), is a protected wild river and one of KentuckyÕs most popular whitewater runs. The scenery is splendid and paddling is both interesting and challenging. To begin with, the run is an exhausting 17 miles long. The Þrst 6 miles are essentially Class I with a fair current, numerous rifßes, and small ledges. Throughout the next 6 miles the river picks up a little gradient and several honest Class II rapids are encountered. While these rapids are not difÞcult, two or three do disappear around boulders or curves. At about mile 12 the river curves hard to the right and then hard to the left, tumbling down a Class II series of ledges and standing waves known as the Stair Steps.

Beyond this rapid, the Rockcastle reverts to long pools punctuated by short Class II drops at the ends. At about mile 15 the river appears to come to a dead end in a large boulder garden, but closer inspection reveals that the whole stream is grunting laboriously between two huge rocks and falling about four feet. This is Beech (Creek) Narrows. Above the drop an ill-placed boulder makes it difÞcult to set up. Below the drop is a very bad, highly aerated keeper hydraulic. Beyond the hydraulic the current washes directly into a large boulder. While this Class IV rapid has been run both decked and open, attempting to run it is considered highly dangerous, with success more a result of luck than skill. A portage trail circles the boulders on the right. If you choose to run, set up a rescue person where you are certain you can reach someone trapped in the keeper on the Þrst throw.

Below Beech Narrows the Rockcastle assumes its normal pool-and-drops for another three-quarters of a mile before entering a second apparent cul-de-sac. Here the river forms a large tranquil pool before cutting hard to the right, churning down a fast chute, and smacking into a rock. This rapid marks the entrance to the Lower Narrows, a three-quarter-mile stretch of tumbling, turbulent whitewater that hits the paddler with every challenge in the book. In this section of the Narrows there are no pools. However, there are some large eddies that let an

Section: KY 490 to KY 80
Counties: Rockcastle, Laurel, Pulaski, Jackson
USGS Quads: Livingston, Bernstadt, Billows
Difficulty: Class IÐII
Gradient: 2.41 feet per mile
Average Width: 30Ð50 feet
Velocity: Moderate
Rescue Index: DifÞcult
Hazards: Deadfalls
Scouting: None required
Portages: None required
Scenery: Pretty
Highlights: Scenery, wildlife
Gauge: U.S. Army Corps of Engineers, (800) 261-5033

Runnable Water Levels	Minimum	Maximum
	75 cfs	2,000 cfs

Additional Information: U.S. Army Corps of Engineers, (309) 529-2604; Sheltowee Trace OutÞtters, (606) 376-5567 or (800) 541-7238

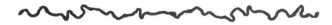

Upper Rockcastle River • Kentucky

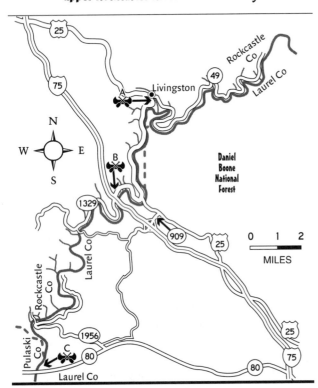

Lower Rockcastle River • Kentucky

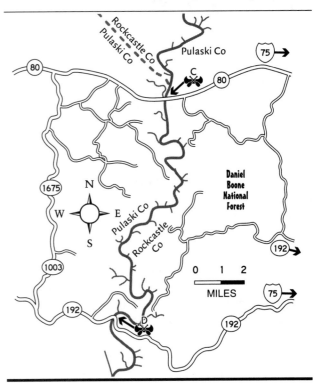

wits, and scramble up the banks to scout whatever lurks ahead. The rapids of the Lower Narrows are all runnable, but they demand considerable expertise in water reading

Section: KY 80 to KY 192
Counties: Laurel, Pulaski
USGS Quads: Bernstadt, Billows, Arno, Sawyer
Difficulty: Class III–IV
Gradient: 5.80 feet per mile
Average Width: 30–60 feet
Velocity: Moderate
Rescue Index: Accessible but difficult
Hazards: Deadfalls, undercut rocks, keeper hydraulics
Scouting: Beech Narrows, Lower Narrows, The Optionals
Portages: Beech Narrows, Lower Narrows
Scenery: Beautiful to exceptional
Highlights: Scenery, wildlife, geology
Gauge: U.S. Army Corps of Engineers, (800) 261-5033

Runnable Water Levels	Minimum	Maximum
	200 cfs	2,000 cfs

Additional Information: U.S. Army Corps of Engineers, (309) 529-2604; Sheltowee Trace Outfitters, (606) 376-5567 or (800) 541-7238

and whitewater tactics. The whole narrows is a series of twisting, turning blind drops, making it impossible to see what lies beyond the next ledge. Thus, each rapid must be scouted individually, entailing a seemingly endless routine of jumping in and out of boats and scrambling up immense boulders to sneak a look at the next rapid.

The scouting and the boulder-hopping are necessary, of course, but also time-consuming. A good running time for the Lower Narrows by an experienced group of four open-canoe tandem teams would be about two hours. The alternative to running the Narrows is portaging via a nice trail on the east bank. This can be reached by climbing the bank at the end of the pool that marks the entrance to the first rapid. When running the lower Rockcastle, time is always a prime consideration. Assuming dark to be around 7:30 P.M. in the spring, a paddler needs to reach the Lower Narrows by 3:00 or 3:30 P.M. to be sure of having enough time to get off the river by dark. Needless to say, a larger group will take longer to get through the Narrows. The portage is long (three-quarters of a mile), but it is much faster than running a group through the Narrows.

Beyond the Lower Narrows are a Class II run and a borderline Class III stretch that contains blind turns and should be scouted. The first rapid has a tendency to trap floating logs in the spring. Downstream from the Class III, it is approximately one mile to the take-out at Bee Rock Boat Ramp.

To shorten the trip there is an alternative put-in a few miles below KY 80 called the Billows. Also, a new road has been established to make a 12-mile run. Call Sheltowee Trace Outfitters for directions.

MARYLAND

Youghiogheny River

The Youghiogheny River in western MarylandÕs Garrett County is the premier whitewater experience among Maryland rivers. The pristine scenery (including the exquisitely beautiful Swallow Falls State Park), the miles of continuous whitewater, the unique play spots, the accessibility to large metropolitan areas (Pittsburgh, Baltimore, and Washington, D.C.), and the dam-released ßows all combine to make this river a classic expert whitewater run.

The Youghiogheny, affectionately known as the ÒYoughÓ (pronounced ÒyockÓ), originates on Backbone Mountain, MarylandÕs highest. Runoff gathers in Silver Lake, West Virginia, from which the Youghiogheny ßows into Maryland. The serious whitewater begins at Swallow Falls State Park north of Oakland. There are two standard runs. The Top Yough is a short, exciting stretch from Swallow Falls State Park (A) to Sang Run Bridge (C, six miles) or to the power plant at Hoyes Run Road (B, two and a half miles). The better-known Upper Yough is a run from Sang Run Bridge to Friendsville (D, nine and a half miles). The Top Yough is described below; a description of the Upper Yough follows that.

Top Youghiogheny River

The Top Yough begins with about two miles of premium whitewater, followed by roughly half a mile of ßatwater to the power plant at Hoyes Run and nearly three and a half more miles of ßatwater to Sang Run Bridge. Adding the 9.5 miles to Friendsville, a combined run on the Top and Upper Yough would be over 15 miles long. Over Þve miles of this, however, is the ßatwater from Hoyes Run on the Top Yough to Warm Up Rifße on the Upper Yough. The Top Yough can be run to Hoyes Run in anything from one and a half hours to more than three hours, depending on the group involved. Add one more hour of ßatwater paddling to reach Sang Run.

The six-mile trip to Sang Run has a total gradient of 280 feet, most of which occurs at Swallow Falls and the drops immediately below. The gauge for the Top Yough is located on the downstream east bridge piling at Sang Run. This gauge can be correlated to the Pittsburgh Weather Service phone gauge reading for Friendsville, (412) 644-2890, which is between 1.2 and 1.3 feet higher than the Sang Run gauge. If the phone reading for Friendsville is 3.4, the reading on the bridge at Sang Run should be approximately 2.1. By subtracting 1.3 feet from the phone gauge reading, you can determine with reasonable accuracy the level at Sang Run without leaving home.

In addition to these gauges, local paddlers and raft guides can often give you a very accurate reading by looking at another gauge on the bridge over the river in Friendsville. The minimum runnable level for the Top Yough is 1.5 feet on the gauge at Sang Run. YouÕll wind up walking if you catch it any lower. Normal runs are in the 1.7- to approximately 2.5-foot range. Above 2.5 feet, extra caution would be in order. Of course, as with any river of this type, the maximum level will be signiÞcantly higher for a skilled paddler who is intimately familiar with the river, or for anyone else with paid-up premiums on his life insurance policy.

The take-out that eliminates most of the ßatwater is located at the power plant near Hoyes Run (B). Take Route 42 south from Friendsville to Route 219. Bear right on Old Route 219 (also known as Deep Creek Drive) just past this junction; very shortly thereafter take a sharp right down Sang Run Road. After less than a mile, turn left onto Hoyes Run Road. The power plant and its road are not open to the public. Take out instead at the Þshing access at Hoyes Run about 0.5 mile below the dam outßow on river right. Seen fom the road, itÕs a small pullover on the Sang Run side of a small creek. A short (100 yards) trail leads to the river.

The put-in for the Top Yough is located at Swallow Falls State Park. This can be reached from Route 219 by

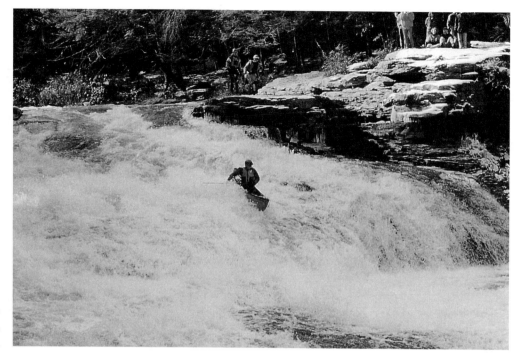

Richard Hopley running Swallow Falls on the Top Yough. Photo by Pete Martin.

left on Sang Run Road and a right on Swallow Falls Road, following the sign to the park. Using the map in this book, you can also reach the park from the power plant take-out.

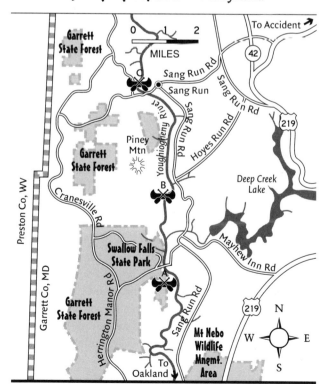

Top Youghiogheny River • Maryland

Swallow Falls is the initial rapid on the Top Yough. This spectacular spot needs no description. You can see

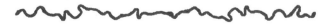

Section: Swallow Falls to Sang Run
County: Garrett
USGS Quads: Sang Run, Oakland
Difficulty: Class II–V with two miles of steady Class IV–V
Gradient: 45 feet per mile; two miles at 100 feet per mile
Average Width: 30–50 feet
Velocity: Fast
Rescue Index: Remote
Hazards: Swallow Falls (100 yards below Swallow Falls Road bridge) and the first ledge just below it (Swallowtail Falls); Class V Suckhole rapids 1.5 miles below this; many Class IV rapids in the first two miles
Scouting: Suckhole; boat-scouting of other rapids recommended when possible
Portages: Swallow Falls and possibly the first ledge just below it (Swallowtail Falls); perhaps Suckhole rapids
Scenery: Beautiful in many places
Highlights: Beautiful wilderness gorge
Gauge: National Weather Service (Friendsville phone gauge), (703) 260-0305 or (412) 262-5290

Runnable Water Levels:	Minimum	Maximum
Sang Run gauge	1.5 feet	2.5 feet
Friendsville phone reading	2.8 feet	3.7 feet

Additional Information: Precision Rafting in Friendsville, (301) 746-5290; Deep Creek Lake State Park, (301) 387-4110

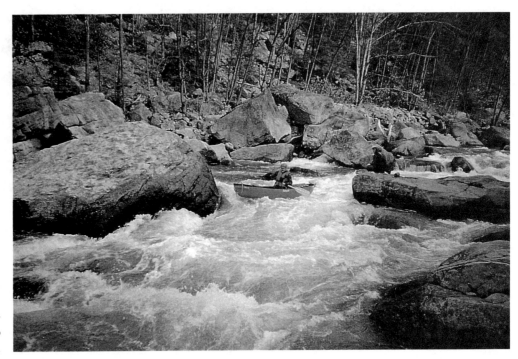

Unidentified paddler in Suckhole on the Top Yough. Photo by Scott Gravatt.

it all from excellent vantage spots in the park. The vast majority of boaters who carefully examine the 18-foot Swallow Falls will elect to put in on river left just below this drop to enjoy the tamer pleasures of the steep creek whitewater that follows. A few hundred yards below is 7-foot-high Swallowtail Falls, which is normally run on the right. It develops a nasty hydraulic at some levels and should be scouted. Carry on the left if needed. Just downstream to the left look up at 70-foot Muddy Falls, Maryland's highest waterfall.

Good, technical whitewater continues from the falls almost without a letup for the first mile or so. Easily the most notorious rapid on this section is Suckhole (Class V) located about 45 minutes (or one and a half miles) into the trip. This rapid can be recognized by the high boulder at midriver with a nasty-looking sieve of timber and trash in the pulsating gap between it and another boulder to its right. An exciting (and true) tale is told of the hapless paddler who went for a swim above Suckhole only to find himself trapped under the debris in this nasty little spot. The story has a happy ending, but it would be a hair-raising swim under the Suckhole rocks and strainers.

To avoid this ugly mess, scout Suckhole from river left and then come down midstream over a series of holes, rocks, and waves that try to push you to the right. Work left against this tendency as you approach the high boulder. You'll find a rock on the left bank just before you reach the high boulder in midstream, a small hole just to the right of this rock, and a good eddy just beyond the rock. You may want to stop in this eddy, but don't drive so close to the rock on the left that you drop in the hole next to it and get disoriented. At lower levels, there's also an eddy on the right of the river not far above the aforementioned trashy sieve. On the other hand, you could continue without stopping in either eddy, going left of the high boulder in midstream and staying in the center of the chute. Continuing on this route, you descend over steep boulder-studded ledges with holes and waves, including a sizable hole at the bottom (Suckhole). These waves and holes (especially the bottom one) should be punched hard. A sharp rock divides the channel just above the bottom hydraulic. If you go to the right of this rock, you won't have to punch the large bottom hole.

If you make it smoothly through Suckhole, it's unlikely that you'll have problems with the remaining whitewater. Take out on river right just below the power plant or for the flatwater trip continue on and take out at the boater's take-out above Sang Run Bridge.

Most of the Top Yough rapids can be scouted from the boat. Suckhole is the exception. Those unfamiliar with the approach to Suckhole would be wise to step out and take a good look. Rescue ropes can be set up at various spots where foul-ups might occur. Keep in mind that the nearest hospital emergency room is in Cumberland, more than an hour away by road from the take-out. If you want to carry, there's an old railroad bed on the right.

Upper Youghiogheny River • Maryland

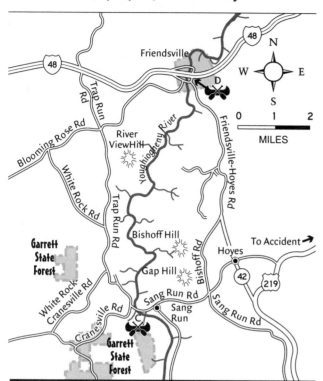

Upper Youghiogheny River

The Upper Yough is the ultimate whitewater run for expert paddlers in Maryland. It is one of the premier streams in the entire eastern United States. Longer and tougher than the Top Yough, it should be attempted only by expert boaters accompanied by someone who knows the river.

The total gradient on the Upper Yough for the entire 9.5-mile run from Sang Run to Friendsville is about 500 feet. From Gap Falls to Friendsville, the gradient is roughly 65 feet per mile, but for the section between Bastard and Heinzerling rapids the gradient is in excess of 100 feet per mile.

A normal run from Sang Run Bridge (C) to Friendsville (D) can take anywhere from three to six hours, depending on the skill levels and the group involved. Local boaters blast down at a much faster pace. If you are dependent on flows released at the power plant (see next paragraph), it would be risky to loiter excessively. Most releases are now three hours, and as long as you catch the beginning of a release and maintain a moderate pace, you will not run out of water.

The Upper Yough is runnable on natural flows throughout the spring and at other times with adequate local rainfall. However, thanks to efforts by local rafting

Section: Sang Run Bridge to Friendsville
County: Garrett
USGS Quads: Sang Run, Friendsville
Difficulty: Class II–V with 4.5 miles mostly steady Class IV–V
Gradient: 53 feet per mile; three miles at 100 feet per mile
Average Width: 30–50 feet
Velocity: Fast
Rescue Index: Remote
Hazards: Class V rapids (National Falls, Heinzerling, Meat Cleaver, Lost and Found); many Class IV rapids. Two dangerous undercuts: Toilet Bowl at second drop on right of Charlies Choice, Tombstone Rock to left of main channel of Lost and Found
Scouting: Previously mentioned Class V rapids; boat-scouting of others is recommended when possible
Portages: Paddlers thinking of many portages should not run this river
Scenery: Beautiful in many places
Highlights: Wilderness gorge
Gauge: National Weather Service (Friendsville phone gauge), (703) 260-0305 or (412) 262-5290

Runnable Water Levels:	Minimum	Maximum
Sang Run gauge	1.5 feet	2.5 feet
Friendsville phone reading	2.8 feet	3.7 feet

Months Runnable: Winter/spring after rain or snow melt; summer/fall on weekdays when water is released into Hoyes Run hydroelectric station
Additional Information: Friendsville Gauge: Penn Elec, (814) 533-8911; Precision Rafting, (301) 746-5290; Mountain Surf, (301) 746-5389

companies and the American Whitewater Affiliation, there are now three-hour releases, generally from 10 A.M. to 1 P.M., every Monday and Friday as well as some Saturdays between April 15 and October 15 (provided Deep Creek Lake is not drawn down too far). At moderate natural flow, it takes the release 1.5 to 2 hours to reach the Sang Run put-in from Deep Creek Lake. So if a three-hour release begins at 10 A.M., it will reach Sang Run just before noon. Occasional releases may also be scheduled at other times. To get the latest information, contact Mountain Surf in Friendsville at (301) 746-5389 or call Penn Elec at (814) 533-8911. Releases are usually 600 cfs (see gauge chart at chapter's end). However, the power plant releasing the water may be sold soon. This could change everything from the phone number to release schedules.

The gauge for the Upper Yough is located on the downstream east (right) bridge piling at Sang Run. (See

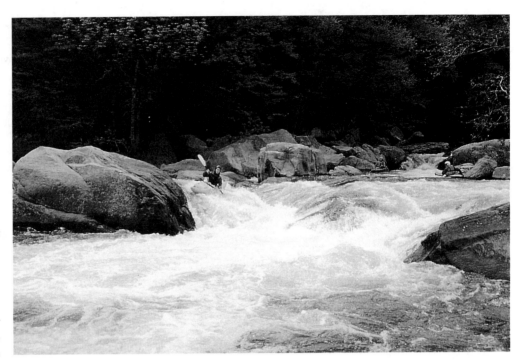

Kia Jacobson running Heinzerling on the Upper Yough.
Photo by Mayo Gravatt.

gauge information for Top Youghiogheny.) Normal runnable levels range from a minimum of 1.5 feet to somewhere around 2.5 feet on this gauge. From 2.5 feet on up, the steeper sections get noticeably more heavy-duty. Do not confuse this gauge with the telephone gauge for Friendsville, which is between 1.2 and 1.3 feet higher than the Sang Run gauge. There is also a river gauge on the upstream left abutment on the bridge in Friendsville that reads 0.1 feet higher than Sang Run. As in the case of the Top Yough, the maximum runnable level is an individual matter of expertise, bravado, and life insurance.

The Upper Yough does not have the stupendous individual Class V falls and drops that characterize the Upper Gauley or the Big Sandy in West Virginia. Instead it has a more narrowly channeled and continuous technical character. Consequently, it is usually accorded an overall Class IV to V rating. Unfortunately, there have been numerous accidents—damaged boats, broken paddles, bruises, and cuts are common. Even broken noses and legs are not unheard of. Exercise good judgment regarding your boating skills and those of the other boaters in your party.

No one should paddle the Upper Yough without being aware of one big problem: politics. Political struggles have continued in the 1990s over the number and reliability of releases to be made from Deep Creek Lake. Because this waterway furnishes recreational opportunities to whitewater paddlers, anglers, and lake users as well as providing power to the citizens of Pittsburgh,

there is no easy answer. The American Whitewater Affiliation continues its struggle and negotiations with Maryland authorities to improve the number and reliability of summer releases from Deep Creek Lake. If you want to help in this effort, send $20 to join the American Whitewater Affiliation, P.O. Box 85, Phoenicia, NY 12464.

The political situation and the pattern of private land ownership used to make it tough to access the Upper Yough. Thanks to the National Lands Trust, which purchased the put-in in 1985 and transferred it to the state of Maryland, things have changed dramatically in the past few years. The state of Maryland now has a very good put-in on the right in a field just upstream of the Sang Run Bridge. Please put in here because it is the only legal access for the public in this area.

The best take-out is on river left just below the Friendsville bridge at John Mason's Mountain Surf whitewater shop. Don't change clothes in the open in Friendsville—it angers the town residents. Please thank Mountain Surf whitewater shop for providing this important public service. Also, if you take a shower and change at his place, please leave a dollar or two for use of his amenities.

If you are doing your own shuttle (see the map), take Route 42 south from Friendsville to Bishoff Road and go right on Bishoff Road to its intersection with Sang Run Road. Turn right on Sang Run Road.

The political mess is the bad news. The good news is that miles of challenging whitewater amidst a pristine

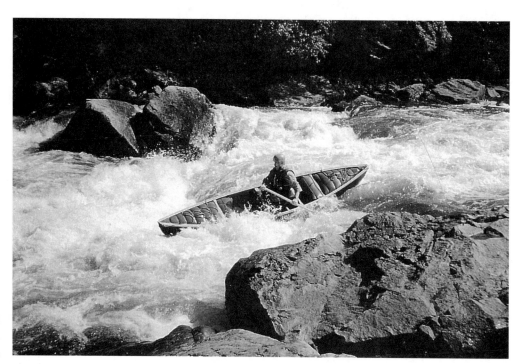

Don Ellis running National Falls on the Upper Yough. Photo by Mayo Gravatt.

mountain setting await you. The river is clear, the shoreline is timbered and covered with rhododendrons, and the rapids are superb. The whitewater ranges up to Class V with at least 13 or more spots that have been given affectionate names, such as Meat Cleaver or Eddy of Death.

A word of caution: this book alone won't get you down the Upper Yough. The descriptions provided here can only give you a rough impression of what to expect. If you have doubts about your ability to handle difficult, steep, or technical whitewater, you should go elsewhere or at least take your first trip with someone who knows the river well.

If there is one rapid that requires a special warning it would probably be Meat Cleaver. A blind drop that cannot be scouted entirely from a boat, it contains some weird currents with the possibility of a broach on sharp rocks in midstream. More paddlers screw up here than anywhere else. Meat Cleaver is worth a few doses of adrenaline, but you will hit lots of good stuff before you get there. The rapids described below are generally Class IV (unless otherwise noted) when the Sang Run gauge is two feet. They are a shade easier at lower levels and tougher at higher levels.

About two to three miles down from the Sang Run Bridge you encounter Warm Up Riffle, a Class II rapid named because it's a good place to goof off and warm up or picnic while getting your trip together. Not far downstream from Warm Up Riffle is Gap Falls, a sizable slide rapid with waves and holes on the way down. Enter

from river left; just before hitting the bigger waves in the middle, angle right and work right to miss the hole at the bottom. As you become more familiar with Gap Falls, at lower levels you may want to try for the Eddy of Death next to the left bank about three-quarters of the way down the drop. It derives its colorful name from the undercut rock guarding its downstream end.

Once you're past Gap Falls things mellow out for less than a mile (III+) before an intense three- to four-mile section begins. Bastard is first. Located on river left, it requires a tight right turn to miss a big hole and pop lightly into a big eddy on the right, behind the boulder that forms the right side of the main drop. The rest of the rapid can be boat-scouted.

Bastard is followed by Charlie's Choice, which can be run in numerous ways. On the right are two tight moves between rocks at the top of two drops, both of which have a pillowed boulder at the bottom. The first one can be quite abrasive at low levels, but the second one has more of a pillow. Don't get too far right on the second drop because of a dangerous undercut called Toilet Bowl. A less exciting sneak is found on river left.

Just after Charlie's Choice is Triple Drop (Class III–V). There is a tricky hole-ledge combination (Snaggle Tooth) that can be run down the right, entering from the eddy upstream on the right or a very small eddy at the very top of the rapid on the left. There are three boulders on the right as you go downstream; for an uneventful descent, you should stay close to these boulders as you go down.

There is a good eddy on river right at the end of Snaggle Tooth before the second phase of Triple Drop, which is nothing more than some Class II ledges. The third part of Triple Drop contains National Falls. The easiest way to run this from the eddy below Snaggle Tooth is to work your way to the far left over the intervening Class II+ ledges. Then, from the eddy just above the main drop on river left, turn left as you ride the curler down. The other route from the right over Class V National Falls is not for the faint of heart. Crank hard if you go this route, and expect to be trashed by the hole at the bottom if you miss your boof.

Beyond Triple Drop lies Tommy's Hole. Located on the left, this hole is tightly packed between an upstream and a downstream boulder. Some small boats with no edges have trouble getting out. A good sneak route exists to the right near the middle of the river, but you should work your way back quickly to river left just below Tommy's Hole.

After a steep sequence just below Tommy's Hole (called Little Niagara) the paddler confronts Zinger, a diagonal wave-hole combination. Enter from the top eddy on river left. There are two routes. You can stay far left as you exit the eddy, heading about two o'clock (cocking your bow sixty degrees to the right of downstream) and go straight, punching the diagonal curler-hole. To take the other route, first go right toward the large boulder that forms the right side of the drop, then surf the diagonal curler from right to left as you pass the large boulder to your right. Sanctuary can be sought in a good-sized eddy next to the left bank below the large boulder. The exit from this eddy is obvious (to the right if you opt not to catch the eddy). Zinger is not a notorious trouble-maker as Upper Yough rapids go, but it has given some paddlers problems. You can sneak Zinger on the far right.

After Zinger and Trap Run Falls (a punchable hydraulic with a rock in its center), and some Class III-type stuff, look for the right-side entrance to Heinzerling, a Class IV-V rapid. If you miss this hard-to-find approach, you will be forced to take a much tougher route down the center and left. To catch the best approach (called Rifle Barrel), cross a shallow rocky area on the right to reach a shady pool upstream and to the right of the initial drop of Heinzerling. The first phase of Heinzerling can be boat-scouted from the bottom of this pool, and it is truly a classic whitewater spot. From the eddy at the top it looks much steeper and more complex than it really is. First you drop several feet over the first ledge and catch an eddy to the right or left to look over the bottom drop. From either eddy you head directly downstream toward the big pillowed boulder visible at the bottom. Ride the pillow on the boulder, bracing right and sliding off it to the left. If you ride high enough on the pillow, you will avoid the nastier parts of the holes just to the left of the big boulder. Going to the right of the boulder may be bumpy. Just below Heinzerling is an interesting little jumble called Boulder Dance.

Meat Cleaver (a genuine Class V) follows Heinzerling. Paddlers used to start from river right, going over a small drop and turning left behind some big boulders. Because of a recent flood, the best way to enter Meat Cleaver now is over a three-foot ledge on the left of the main channel entering the rapid. You can then see the final drop with two shark-teeth rocks more or less in the center of the drop. Thread your way between (or to one side of) these sharp rocks (the route between the two rocks is preferable). If you eddy out on the left above the shark teeth, your trip will become more exciting because it is more difficult to thread the proper course without broaching. Broaching on the Meat Cleaver rocks is not recommended.

After a few Class III rapids beyond Meat Cleaver, the paddler encounters Powerful Popper, a Class III–IV rapid marked by three midstream boulders. A pop-up–and–squirt stop is in order here. Be sure to work hard enough right to avoid the Death Slot to the left of the big boulder forming the left side of the main drop.

The next major rapid follows quickly and is one of the more technical drops on the river: Lost and Found (Class V). Some choice surfing holes are immediately upstream, so enjoy them while you can. Lost and Found consists of a maze of congested offset rocks. As with almost everything on the Upper Yough, it can be run in different ways. The various possibilities can be boat-scouted to some degree from an eddy just above the rapid. The cautious boater on an initial run may want to look it over from the island on the right side of the main drop. A sneak route is available from the eddy around on far river right; this involves dropping off a four-foot ledge into the pool below all the messy stuff. There are several routes through the hard stuff if you elect to try that. If enough water is available, the easiest route is to squeeze between the round rock on the upper right at the beginning of the rapid and the adjacent rocky island. This approach offers a reasonably straight shot downstream. With this approach you will be less likely to get lost when slaloming right and left around the rocks in midstream. You also will not go so far left as to get tangled up in "F— Up Falls" at the bottom. Also lookout for Tombstone Rock lurking by the left side of the main channel—it is dangerously undercut.

If you have made it this far without incident, you'll probably have few problems with the remaining Class

IVs: Cheeseburger Falls, Wright's Hole, and Double Pencil Sharpener. Except for Cheeseburger Falls (a blind drop on river right), these can all be scouted from the boat. Try to run the main drop at Cheeseburger at least one boat length out from the right bank to avoid a submerged rock at the bottom of the ledge that forms Cheeseburger Falls. This submerged rock has broken several paddles. You can sweep into the eddy on river right just past this hole. Sticky Wright's Hole can be punched at the usual summer-release water levels by driving hard through the left side of the hole. The hole can also be sneaked on far river left or circumvented on river right by surfing down some diagonal waves. Double Pencil Sharpener is just below Wright's Hole and can be boat-scouted from an eddy on river right. After these rapids, three to four miles of less distinguished small stuff and flatwater remain until Main Street in Friendsville.

There is one final item of interest about this spectacular river. Starting in 1981, there has been an annual downriver race on the Upper Yough in August by expert paddlers who know the river intimately. The race continues to draw boaters who are on the cutting edge of paddling. National Falls is one of the best places to view the race. Contact Precision Rafting in Friendsville for details. (Roger Zbel, owner of this raft company, has won the race 16 out of 17 times as of 1997.)

Friendsville USGS Gauge

Procedure to get Sang Run Gauge reading from natural flow plus Penn Elec release from Deep Creek Lake.

1. From the table below, determine the cfs of the early-morning Friendsville natural flow gauge reading.
2. Add 600 cfs (from the Penn Elec release) to this amount.
3. Determine the revised Friendsville gauge level.
4. Subtract 1.3 feet from this revised Friendsville level to get the Sang Run gauge level.

Note: When comparing natural flows, Friendsville is generally 1.3 feet higher than Sang Run at lower flows and 1.2 feet higher at medium and higher flows. At two feet on the Sang Run gauge, the Friendsville gauge is usually 3.25 feet.

Level (feet)	Flow (cfs)
2.0	45
2.1	60
2.2	77
2.3	100
2.4	130
2.5	168
2.6	211
2.7	261
2.8	317
2.9	380
3.0	449
3.1	526
3.2	610
3.3	713
3.4	826
3.5	952
3.6	1,077
3.7	1,211
3.8	1,355
3.9	1,509
4.0	1,673
4.1	1,847
4.2	2,032
4.3	2,213

Chart from Youghiogheny River Recreational Capacity Study by A. Graefe, et al., December 1989, courtesy USGS.

Savage River

The Savage is a little brawling river that certainly lives up to its name. Here you have four miles of jam-packed continuous whitewater for the advanced paddler. At very low levels (below 2.5 feet on the recorded gauge), strong intermediate paddlers can try the last two miles of this section to see if they're ready for the tougher upper half. However, be warned: There are very few eddies on the relentless downhill scramble to the North Branch of the Potomac. Also, because of the cold, dam-released water averaging 46 degrees Fahrenheit, wet suits should always be used—even in summer months at this elevation of 1,300 feet. One important safety feature is that the Savage River Road closely follows the river. It provides first-timers with the chance to see what they are up against and a take-out is relatively easy if problems develop. However, some of the major rapids can't be seen from the road, so these will need to be scouted from the river. At moderate levels (800–900 cfs or 3.2–3.4 feet on the recorded gauge) the river is a continuous heavy Class III with a couple of Class IV rapids thrown in for added excitement. This is the level described below. However, at higher levels, the run gets much tougher because of the relentless 75-foot-per-mile gradient.

The best action and scenery are found within the first two miles of the trip. Here the clear, clean river drops through a small, pretty gorge, and the riverbanks are festooned with rhododendrons, maples, mountain ashes, tulip poplars, and hemlocks. During the second two miles the rapids calm down to an easier, steady, Class III dull roar, and the scenery beyond the riverbanks slowly gets worse as one nears the take-out. Trash is increasingly scattered near the riverbank on the right, and big excavations scar the land beyond the riverbank on the left.

Nevertheless, this river is a gem of whitewater brilliance. The easiest put-in is just over four miles up Savage River Road (A). It is on river right from a very short dirt-road spur about 100 yards upstream of a white concrete bridge. Or you can put in on river left half a mile

farther upstream from a dirt road that leaves the camping area just downstream from the same bridge. The description that follows covers the trip from the put-in by the white concrete bridge.

Incidentally, the Savage River Dam is worth a peek if you have the time and don't mind listening to the noisy pumping station. Only three-quarters of a mile upstream from the white concrete bridge near the put-in, this earth-and-rockfill dam is over 1,000 feet wide and nearly 200 feet tall. Its capacity is 6.5 billion gallons of water. Fishermen enjoy the lake formed by the dam and can often be seen casting from the dam's rocky face. Bass, crappie, and brown and rainbow trout can be caught here. Fish are also stocked downstream in the spring for the fishing season. Even if you don't want to fish, Savage Lake is a very scenic flatwater paddle.

About 20 to 30 yards downstream from the put-in is a good 25-yard Class III rapids over two ledge-like drops. This will wake you up immediately—even if the cold, dam-released water does not. You may want to peek at this rapid before running it. A river gauging station used to be found right below this rapid, on the left about 30 yards upstream from the white concrete bridge. Unfortunately, this gauge was washed away by high water in recent years. As a result, you should rely on the recorded message at (703) 260-0305—with one exception. On whitewater race days you should check with race officials or call the Savage Dam to determine the timing and level of cfs released.

Next to the old gauge site and immediately before passing under the bridge, the paddler will encounter a two-foot ledge. A half-mile of continuous Class III waves and boulder-garden action follows, until the paddler reaches a pool 100 yards or so long—the only sizable pool encountered before the paddler is disgorged at the take-out on the North Branch of the Potomac. This pool is formed by the five-foot Piedmont Dam.

The dam can be run in two ways. First there is a two-yard notch (exciting) in the dam a few yards from the left

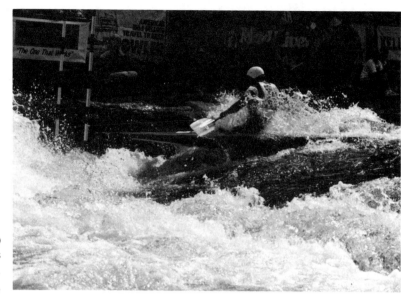

John Lugbill at the 1989
World Championships
on the Savage.
Photo by Ed Grove.

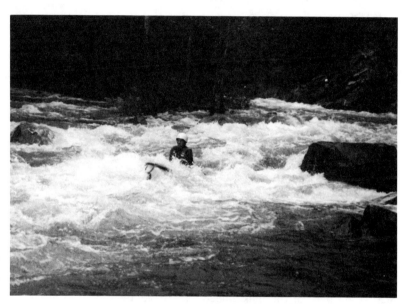

Paul Possinger in the middle of
Island Rapid on the Savage.
Photo by Ron Knipling.

bank, or a challenging jumble of rocks on the extreme right (runnable only by experienced boaters with great care and attentive scouting). At low levels (500 cfs or 2.8 feet on the put-in gauge) there won't be enough water in the notch. At 1,000 cfs a nasty hydraulic develops below the notch on the left side of the river. Nervous boaters can carry on the left. Just below the dam (where the whitewater slalom course is usually set up for regional and national competition) continuous Class III waves and boulder-garden action continue for another good half-mile, then the river flows toward the road, which has a

nice, white stone face on its other side. As the Savage turns right and away from the road, get ready for the first drop of Triple Drop, also known as Crisscross.

At moderate levels this rapid is a low Class IV consisting of three drops. Scout from the left. The first can be run next to a rock on the right side; the second has a nice tongue in the center; the last drop, which can develop a strong hole, is best run on the right. It should be mentioned that trees often fall across this small river. On one trip a tree blocked the third drop, and one boater (who had fallen out of his boat upstream) briefly suffered a

Section: Below the Savage River Dam to confluence with the North Branch of the Potomac

County: Garrett

USGS Quads: Westernport, Barton, Bittinger

Difficulty: Class III–IV up to 800 cfs (up to 3.4 feet on gauge); Class IV from 800 to 1,200 cfs (from 3.4 to 3.8 feet on gauge); Class IV–V above 1,200 cfs

Gradient: 75 feet per mile

Average Width: 20–40 feet

Velocity: Fast

Rescue Index: Accessible

Hazards: Trees down in river, large holes at high levels, few eddies

Scouting: Advisable for Class III–IV Triple Drop, Class IV Memorial Rock, and Class III–IV Island Rapid

Portages: None

Scenery: Pretty to beautiful at the put-in, slowly changes to fair at the take-out

Highlights: Beautiful small gorge for most of the trip; dam-release river

Gauge: Savage Dam, (301) 359-0361

Runnable Water Levels:

	Minimum	Maximum
	2.5 feet (350 cfs)	4 feet (1,400 cfs)

Months Runnable: Generally a dam release for races and in winter and spring after hard rains and snowmelt

Additional Information: Corps of Engineers recording, (410) 962-7687

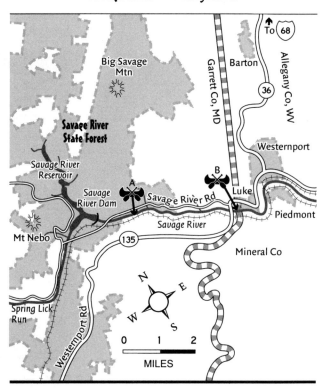

Savage River • Maryland

body pin on the trunk of this tree.

Following Triple Drop, the paddler reaches the toughest single drop on the river, fittingly called Memorial Rock. At moderate levels this low Class IV can be recognized by a large, pointed boulder sticking out of the water about 10 feet off the left bank. Generally, one should run just to the right of the rock angled left to avoid a submerged rock and a mean hole covering the river on the right. Be ready to punch a few holes just below. If there is enough water, you can sneak on the extreme left on the other side of Memorial Rock. No wonder things are so busy during this part of the trip: the gradient is 100 feet per mile!

Below Memorial Rock, go left of an island to run the best part of Class III–IV Island Rapids. At higher levels you may want to scout this turbulent passage from the left. There are a couple of good holes to avoid or punch as the river closely follows the road again. Then, two miles into the trip, you'll reach a white clapboard church. Just before the church at lower levels, a super surfing hydraulic extends over three-quarters of the river from the left

and has a nice small recovery pool. This used to be the take-out for those only wanting to run the tougher upper part of the Savage and the put-in for more nervous souls who did not want to challenge the upper section. However, if you want to use the church (or another spot downstream 100 yards) for access, get permission first.

For the last two miles the Savage continues at a calmer pace. The main items to note on this lower section include a two-foot diagonal ledge just upstream of a bridge a mile below the church, followed about three-quarters of a mile later by a pool where paddlers can regain composure before the final quarter mile to the North Branch. At press time, the last mile of the Savage had many strainers. Therefore, you may want to consider taking out at the bridge one mile above the take-out. Once you reach the North Branch, you can either take out river left on the Savage or you can paddle 100 yards upstream for a river left take-out on the North Branch.

The Savage is not a river for the inexperienced or unwary. Kayakers should have a bombproof roll under rocky conditions and open boaters should have full flotation, helmets, and wet suits—even in summer months. Swims are generally long and cold despite the small size of this river. Boat recovery is difficult because of the ceaseless nature of the rapids.

As mentioned earlier, this description reflects 800 cfs or 3.2 feet on the put-in gauge. When the level goes from 800 to 1,200 cfs the river becomes much pushier. Although the rocks are covered and padded, the hydraulics become grabbier and the waves much more powerful. It gets more difficult to catch the few eddies available along the shore because by this time the river is running through the rhododendrons on the banks. Consider this a solid Class IV run. At 1,200 cfs and higher the river becomes very nasty with very dangerous hydraulics and should be considered a Class IV–V trip for expert boaters only.

Unfortunately, running this river is dependent on getting releases from the Savage River Dam through the cooperation of the Upper Potomac River Commission. These releases are scheduled sporadically in the spring and summer, particularly if races are scheduled, but sometimes heavy rains will allow the dam keepers to release unspecified amounts in an unscheduled manner.

On the other hand, exciting things have happened to the Savage. The 1989 International Canoe Federation World Championships in Slalom and Whitewater (for decked boats) was held here in June 1989. This was the first time world championships were held in the United States. Our team won several medals—including Jon Lugbill, who won the gold medal, and Davey Hearn, who won a silver medal, both in C-1 slalom.

Savage River Water Level Conversion (Correlation) Table

Savage River Gauge (0.7 miles below Savage River Dam)

Height (feet)	Flow (cfs)
0.6	2.0
0.8	6.8
1.0	15.3
1.2	28.0
1.4	61.0
1.6	93.9
1.8	135.9
2.0	187.8
2.2	250.4
2.4	324.3
2.6	410.2
2.8	508.8
3.0	620.8
3.2	746.6
3.4	887.0
3.6	1,043
3.8	1,214
4.0	1,401
4.2	1,605
4.4	1,8Z7
4.6	2,066
4.8	2,323
5.0	2,600
5.2	2,895
5.4	3,211
5.6	3,546
5.8	3,902
6.0	4,279
6.2	4,678
6.4	5,099
6.6	5,542
6.8	6,008

Source: The above data, obtained from the Maryland District Office of the USGS, are based on 1984–86 measurements.

North Branch of the Potomac

Steyer to Shallmar

The run from Steyer to Shallmar is the classic section of the North Branch of the Potomac River and is for advanced to expert paddlers only. Be warned that the length and continuous nature of this trip give it an expedition-like quality. Here the North Branch drops at a giddy gradient of over 50 feet per mile, quite a drop for a reasonably sized river. There are no midway take-outs, and the only solace is a set of railroad tracks next to the river, which can be used for emergency walkouts (with or without boats). For the first third of the trip, the tracks are on your left; for the remainder, they are on the right.

Do not venture on this river unless you are very competent and in good physical and mental shape. The whole run is long and strenuous, and a full day should be allowed to complete it by those running this section for the first time. Even highly experienced boaters who know the river well should allow six hours of daylight on the river. Except for the very beginning and the very end you will be working continuously. Throughout most of the trip quiet stretches of water are not more than fifty yards long. Each decked boater should have a strong roll; each open boater should be capable of self-rescue in continuous Class III rapids. Naturally helmets and flotation are mandatory for all boats. Rescue is very difficult, particularly at upper levels, and you're on your own because of the relentless nature of this run. There have been quite a few hairy experiences for intermediate paddlers who have found this river too much to handle. Advanced and expert paddlers have also had real trouble when the river was too high.

To avoid an excessive case of white knuckles or a long walk on a railroad track, pay careful attention to the gauge at Kitzmiller. A reasonable absolute minimum is 4.7 feet. An extra foot of water on this gauge (say, moving from five to six feet), can change this from a demanding Class III–IV trip to an extremely difficult Class IV–V run. A level of five and a half feet on the Kitzmiller gauge would be very taxing for highly experienced open boaters with full flotation. Expert decked boaters should think of six and a half feet as an upper limit, primarily because of the countless hydraulics and the relentless gradient. Clearly, when the water get higher, the hydraulics get grabbier, with many becoming absolute keepers at levels over seven feet.

Besides checking the Kitzmiller gauge at the take-out, paddlers should also check Stony River where it crosses Route 50 to determine the volume of water from this river. The Stony joins the North Branch a third of the way into the trip and nearly doubles the volume of the North Branch.

About a half mile downstream from the put-in at Steyer (A), look for a Steyer river gauge on the left. It should be between 2.9 (very scrapy) and 4.2 feet. Unless you are really into rocks, however, this gauge probably should be a good three feet. If the gauge is underwater, perhaps you shouldn't be here at all.

After a mile or two of placid Class I–II rock garden rapids (quite scrappy if the river is low), the drops become more abrupt and interesting. The first island below Steyer should be run to the right and has a good drop into a hole.

When you reach the second island, get out on the left bank, climb up to the railroad tracks, and scout Corkscrew—an aptly named Class III–IV rapids. Corkscrew is basically a four-foot horseshoe ledge (prongs downstream) and is best entered left of center, headed toward the right. At lower levels, most of the water is channeled to the right of this second island, providing an exciting alternative to Corkscrew. Here a fairly steep drop climaxes in a large but punchable hydraulic. If you have any real problems to this point, strongly consider the three-mile carry back to the put-in. A seemingly interminable walk with a boat is vastly preferable to a seemingly interminable flush down the river without it.

From here to its junction with the Stony, the narrow and rocky North Branch continues falling away at a steep and respectful pace. If you haven't noticed by now, this is probably the ledgiest river you have ever paddled. Surf

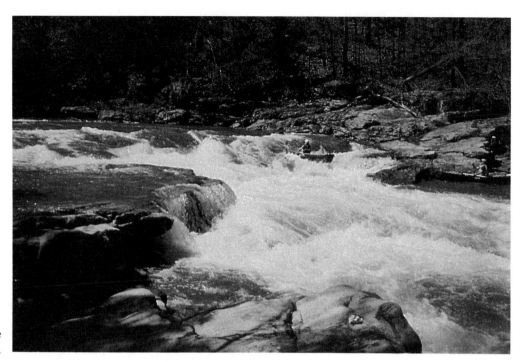

Ron Knipling on Rattlesnake
Rapid. Photo by Bob Maxey.

away if you wish, but make sure you save enough energy to complete this long, demanding run. A half mile before the North Branch joins the Stony, look out for steep rapids that feature two powerful offset diagonal holes.

When the Stony joins the North Branch four miles below Steyer, not only does the water volume nearly double but the color generally changes for the better, too. The brown foamy North Branch, usually muddy from strip mines, is diluted by the clearer waters of the Stony. Unfortunately, both rivers are sterile and polluted with mine acids. Once the Stony merges with the North Branch, the river becomes more powerful and pushier. About a half mile below the confluence of these rivers you will pass under a railroad bridge. Get ready, because just below this bridge lies the biggest action of this trip— three large ledges located fairly close together.

The first and perhaps most difficult ledge is Rattlesnake Ledge, a Class IV at moderate levels. It has been given a very salty name by old-time paddlers—"MF" is their abbreviation for this name. Get out and scout this rapid on the left. It is a large, complex sloping ledge of roughly six feet. Enter left of center and move farther left to skirt an impressive roostertail, then punch or miss (to the left) a deceptively nasty hole at the very bottom. Many a paddler has concentrated his attention on the roostertail and breathed a sigh of relief when safely past it, only to be nailed by the hole, whose viciousness can escape a casual glance. This hole is called "Lady Kenmore" by local paddlers.

Fortunately, at moderate levels you'll find a nice pool in which to pick up the pieces. Set throw ropes and rescue boats just below this large ledge and Lady Kenmore on river left. At about 4.8 feet on the Kitzmiller gauge a passage opens on the right that is probably the best shot for open boaters.

Although your attention will be focused totally on the river at this point, do look out for timber rattlesnakes here and elsewhere along the banks, particularly on warm, sunny days. A paddler who was once walking on the bank by this ledge thought the timer in his camera was buzzing, but it turned out to be a three-and-a-half-foot rattlesnake lying in front of him sounding its own built-in buzzer.

Not too far downstream is the second big ledge, the steepest of the three and perhaps the most fun. At reasonable levels, this sharply sloping six-foot ledge is a Class IV rapids. It is a straightforward drop best run with good speed down the center of the ledge into a generally forgiving mass of foam and water.

The third ledge (Class IV) of over five feet also appears very shortly. It should generally be run on the right—a sloping and jagged complex drop with some scraping. At low levels this last ledge has been run on the far left with a turn to the right.

First-timers should scout all three ledges and even experienced paddlers who know the river should look them over—particularly at higher levels such as five and a half feet on the Kitzmiller gauge. Above six and a half

Section: Gormania, WV (Steyer), to Kitzmiller, MD (Shallmar)

Counties: Garrett (MD), Mineral (WV), Grant (WV)

USGS Quads: Gorman, Kitzmiller, Mount Storm

Difficulty: Class III–IV (Kitzmiller 4.7–5.2 feet); Class IV (Kitzmiller 5.2–5.5 feet); Class IV–V (Kitzmiller 5.5–6.5 feet)

Gradient: 55 feet per mile

Average Width: 30–70 feet

Velocity: Fast

Rescue Index: Remote

Hazards: Occasional trees in river, three large ledges, old bridge pier and Maytag rapids near the end of the trip, continual hydraulics, heavy water at high levels

Scouting: Corkscrew rapid above confluence with the Stony (Class III–IV), three big ledges (Class III–IV) at moderate levels, Maytag rapids (Class IV)

Portages: None

Scenery: Pretty or beautiful in spots

Highlights: Heavy continuous whitewater through reasonably scenic gorge

Gauge: National Weather Service for Kitzmiller gauge (703) 260-0305

Runnable Water Levels:	Minimum	Maximum
Kitzmiller	4.7 feet	6.5 feet
Steyer	2.9 feet	4.2 feet

Additional Information: The Steyer gauge is a half mile downstream from Steyer put-in; Potomac State Forest, (301) 334-2038

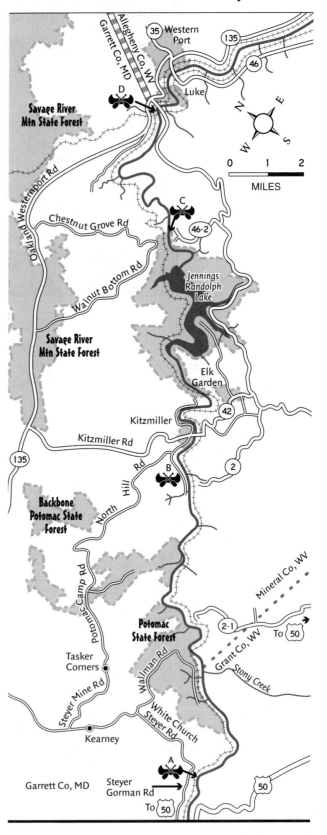

North Branch of the Potomac • Maryland

feet on this gauge some of the holes below these three ledges become absolute keepers.

Following these drops the river broadens, and for a short distance the rapids become straightforward wave trains. Then the river narrows and again takes on a serious nature with a seemingly endless series of Class III ledges, boulder gardens, and crosscurrents at moderate levels. Surfing freaks can go bonkers again. Constant maneuvering becomes the order of the day. At higher levels—say, five and a half feet on Kitzmiller gauge—this turns into Class IV stuff. At six feet and above, one rockets along through big waves while avoiding some keeper holes.

Roughly three-quarters of the way through the run, be alert for two dangers: first, a toppled concrete bridge pier, which should be run far left; second, an innocent looking rapid that contains several powerful holes and a series of sizable offset waves, appropriately called Maytag. More paddlers seem to swim here than anyplace else, perhaps due to fatigue and the fact that Maytag resembles an approach to several other, much easier upstream rapids. There are two ways to know when Maytag is imminent. First, it is located on the third left turn as the river winds close to the railroad tracks on the right. Second, look for a tall, sheer rock cliff on the left reminiscent of the wall above High Falls on the Cheat River in West Virginia. This cliff has a man-made stone wall in the center that distinguishes it from other cliffs on this trip. Maytag is the next rapid downstream from this cliff. It begins as a gentle left bend that looks easy but soon becomes a monster. Approaching six feet on the gauge, this rapid has several large holes in the first half of a long train of big waves. Paddling on the extreme left is generally the way to miss the worst of the holes, but you will still have to keep your balance through some powerful offset waves. Maytag is Class IV at five feet on the gauge and tougher at higher levels. Scout it.

After you have paddled about 11 miles and are panting from maneuvering and playing (if you still have any energy), look for the take-out at the old mining town of Shallmar on the left (B). Abram Creek joins the North Branch on river right just opposite the take-out. By taking out at Shallmar you can avoid two miles of less interesting rapids (dredged channel) and scenery (strip mines) before you get to the Route 42 bridge in Kitzmiller. At five feet and below on the Kitzmiller gauge, parts of the last two miles become almost too shallow and picky to paddle.

Except for the water quality and railroad tracks, this is a very scenic trip when you can get your head out of the rapidly unfolding rapids and look around. There are pretty cliffs, hemlocks, rhododendrons, and forested canyon walls to make you forget your increasingly aching muscles.

For more experienced paddlers who are really in shape, a tougher trip can be had by putting in on the Stony River (with its gradient of 75 feet per mile) at Route 50. This makes the trip two miles and perhaps two hours longer and considerably more demanding. The Stony is somewhat more difficult than the North Branch and consists of many sharp, blind drops throughout its boulder-choked descent. Downed trees are also a particular risk on this narrow stream. Several years ago an experienced paddler was trapped and killed underneath a log hidden just below water level. Paddlers who brave the Stony (a solid Class IV river at even moderate levels) will usually welcome the relatively open and larger nature of the North Branch.

The main negative aspect of this trip is that the North Branch is not up very often. The prime times are during winter and spring two to four days after a hard rain. But, keep the faith: It has been run on Labor Day after a humongous rain a couple of days earlier.

The shuttle is straightforward, if somewhat long. From Shallmar drive downstream to Route 38, turn right, and cross the Potomac into West Virginia. Climb to the top of a high plateau. Enjoy the outstanding views before turning right onto WV 42 at Elk Garden, then right again onto US 50. This road crosses over the Stony River and makes a steep run down the mountain into Gormania. Cross the Potomac back into Maryland, take the first right, and follow the river downstream. Stop at a rough parking lot on the right, next to the tracks, where the road heads away from the river.

Barnum to Bloomington

The six-mile section of the North Branch of the Potomac River from Barnum (C) to Bloomington (D) is a solid intermediate run. It is basically composed of long, strong Class II+ wave action and rock gardens interspersed with long pools. At 1,000 cfs, a few of these wave trains approach Class III. To break this delightful monotony, however, a short but strong Class III double ledge appears midway through the trip. It should be scouted the first time. For those who like to play, surfing spots galore during the first third of the trip provide many opportunities.

This section of the North Branch is much gentler than the smaller Savage River, which joins the North Branch at the Bloomington take-out. It is also easier than the tougher big-brother section of the North Branch from Steyer to Shallmar, which ends about ten miles upstream from the Barnum put-in. However, the steady gradient and general feeling of going downhill often remind one of these other two sections.

The trip is very scenic. The North Branch flows through a beautiful gorge broken only by the occasional appearance of railroad tracks and, near the end, large industrial buildings and logging trucks. The hardwood forest generally extends right down to the river—maples, sycamores, and sometimes oaks are found near the banks, and evergreens such as hemlocks are also seen here and there. The clear waters used to be sterile from earlier mining operations, but now fish and other life appear in the river.

Just below the Barnum bridge abutments you will encounter a 50-yard Class II rapid with a two-foot ledge, followed shortly by a 100-yard-long Class II rapid and a railroad bridge. This bridge is followed by a pool, 100 yards of good Class II–III standing waves, another pool,

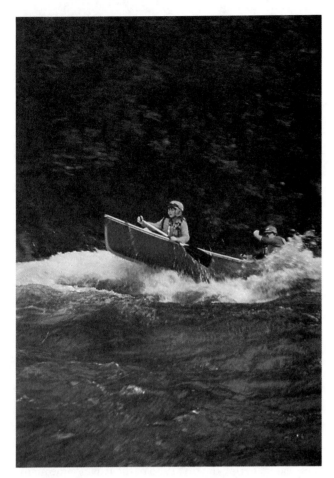

Top of the World Rapid on the North Branch of the Potomac.
Photo by Ron Knipling.

Section: Barnum (WV) to Bloomington (MD)
Counties: Garret
USGS Quads: Kitzmiller, Westernport
Difficulty: Class II–III with two solid Class III rapids
Gradient: 35 feet per mile
Average Width: 40–70 feet
Velocity: Fast
Rescue Index: Remote
Hazards: None
Scouting: Class III Double Ledge
Portages: None
Scenery: Beautiful at start, pretty in spots at end
Highlights: Beautiful gorge, dam release trip
Gauge: U.S. Army Corps of Engineers (Randolph Jennings
    Dam on Bloomington Lake), (410) 962-7687
Runnable Water Levels: Minimum   Maximum
                                300 cfs   1,250 cfs
                                (600 is good)   (max release)
Months Runnable: Several dam releases each year
Additional Information: Bloomington Dam, (304) 355-2346

and then another spot of standing waves. The relaxing monotony of the run continues with yet another pool and still another 100 yards of Class II–III standing waves. However, here there is a difference. At the end of these last waves two major surfing ledges appear with several minor surfing places adjacent or downstream. At 1,000 cfs, one of these ledges brings to mind Swimmer's Ledge on the Lower Youghiogheny in Pennsylvania except that the runout here is not nearly as clean if one flips. At higher levels these two ledges can create stopper hydraulics.

A couple of minutes and another set of standing waves later, take note of the rock face and pretty evergreen tree on the left. This pool is called Blue Hole. Ahead, when the river splits, take the larger right channel (if there is sufficient water) and you'll find yourself dropping down a Class II rapid with a cobble bar on the left and a smooth concrete rock face on the right supporting the railroad tracks above. Two nice surfing spots are encountered at the end of this rapid. At 1,000 cfs, the second of these is a particularly enjoyable kayak-sized hole in the middle of

the river. A kind but firm teacher, it does not discriminate against open boats. The cobble bar here also makes a nice lunch stop.

Past the cobble bar the long sections of standing waves and pools alternate again. One of these Class II standing wave fields is about 300 yards long. After a few more rock gardens and pools the river splits again around an island and you should take the much larger main channel to the right. About a quarter mile later, when the first island ends and another small river channel on the left creates a second island, continue on the right, but be alert because the one strong Class III rapid of the trip is approaching.

After three wave patches, the river bends left into a horizon line and a major-sounding rapid. Quickly catch the last-chance eddy on the left. Get out on the island and scout this rapid, which consists of two ledges about 25 yards apart. The first ledge should be run center or left of center because at 1,000 cfs the hole formed by the ledge gets nasty toward the right. This will also set you up to run the second, larger ledge center or left of center. At 600 cfs good tongues mark the routes over these two ledges, but at 1,000 cfs the routes are less obvious. The second island ends shortly after the rapids.

This spicy change of pace is followed by a couple of long rock gardens and a long pool. At the end of this pool, look for a railroad trestle on the left and the point where the river necks down on the right. You have reached Top of the World Rapid with its Class III twisty waves on the right at 1,000 cfs and a vigorous, punchable hole at the end.

After another pool the river necks down slightly on the left and you're faced with a second helping of standing waves not quite as dynamic as those just upstream. However, there is a vigorous surfing hole and two good surfing waves at the end of this rapid. Next, there is a long pool and another island. If there's enough water, go right. Pools and long Class I–II rapids alternate until you reach a railroad bridge a half mile from the take-out. The bridge is followed by another Class I–II rapid, a long pool, and then the river splits. Go left this time. About five minutes later you will approach a high concrete-and-stone-block railroad bridge. The concrete is located on the upstream face of the bridge and the stone block on the downstream face.

The best take-out is above this bridge on river left. To reach it from WV 46, go west on Route 135 for a long block and take the first left turn. Then take the next left turn that goes down a rutted road to a county park with plenty of parking. When you are on the river, it is hard to see the take-out because of the foliage, so walk down to the ruin so you can recognize where the take-out trail starts before heading to the put-in.

It's a shame that sufficient water on this delightful section is now solely generated by dam releases. As of this writing, water is released several weekends a year from early spring until fall. Remember, this water comes from the bottom of a big dam and therefore is very cold. Decked boaters in particular should pay attention if the day is brisk and cloudy.

As described above, this section of the North Branch at 1,000 cfs makes for a very pleasant trip. At 600 cfs the river is somewhat gentler and pickier. All rapids except one are no more than straightforward Class IIs, and even the double-ledge exception softens to an easier Class III. Conversely, at 1,250 cfs the river is clearly pushier, and some of the wave trains develop more of a Class III character.

To reach the put-in at the remains of the Barnum bridge, proceed for about five and a half miles, making several careful right turns, on WV 46, a Class III dirt road (Class IV when it's raining). Look for a right turn by three churches, which will take you about two and a half miles down to the river. Here you will find an elaborate parking area with a changing room. There is a nominal fee to park during scheduled release days. After putting in don't hurry downstream. There are two small surfing spots about fifty yards upstream on the left for the wide awake and adventurous to warm up on.

Normally the U.S. Army Corps of Engineers conserves lake water, releasing it gradually to serve the needs of downstream communities and industries. These 400 cfs flows are less than boaters prefer. A series of recreational releases are scheduled for April and May, and there are periodic "flushes" to improve downstream water quality. These 800–900 cfs "events" put the river at a very enjoyable level. Scheduled releases are publicized through club newsletters and Web sites. For daily flows, call the U.S. Army Corps of Engineers in Baltimore, (410) 962-7687. For more information call the Bloomington Dam, (304) 355-2346. You can also get this information from the National Weather Service in Washington, DC, (703) 260-0305.

Sideling Hill Creek

This section of Sideling Hill Creek is a Class I–II pure delight for good novice paddlers. However, the scenery and frequency of mild whitewater action on this 13-mile trip are sufficient to attract more experienced boaters. The rapids are gravel bars and broken ledges that can be rather spicy when they occur on tight turns. Reasonable boat control and a solid brace are important in these situations. Most of the trip wanders near the base of 1,600-foot-high Sideling Hill, which has 200- to 400-foot-high cliffs and sharp slopes made of crumbling shale, a soft sedimentary rock. Because of the poor shale soil with nutrients leached away by quickly draining precipitation, only the toughest trees grow here—pines and eastern red cedar. Sharp-eyed paddlers can spot columbine as well as prickly pear cactus along the way. In early May red columbine flowers give a bright touch while the yellow prickly pear flowers add their own bit of dazzle in late June.

The first half of the trip passes primarily through woods and a gorge that are partially included in the Sideling Hill Wildlife Management Area. In the latter half, the river skirts abandoned farms and traverses the Boy Scouts of America's Lillie-Aaron Straus Wilderness Area. The main hazard of note is a deteriorating low-water bridge about a mile below Zeigler Road near the take-out by Lock 56 at Pearre. Other hazards include the occasional log in the river and sometimes anglers, particularly during spring.

The put-in for this trip is located at the Old US 40 bridge (A), just downstream or south of the new I-68 interstate. On the downstream side of the bridge you can find the canoeing gauge. Shortly below the put-in you'll wander through a pretty gorge of woods and scenic shale cliffs. Roughly a mile into the trip, after a bend to the right and a nice Class I–II rapids, a pretty waterfall appears on the left. The only real sign of civilization in this gorge is a telephone line two miles or so after the put-in. The cliffs and Class I–II rapids on this winding stream continue with a pleasing frequency until one reaches a Class II ledge just as the river turns sharply left, roughly four miles into the trip. This ledge should be run on the left. Here in the gorge, the gradient is a bit steeper—up to 25 feet per mile at one point. Following the ledge, cliffs and Class I–II rapids continue for another mile or so. After five miles the gorge ends and you'll soon reach Norris Road, a rough, ford-type take-out not recommended except in emergencies.

Just below Norris Road the creek splits around a couple of islands, and more nicely spaced Class I–II rapids continue for a mile or so. You will see farmland on the right and Sideling Hill above on the left, followed by a pretty rock wall on the left. Over a mile later, past three bends and Stottlemeyer Road on the right, you'll encounter another Class II rapid. At that point you will paddle almost due east—straight toward Sideling Hill— for about a mile. After a right turn below a high bluff is another Class II rapid, followed by high cliffs on a second right turn.

Below the cliffs you cross Zeigler Road. You can take out here if you are pooped and want to avoid a portage downstream. Immediately following Zeigler Road is an easy Class II weir. If you haven't yet seen the Randy Carter gauge upstream, there is enough water for the trip if the weir is runnable. About a mile below Zeigler Road lies the previously mentioned disintegrating low-water bridge that must be approached with care and carried on the left. Roughly a quarter mile below the low-water bridge is the 110-foot arch of a picturesque C & O Canal Aqueduct built in 1848. Just past the aqueduct, Sideling Hill Creek enters the Potomac. The take-out is about a half mile downstream opposite Lock 56 of the C & O Canal at Pearre.

Because much of the Sideling Hill Creek area is remote, this is a good opportunity to spot wildlife. Deer are often seen, as well as beaver, muskrats, raccoons (early morning), and squirrels. Bird life includes wild turkeys, turkey vultures, hawks, and an occasional bald eagle.

Incidentally, if you prefer a big winding river to a lit-

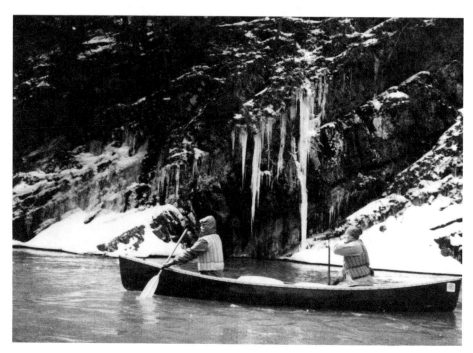

Icicles on the bank of Sideling Hill
Creek. Photo by Ed Grove.

winding stream, you should consider the serpentine, 25-mile section of the Potomac from Paw Paw to Pearre

Section: Old US 40 to Potomac River (Pearre, MD)
County: Allegany
USGS Quad: Bellegrove
Difficulty: Class I–II
Gradient: 16 feet per mile; one mile in gorge 25 feet per mile
Average Width: 15–30 feet
Velocity: Moderate
Rescue Index: Remote
Hazards: Deteriorating low-water bridge one mile below Zeigler Road, occasional logs in stream
Scouting: Approach the low-water bridge carefully
Portages: Low-water bridge one mile below Zeigler Road
Scenery: Beautiful for most of the trip
Highlights: Bluffs and cliffs, Sideling Hill, 1848 C & O Canal Aqueduct
Gauge: Visual only at put-in gauge
Runnable Water Levels:

	Minimum	Maximum
	Weir runnable below Zeigler Rd.	Flood stage
	0 feet on put-in gauge	

Additional Information: 3.2 feet on Saxton gauge (Raystown Branch of Juniata River) is a very rough correlation to zero on put-in gauge—call the U.S. Weather Bureau in Harrisburg (717) 234-6812.

(Class A-1, see note bottom of next page), particularly for low-key paddlers who like weekend canoe camping. There are periodic "hiker-biker" stops provided on the C & O Canal along the way with such colorful names as Sorrel Ridge, Stickpile Hill, Devils Alley, and Indigo Neck.

Sideling Hill Creek • Maryland

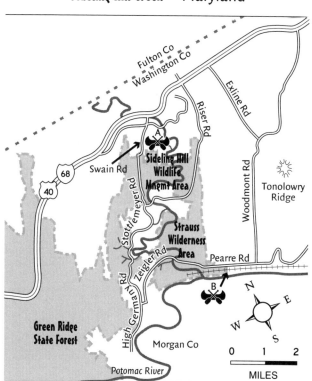

Sorrel Ridge is near the scenic Paw Paw tunnel on the C & O Canal and is mostly preferred by canoeists. These stops provide camp sites, outdoor restrooms, and potable water as the Potomac snakes its way between Paw Paw and Pearre. There is also a 14-mile canoeable stretch above this section of Sideling Hill Creek, which is almost as pretty, but the rapids only reach Class I in difficulty.

Finally, when you run this creek the first time, try to go with someone who has run it before. You will need some intelligent help to guess the water level before arriving at the put-in. Although Sideling Hill Creek is up several times during the year, there are no gauges that reasonably correlate to those on the river. Also, the shuttle roads on the western side of the creek are not marked and one can easily make a wrong turn. The shuttle roads on the eastern side of the creek are much easier to follow but are longer and require the substantial effort of crossing Sideling Hill.

Note: Class A is a flatwater classification. Class A denotes standing or slow flowing water, Class B denotes current between 2.5 and 4.5 miles per hour, and Class C denotes current that exceeds 4.5 miles per hour.

Antietam Creek

Because of the numerous bridges crossing Antietam Creek from Oak Ridge Road (A) in Funkstown to Harpers Ferry Road in Antietam (E), this is a roll-your-own Class I–II novice trip that depends on how many of the 23.5 miles between these two towns you wish to paddle. The Class Is are numerous riffles formed by gravel bars and small ledges. The Class IIs are primarily the remains of old mill dams, thoughtfully spaced over much of this section. The only hazard is located in the Devil's Backbone Park area: a six-foot dam. Also, you should scout the rapids at each bridge and dam; high water will occasionally carry trees into the entrances of rapids around the bridges, making them hazardous. Paddlers should watch for trees in the river (strainers) below some rapids when the water is high.

On this 23.5-mile stretch, farmhouses, bridges, old mills, and stone walls complement rather than detract from the rural setting. There are scenic lunch stops galore. The remains of dams used to provide water power for the mills have formed good Class II rapids at Poffenburger Road, Wagaman Road, and Roxbury Road during the first third of the trip. There is also a triple ledge two and a half miles downstream from Wagaman Road.

After this ledge and about 10 miles below Funkstown, paddlers must portage the six-foot dam at Devil's Backbone Park just upstream of Route 68. The Antietam

Antietam Creek • Maryland

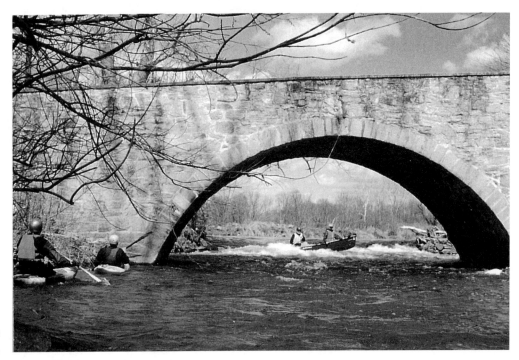

Stone bridge across Antietam Creek. Photo by Ed Pilchard.

Section: Oak Ridge Road to Harpers Ferry Road

County: Washington

USGS Quads: Funkstown, Keedysville

Difficulty: Class I–II

Gradient: Seven feet per mile

Average Width: 50–100 feet

Velocity: Moderate

Rescue Index: Accessible

Hazards: Six-foot dam at Devils Backbone, three-foot dam one mile downstream

Scouting: Recommended if running three-foot dam and at rapids formed by bridges/dams, look for trees in chutes

Portages: Six-foot dam at Devils Backbone

Scenery: Pretty to beautiful in spots

Highlights: Picturesque bridges, old mills and farms, Antietam Battlefield, wildlife

Gauge: National Weather Service (Antietam Creek gauge), (703) 260-0305, or visual at Burnside Bridge

Runnable Water Levels:	Minimum	Maximum
Burnside Bridge	3.2 feet (upper)	5.0 feet (upper)
	2.7 feet (lower)	6.5 feet (lower)
Antietam Creek	about 3.0 feet (upper)	5.0 feet (upper)
	2.5 feet (lower)	6.5 feet (lower)

Additional Information: Antietam Creek Canoe livery, (301) 582-1469; Antietam National Battlefield, (301) 432-5124; C & O Canal National Historical Park, (301) 739-4200

Creek Canoe livery is just below the Route 68 bridge (B) on the right. A mile below the six-foot dam is a broken three-foot dam that is breached on the sides; the right side can be run with care.

The next five and a half miles from the Route 68 put-in to Keedysville Road (C) are easily paddled and isolated, giving you the opportunity to watch for ducks, beavers, and your favorite songbird. The minimum level for the 14-mile upper stretch is three feet on the Burnside Bridge gauge (D) farther downstream.

The last seven and a half miles below Keedysville Road (Hicks Bridge) are quite interesting. To begin with, a beautiful waterfall appears on the right about one mile below Hicks Bridge, and then you enter that stretch of the river wandering through Antietam National Battlefield. Roughly two miles below Hicks Bridge you will reach Route 34 and a nice Class II ledge formed by the remains of an old mill dam. For those who don't have a lot of time or for winter paddlers, the remaining five miles or so downstream from Route 34 make for a scenic short trip.

A mile below Route 34 is Burnside Bridge, where paddlers can admire Antietam Battlefield and its striking markers some more. Also, there is a surfing wave formed by a two-foot, V-shaped dam that is easily run. The Burnside Bridge gauge is located just above the dam on river left below the bridge and should read at least 2.7 feet for the lower section. Before running the upper or lower sections of this creek, check this gauge even though the Antietam gauge gives a good correlation.

Only four miles remain to the take-out. The main Class II+ rapid on this final stretch is the rock garden slalom just above the Harpers Ferry Road take-out on river right after going under the bridge.

Sharp-eyed folks can spot a surprising amount of domestic and other wildlife on this trip. In addition to cows in the pastures along the riverbanks, there are great blue herons, ducks, woodpeckers, kingfishers, quail, deer, rabbits, beavers, and signs of river otters. One other interesting feature about this creek is that it continues to flow after other rivers ice up. If you crave some winter paddling when ice has your favorite river in its frosty grip, check out Antietam Creek.

The best access points on public land with reasonable parking are Oak Ridge Road in Funkstown, Route 68, Burnside Bridge Road, and Harpers Ferry Road in Antietam. All other access points are privately owned and permission should be obtained before using them. You can paddle this scenic run at levels lower than the suggested minimums, but you may have to occasionally get out of your boat to get over shallow areas.

Shenandoah and Potomac Rivers

Bull Falls and the Staircase

One of the true classic Class II–III trips for accomplished intermediates and shepherded novices who want to sharpen their paddling skills is Bull Falls and the Staircase. If you are willing to pay the admission price of two to three miles of flatwater, the remaining three and a half miles of whitewater make the trip worthwhile. The flatwater does have a positive side: It's a lazy start for rafters, boaters, and experienced tubers as well as a perfect opportunity to sharpen novices on whitewater strokes they'll soon need.

Almost halfway through the trip, Bull Falls (Class III) starts off the more serious whitewater with a bang. Below Bull Falls are fairly continuous Class I and Class II rapids through the Staircase until an emergency-only take-out at Harpers Ferry is reached. Below this point there is still Whitehorse Rapids (Class II–III) before the final take-out at Sandy Hook.

The trip from Millville to Sandy Hook is very scenic. The low hills where the Shenandoah and Potomac Rivers merge are very pretty, and there is the charming and historic town of Harpers Ferry to explore after the trip. Also, this is a dependable trip because the rivers hold their water for virtually the entire year. The only dangerous time is when the river is too high on occasion in winter and spring and rarely during other times of the year.

For the put-in on Bloomery Road (A), launch underneath the power lines by the transformer station on the outskirts of Millville, or, to avoid some of the flatwater, put in farther downstream. The last good put-in is River and Trail Outfitters, a quarter mile below the transformer station. However, you should get permission from the Outfitters and join an organized club trip if possible. Finally, be careful about leaving shuttle cars at isolated spots on Bloomery Road; thieves have broken into unattended cars on numerous occasions. Having a gracious camper or outfitter keep an eye on your shuttle cars would probably be very wise.

Wherever you put in along this stretch, notice the many camping spots on river left. Also, silver maples, sycamores, cottonwoods, box elders, and occasional ashes line the riverbanks. The Route 340 shuttle road is lined with royal paulownia trees that are breathtaking in midspring when they are covered with large, light purple flowers. From the put-in to Bull Falls two to three miles downstream, the river is popular for fishing in canoes, johnboats, and other watercraft. Smallmouth bass, bluegill, channel catfish, and the omnipresent carp are the primary fish that swim these waters. Also, be alert for bird life: great blue herons, turkey vultures, ducks, geese, and swallows are most common, and you may even see an occasional majestic pileated woodpecker.

Just below the power-line put-in the paddler has the choice of running a Class I channel between two islands in the center of the river or continuing down the left to Class I riffles at the end of the second island. About a half mile downstream, you will pass the Millville gauge on the left, followed by the put-ins for various outfitters on the left and summer homes on the right. The river is about 100 yards wide here.

Over two miles from the power-line put-in, some small islands appear on the right, and you will be heading straight toward a hill roughly 200 feet high. Approaching this hill several minutes later, you'll see rocks across the right and center of the river with a long Class II rock garden on the left. Notice the nice stone wall supporting the railroad track and the interesting rock formations on the left when passing through this rapid. There are also one or two mild surfing spots near the bottom of this slalom.

Then, in the pool below this rapids, look for an exposed broad, flat ledge blocking most of the river. Stop on this 50-foot-long section of the rock ledge between the current flowing through a narrow notch on the right and diagonally from right to left over a more powerful drop to the left. Congratulations! After three miles of warm-up you have arrived at Bull Falls. Novices can now start quivering. At low and medium levels the long, low ledge here is a perfect place to beach boats, rafts, and tubes

Section: Millville, WV, to Sandy Hook, MD

Counties: Washington (MD), Jefferson (WV)

USGS Quads: Charles Town, Harpers Ferry

Difficulty: Class III–III at moderate levels, Class III–IV at high levels

Gradient: 10 feet per mile, 3.5 miles at 15–20 feet per mile

Average Width: 250–1,000 feet

Velocity: Moderate to fast

Rescue Index: Accessible

Hazards: Occasional trees in river

Scouting: Bull Falls (Class III)

Portage: None

Scenery: Pretty to beautiful in spots

Highlights: Scenic confluence of Shenandoah and Potomac Rivers, historic town of Harpers Ferry, wildlife and birds

Gauge: National Weather Service (Millville gauge), (703) 260-0305

Runnable Water Levels	Minimum	Maximum
Millville Gauge	1.8 feet	5.5 feet

Additional Information: Harpers Ferry National Historic Park, (304) 535-6223; River and Trail Outfitters, (301) 695-5177

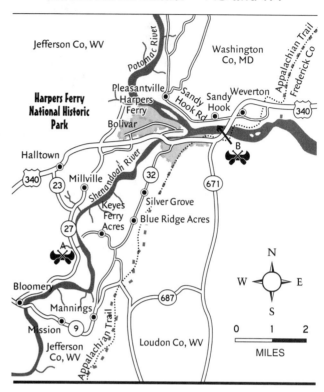

Bull Falls and The Staircase • MD and WV

ous parade of boats and bodies go over the fall.

The most classic route here is the three- to four-foot Class III drop immediately to the left of the large, low scouting ledge. The paddler should start this run reasonably close to the scouting ledge to prevent being carried too far left by the current. On reaching the drop, see if there is a just-exposed rock (low water) or a roostertail (higher water) about five feet from the scouting ledge. Turn hard right ninety degrees and run this drop on the tongue just to the left of this rock/roostertail. The reason for running this drop tight right is simple: The farther left one goes the greater chance of hitting a submerged rock in the channel.

After running this drop, keep your boat parallel with the current because at lower levels a hydraulic about 25 feet below can flip those who drop into it sideways. Incidentally, this hydraulic is a great teacher for those who want to explore the world of sideways hole surfing. It is gentle enough not to be a keeper but tough enough to bounce boaters around a bit; sometimes considerable effort is required to exit. If you plan on sitting in it sideways, have flotation in your boat and wear a helmet—the ledge is shallow. Also, have a rescue boater nearby to pick up the pieces in the pool below. As the Millville gauge reaches three feet, this hole starts to wash out and is not as grabby.

Getting back to Bull Falls, the classic drop described above is actually the third runnable slot from the left bank. To run the other two, either scout them from below after running Bull Falls the classic way or look them over from the railroad tracks on the left after beaching your boat upstream. The drop closest to the railroad tracks is basically two drops (Class II–III) that can be run center. The second drop from the left (low Class III) can also be run, but scout it first to avoid a nasty rock near the bottom.

The fourth slot (on the right of the scouting rock) is a Class II–III rapid with a one-foot ledge on the top into a narrow slot below that drops two to three feet. Novice paddlers and tubers too nervous about the classic drop just to the left of the scouting rock can run this one if they have some boat control. Incidentally, this slot also has a small surfing spot near the end at moderate levels.

The adventurous can explore other drops farther to the right on this riverwide ledge. The first of these is a straight drop that used to have a tree lodged in the normal runout. The next drop is a narrow slot with a nasty rock to dodge immediately below entry. There are perhaps four other possibilities farther to the right that are unrunnable at low water but may be possibilities at high water—particularly a rocky slalom on the extreme right.

The great thing about Bull Falls is that the easy carry

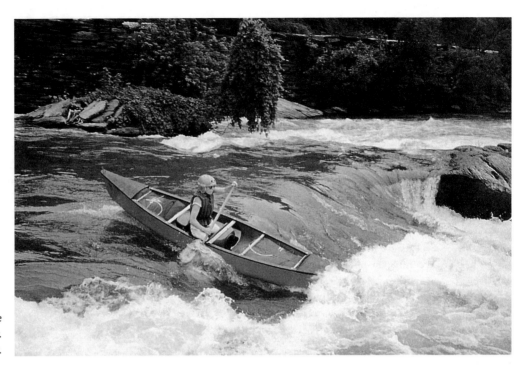

Bull Falls on the
Shenandoah River.
Photo by Ron Knipling.

over the scouting rock allows paddlers many opportunities to run this rapids. They can either take alternate routes or try again if they don't run it right the first time. However, at really high levels, this riverwide ledge is covered and parts of Bull Falls take on Class IV characteristics.

After a hopefully invigorating stop at Bull Falls, one reaches a 50-yard pool before hitting 50 yards of Class I–II standing waves. These are followed by another 50-yard pool and a Class II ledgy drop best taken on the far right at lower levels. A nice long pool follows and then the river splits in several places. Going from right to left, the first three splits are straightforward Class I–II drops over covered cobbles with some riffles below. The last alternative on the extreme left, a small Class I–II slalom, gives one the feeling of running a creek.

From the long pool located below the splits you can clearly see the first Route 340 bridge. You are now about to begin the well-known Staircase—named so because it is a stairstep-like series of ledges that continue for a good mile. At lower levels this mile is generally Class II; at high levels it starts taking on Class IV characteristics because of its length, strength, complexity, and the big holes that develop.

The Route 340 bridge marks four and a half miles from the transformer station put-in and is about halfway down the Staircase. At low levels the upper half of the Staircase tests one's water-reading ability because it is very picky. Perhaps the best route at lower levels is to start on the

left and then work toward the center. Just above the center abutment of the bridge is a one-and-a-half-foot ledge that can be run to the right or left of the abutment. The ledge also offers surfing opportunities.

After getting a breather by the center bridge abutment, paddlers can continue their Staircase descent. Just below the abutment to the right is another nice one-and-a-half foot ledge followed by 100–200 yards of little ledges. Then there is a spicy Class II–III double drop in the center over two one-and-a-half-foot ledges called Hesitation Ledge by local paddlers. Another 100 yards of small ledges follow, and you'll find yourself in a series of nicer Class II ledges and surfing spots until you reach a 10-foot-high wall with a 10-foot circular hole in it on river left. These are the ruins of an old cotton mill. Just below this wall is the Harpers Ferry beach.

Having come five miles below the transformer put-in, you can no longer take out at the massive parking lot on the left in scenic Harpers Ferry. Instead, continue downstream and within a half mile you will reach the confluence of the Potomac and the Shenandoah. Greeting you at this confluence are the abutment remains of an old bridge on the Shenandoah, a working railroad bridge over the Potomac, a striking hill 1,200 feet above the river, and a railroad tunnel. Once past the confluence, look back upstream at the pretty village of Harpers Ferry nestled in the trees.

The last mile begins with an easy set of Class I waves with a good surfing spot on the left. A few minutes later you'll encounter a pleasant 50-yard run of Class I–II waves. Shortly below these waves the river flows between two large rocks on the left with some impressive waves below. This is Whitehorse Rapid. At the top left are a couple of surfing possibilities at reasonable levels and below are about 50 yards of vigorous Class II–III waves, which become Class III at higher levels. There are also two routes to the right of Whitehorse that you should look at before running.

Just below Whitehorse, pick up any errant boats and boaters and begin looking for a wall on the left. The second Route 340 bridge looms just below. After several minutes, you'll notice a sandy beach and a three- to four-foot sandy hill instead of a wall. This is the first possible take-out at Sandy Hook (B), but if you go a couple of minutes farther downstream and remain about 100 yards or so upstream of the bridge, you will find another beach. This spot is the preferred take-out because the walk takes you over more gradual terrain. This 125-yard portage first goes over the C & O Canal towpath (which is also the Appalachian Trail here), then continues down across a new, rustic-style bridge over a muddy stream (the old canal), and finally over the railroad tracks to Sandy Hook Road. Be very careful when crossing the tracks here; freight trains pass frequently at a good clip.

Patoma Wayside is on river right just above the Route 340 bridge, but you can't leave cars here. On the other hand, a nice little cascade from a nearby stream provides welcome wet relief on hot days. Unlike the take-out at the Harpers Ferry parking lot, it is hard to find a place to park cars at Sandy Hook. You basically have a few sloping places next to the railroad track or in people's driveways on the other side of Sandy Hook Road, but parking in driveways is not recommended unless you get permission. So leave as few cars as possible and watch your valuables; there have been some thefts here, too. Perhaps the best way of dealing with the shuttle for this trip is by convincing a couple of shuttle bunnies to do the chore.

While you meander down the river, they can visit scenic Harpers Ferry and pick you up later in the day.

Harpers Ferry is rich in history. The first settler, a trader named Peter Stephens, arrived in 1733 and set up a primitive ferry service at the junction of the Potomac and Shenandoah rivers. Robert Harper, a miller and the man for whom the town is named, settled here in 1747 and built a mill. The original ferry and mill are long gone. In the 1790s George Washington was instrumental in establishing a national armory here. By 1801, the armory was producing weapons; arms produced at Harpers Ferry were used by Lewis and Clark on their famous westward expedition of 1804–1806. The arrival of the C & O Canal and the B & O Railroad in the 1830s generated prosperity, and by the 1850s Harpers Ferry had 3,000 residents.

In 1859, however, John Brown's raid on the eve of the Civil War thrust the town into national prominence and set the stage for its eventual decline. When the Civil War began in 1861, the armory and arsenal buildings were burned to prevent them from falling into Confederate hands. Because of the town's geographic location and railway system, both the Union and Confederate forces occupied the town intermittently throughout the war. Discouraged by war damage and fewer jobs, many people left. The finishing blow to the town was dealt by a series of devastating floods in the late 1800s.

Harpers Ferry has since been restored by the National Park Service and today is a delightful place to visit. Besides restored streets, shops, houses, and public buildings, there are other points of interest. On the Shenandoah side above the town is Jefferson Rock. Here, in 1783, Thomas Jefferson was so taken with the view he thought it was "worth a voyage across the Atlantic." Not far from this rock is the grave of Robert Harper and a very interesting cemetery. On the left side of the Potomac River across from Harpers Ferry is the Appalachian Trail and the C & O Canal towpath for day hikers and backpackers.

Gunpowder Falls

Gunpowder Falls is a pleasant Class II–III trip at moderate levels for good intermediate boaters. A 3.3-mile run from Route 1 (A) to Route 40 (B), it passes through a pretty but shallow wooded gorge and has only one drawback: It's too short. One can put in at Lower Loch Raven Dam upstream, but this would mean an additional seven-mile scenic paddle over flatwater with only occasional riffles.

The falls line of Gunpowder Falls begins just below Route 1. You can warm up by running the Class II rapids at the put-in and doing some elementary surfing at the bottom of this rapids. About a quarter mile below is Pot's Rock, a nice long Class II–III rapids entered by way of a rock garden 50–100 yards long. Then, move right with a quick cut back to the left just before dropping over a two-

Section: Route 1 to Route 40
County: Baltimore
USGS Quad: White Marsh
Difficulty: Class II–III at moderate levels, Class III–IV at high levels
Gradient: 20 feet per mile; a half mile at 40 feet per mile
Average Width: 50–100 feet
Velocity: Moderate to fast
Rescue Index: Accessible but difficult
Hazards: Occasional tree in river
Scouting: Long rapid just below Route 7 is Class III (moderate level) or Class IV (high level)
Portages: None
Scenery: Pretty in most spots
Highlights: Nice wooded gorge
Gauge: Visual only

Runnable Water Levels:

	Minimum	Maximum
	Class II rapid at put-in, cleanly runnable	5 feet of water over put-in rapid

Additional Information: None

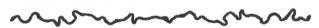

foot ledge. Adding spice to Pot's Rock is a fun surfing spot located just below the ledge. Decked boaters can get enders here at one and a half to two feet on the Route 1 gauge. Shortly below Pot's Rock is a Class II rock garden.

The next rapids of significance occurs as the paddler reaches the I-95 bridge. Here a 100-yard Class II rock garden (Class III in high water) appears just above the bridge and continues well beyond. The rock garden ends and a pool is reached just as you pass under the nearby Route 7 bridge. You'll also hear an impressive roar at this point, which is your signal to get to river right and scout because you have a long, strong, Class III rock garden of over 100 yards to run. There are surfing spots toward the end of the rapid. At higher levels it gets tougher because of its length, strength, and complexity.

One can take out at the Route 7 bridge, the most convenient take-out, but this makes the trip only a couple of miles long. Also, the long, Class III rock garden and a couple of other nice rapids will be missed.

Below Route 7 there are two good drops. The first is a relatively short Class II rock garden known as Finger Rock. The second is a Class II–III drop with a ledge on the left and (with enough water) a tight S turn on the right. First-timers should scout from river right. The second rapid also has reasonable surfing opportunities here and there.

The Route 40 bridge take-out follows. Take out on river left, and you'll encounter the only problem with this otherwise pleasant trip: no legal parking near the bridge. The nearest place is a quarter- to a half-mile southwest of the bridge, so have a shuttle driver meet you or be willing to hike.

Unfortunately, things have changed at the Gunpowder Falls put-in. The new Route 1 bridge is much higher than the old bridge, so the portage to the river is more difficult. Also, parking is in a state of flux. Finally, the gauge for this trip disappeared along with the old Route 1 bridge. Consequently, paddlers must use their best judgment concerning water levels. If the Class II rapid at the put-in

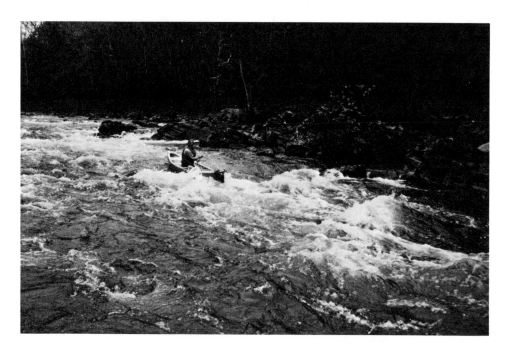

Ed Grove on Gunpowder Falls.
Photographer unknown.

Gunpowder Falls • Maryland

is cleanly runnable, there should be enough water.

The Gunpowder is basically a winter or spring trip following a recent rain when the Loch Raven reservoir is full of water. This will usually produce runnable levels for a week. There is reasonable bird life along the river, such as herons and turkey vultures, and the scenic gorge is restful. It's too bad this delightful trip isn't longer.

NORTH CAROLINA

Big Laurel Creek

Big Laurel Creek is a fast, wildwater stream in Madison County that cuts a gorge 1,200 feet deep between Mill Ridge on the north and Walnut Knob on the south. This is truly a spectacular run. Unfortunately, as with many trips of this type, you aren't able to raise your eyes from the job at hand long enough to have a chance to enjoy nature's wonders to the fullest.

Big Laurel Creek flows into the French Broad three and a half miles above Hot Springs. This section must be run unless the paddler goes upstream a quarter mile to the community of Stackhouse (see the section on the French Broad River). The run begins at the US 25-70 bridge (A), with the usual take-out being the US 25-70 bridge over the French Broad at Hot Springs (B).

There is a gauge on the east side of the bridge at the put-in. A reading of six inches below zero is minimum for a solo run; at this level two rapids must be carried. A reading of three inches above the bottom of zero is the maximum level recommended. The great increase in difficulty with the slight increase in level is due to the constricted course. Big Laurel is runnable except in extremely dry seasons.

In terms of difficulties, many rapids should be scouted, the first of which is a quarter mile below the put-in. An innocuous-looking two-foot ledge, which is run on the left, pushes the bow squarely into a pointed rock at the bottom of the chute. This ledge can be recognized by the cottage just below it on the left bank, the last sign of habitation until the railroad bridge 100 yards

Big Laurel Creek • North Carolina

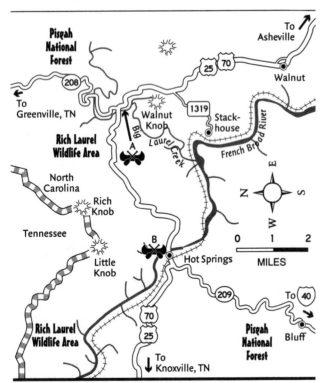

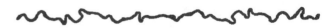

Section: Madison to Hot Springs
County: Madison
USGS Quads: White Rock, Hot Springs
Difficulty: Class III–IV
Gradient: 50 feet per mile (0.5 mile and 80 feet per mile)
Average Width: 20–40 feet
Velocity: Fast
Rescue Index: Remote
Hazards: Rapids
Scouting: Suddy Hole and the Narrows—scout on left (see French Broad)
Portages: None required
Scenery: Beautiful
Highlights: Scenery, whitewater, geology
Gauge: Visual only; gauge at put-in bridge
Runnable Water level:

	Minimum	Maximum
	6 inches	3 inches
	below 0	above bottom of 0

Months runnable: January through June and after heavy rains
Additional Information: Nantahala Outdoor Center, (704) 622-7260

above the confluence with the French Broad. This ledge is a warning of bigger and better things to come.

Some other rapids worth mentioning include Stair Steps, a tightly constricted series of three drops of three feet each, which becomes quite hairy at even two inches below zero on the gauge. There's also Suddy Hole, an eight-foot ledge that can be run on the left at water levels above the bottom of zero, and on the right by those with suicidal tendencies. The Narrows is easily recognized and certainly should be scouted to determine the best passage. The bed of an old railroad runs on the south side the entire length of the creek, which can help one in scouting.

The previously mentioned railroad bridge marks the end of the Big Laurel run and the beginning of big water on the French Broad (see the French Broad River).

North Fork of the French Broad River

The North Fork of the French Broad River heads up on the eastern edge of the Nantahala National Forest. The stream originates in the vicinity of Devil's Courthouse off the Blue Ridge Parkway. Its protected watershed ensures excellent water quality. High in the mountains it tumbles over Courthouse Falls, a stunning 50-foot drop. Below the falls it remains a steep mountain rivulet for some miles before entering the flat valley at Balsam Grove. Downstream of Balsam Grove are several beautiful falls—most notably Birdtown Falls, a runnable 20-foot drop. Flatwater follows Birdtown Falls down to the section described. The North Fork drains a small area, so extended rainfall is necessary to be able to paddle it.

Also worth mentioning here is the current interest that Rosman farmers have for a dam in the Balsam Grove area, which would essentially inundate the North Fork gorge. The main issue is flood control—Rosman is on the French Broad flood plain. Things are only in the talking stage at this point, but paddlers need to be aware of this possibility and respond to it if it goes any further.

The basic run is from the Route 1326 bridge (A) to the US 64 bridge (B). To reach the put-in go north on NC 215 off US 64, one mile west of Rosman, then go west on Route 1326. The takeout at the US 64 bridge is 1.1 miles west of Rosman. A gauge can be located on the south side of the center piling of the US 64 bridge.

The rapids of consequence start at the end of the first mile, where a slide drops 12 feet, followed by a Class III. Scout on the left. The next rapid of consequence, Boxcar Falls, is named because of a mishap that occurred when

North Fork of the French Broad River • North Carolina

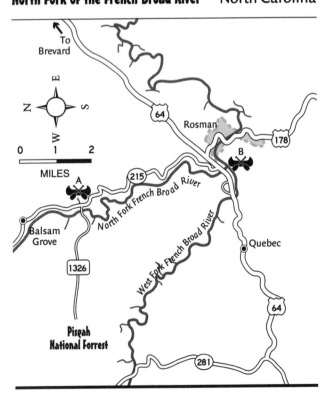

Section: Route 1326 bridge to US 64 bridge
County: Transylvania
USGS Quad: Rosman
Difficulty: Class IV–V
Gradient: 54 feet per mile (1 mile at 145 feet per mile)
Average Width: 15–40 feet
Velocity: Fast
Rescue Index: Accessible but difficult
Hazards: Difficult rapids, waterfalls
Scouting: Several rapids require scouting—scout from old railroad bed
Portages: Strongly consider Boxcar Falls
Scenery: Beautiful to spectacular
Highlights: Scenery, whitewater, geology
Gauge: Visual only. Gauge on south side of US 64 bridge
Runnable Water Level: Minimum   Maximum
                        Bottom of 0   6 inches above 0
Months runnable: March through May and after heavy rains
Additional Information: Headwaters Outfitters, (704) 877-3106

the narrow-gauge railroad was in operation. Legend has it that a boxcar fell in the narrow, deep sluice at the base of the falls. Boxcar Falls drops about 22 feet into a narrow rock trough. There are two obvious routes over the drop, neither of them pleasant, both with a certain potential for injury. Scout or portage on the old railroad bed on the right. Below here is good Class IV gradient for several hundred yards. Razorback comes at the end of this stretch. Below Razorback is the Clog, a steep Class V boulder garden of a hundred yards. Scout or carry on the left. More interesting Class IV rapids follow, leading into Submarine, a nine-foot slide on the far left. The gradient starts to slow progressively from Submarine to the take-out. For those interested in cutting some flatwater out of the run, take out at Alligator Rock. Alligator Rock (named because of a jaws-like formation above the road on the right) pull-off is 1.7 miles north on NC 215 from the intersection at US 64.

French Broad River

The French Broad River is formed in the vicinity of Rosman, in Transylvania County, where the North Fork, West Fork, Middle Fork, and East Fork join together. The upper reaches of the river are primarily flat, flowing over shallow shoals alternating between farmland and wooded areas. It is ideal for quiet floating trips.

From Asheville downriver to Hot Springs the river cuts through a more mountainous area and changes complexion greatly as the volume and gradient increase. It becomes a wide, powerful force, flowing through scenic gorges, over series of ledges, and through large boulders. The river here requires a much higher level of skill from paddlers.

Beyond Hot Springs the river slows down to flat stretches interspersed with rapids, along with some outstanding rock formations such as Paint Rock and Chimney Rock.

The upper 76 miles of the French Broad (from the US 64 bridge over the North Fork west of Rosman to the North Carolina Electric Power Dam on NC 191) consists primarily of flat, scenic Class I floats with an occasional Class II shallow or shoal. The water quality is fair and the only significant hazard is the 10-foot Electric Power Dam. Numerous access points afford the paddler a variety of possible trips in this upper section. The river is runnable all year except for periods of extreme dryness.

Below the dam (A), six and a half miles down to the Buncombe County Route 1620 bridge (B) at Alexander, difficulty increases to Class II–III as the river begins to drop over a series of ledges and heavier shoals and the current picks up speed. On the far right about a mile below the dam, a Class III chute with heavy water presents the experienced paddler with an exciting run. This can be bypassed by working through the rock gardens in the center. With the increased gradient and widening of the river, this section can become quite difficult in higher water. The Metropolitan Sewage Treatment Plant empties just below the put-in, which might give one added incentive to stay upright.

Downstream of Alexander the river shows its tamer side, reverting to Class I and mild Class II. At Marshall (C) an eight-foot dam can present problems. If you take out, you would do well to pull out on the right bank in the vicinity of the intersection of NC 213 and US Business 25-70, which will cut about a half mile off the trip. If continuing, a carry of some 400 yards to below the Route 1001 bridge will be necessary due to the bulkhead built along the banks below the dam. About one and a half miles below Marshall, 25-foot-high Redmon Dam should be approached very cautiously. A carry of some 200 yards on the right side is necessary. Beyond the dam the river really begins to flex its muscles. A constant gradient presents the paddler with steady Class II water and practically no flatwater. Those putting in to run this section can do so below the dam and above the Route 1135 bridge on the right bank.

Section: Woodfin to Barnard
Counties: Buncombe, Madison
USGS Quads: Asheville, Weaverville, Leicester, Marshall
Difficulty: Class I–II (III)
Gradient: 15 feet per mile
Average Width: 250–600 feet
Velocity: Moderate to fast
Rescue Index: Accessible to accessible but difficult
Hazards: Difficult rapids, dams
Scouting: None required
Portages: 8-foot dam at Marshall, 25-foot dam below Marshall on right
Scenery: Pretty to beautiful
Highlights: Scenery, geology, whitewater
Gauge: TVA, (800) 238-2264

Runnable Water Level	Minimum	Maximum
	800 cfs	4,000 cfs

Months runnable: All
Additional Information: Nantahala Outdoor Center, (704) 488-2175, or during raft season, (704) 488-2176 x426.

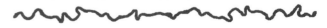

French Broad River • North Carolina

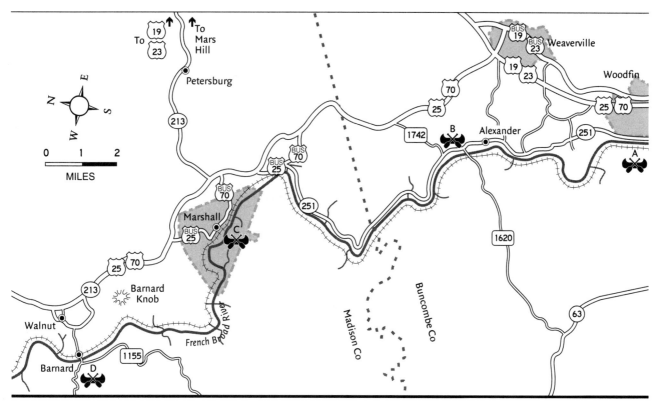

By far the most celebrated run on the French Broad is the Class III–IV (V), seven-and-a-half-mile run from the Madison County Route 1151 bridge at Barnard (D) to the US 70-25 bridge in Hot Springs (E). Beautiful scenery combines with some of the southern Appalachians' foremost whitewater to offer a year-round paddling experience.

The increased gradient combined with greater width and heavier water makes for an exciting trip through this section. Scouting becomes very difficult but quite necessary. For those who don't have a very dependable eddy turn in their repertoire, this stretch simply "ain't the place to be." Generally, the rule to follow is to stay to the left of all islands of any size.

There are seven major rapids in this section, all of which should be approached cautiously. The third of these rapids, Big Pillow, will be found on the left side. The main flow of the river runs left, as the right side is clogged with boulders. The entrance rapid, a fast chute, flows diagonally left and requires the boater to fight to get back to the right in order to get by the large pillow and souse hole below it. There is, however, a narrow chute on the immediate left of the pillow, which can be negotiated in the event that one ends up too far to the left. Both the entrance and the pillow should be scouted carefully. Big Pillow is located approximately one and a half miles below the put-in. The next two rapids should be scouted on the left and right, respectively.

The town of Stackhouse, located about halfway through this section, can be recognized by the second island on the right. Move to the far left as soon as the island is observed. From this island a row of iron rods extends diagonally upstream about two-thirds of the way across the river. These rods can be seen at levels below 4,000 cfs.

Big Laurel Creek joins the French Broad about a quarter mile downstream from Stackhouse. Another three-quarters of a mile downstream is Needle Rock, a sliver of shining rock located on the left bank high above the island separating the main channel. The main channel, which is on the left, has big standing waves that can easily swamp an open boat. It can be scouted best from the island. A small, protected chute just left of the island drops rather quickly but can be run without too much danger. For those into running drops, Kayak Ledge, a five-foot vertical ledge, lies on the right of Needle Rock. Scout from below the railroad tracks on the right bank.

The next large island in the middle of the river below

French Broad River • North Carolina and Tennessee

Needle Rock will indicate a Class V rapid, the last rapid of any consequence on this section. The rapid, on the right, has become known as Frank Bell's Rapid by canoeists in the area. It consists of three concentric

ledges that funnel the river into a giant whirlpool at the bottom. The passage to the left of the island is safest but certainly not unexciting. Both sides can be best scouted

Section: Barnard to Hot Springs
County: Madison (NC)
USGS Quads: Spring Creek (NC), Hot Springs (NC)
Difficulty: Class III–IV (V)
Gradient: 28 feet per mile
Average Width: 250–500 feet
Velocity: Moderate to fast
Rescue Index: Accessible but difficult
Hazards: Difficult rapids
Scouting: All difficult rapids
Portages: None required
Scenery: Poor to beautiful
Highlights: Scenery, whitewater
Gauge: TVA, (800) 238-2264

Runnable Water Level	Minimum	Maximum
	800 cfs	4,000 cfs

Additional Information: Nantahala Outdoor Center, (704) 488-2175, or during raft season, (704) 488-2176 x426.

Section: Hot Springs to US 25-70 bridge
Counties: Madison (NC), Cocke (TN)
USGS Quads: Hot Springs (NC), Paint Rock (TN-NC), Needy Mountain (TN)
Difficulty: Class II–III
Gradient: 12 feet per mile
Average Width: 250–400 feet
Velocity: Moderate to fast
Hazards: Moderate rapids, hydraulics
Rescue Index: Accessible to accessible but difficult
Scouting: Unfamiliar rapids
Portages: None
Scenery: Good to excellent
Highlights: Scenery, whitewater
Gauge: TVA, (800) 238-2264

Runnable Water Level	Minimum	Maximum
	800 cfs	4,000 cfs

Additional Information: Nantahala Outdoor Center, (704) 488-2175, or during raft season, (704) 488-2176 x426.

from the island. (The late Frank Bell, owner of Camp Mondamin in Tuxedo, NC was fortunate enough to be around before dams were the answer to all problems. He paddled the French Broad from its headwaters to the Gulf of Mexico. An attempt to run down the right side below Needle rock ended with his canoe remaining in the whirlpool for some ten minutes; he got out only after great difficulty.)

Below Hot Springs to the US 25-70 bridge in Tennessee the river broadens and settles back to Class II–III as it flows out of North Carolina into Tennessee. At normal water levels there are several rapids where standing waves build up enough to give tandem paddlers problems. All can be "sneaked" by scouting carefully and generally staying to the inside on the bends. Below the second railroad bridge a four-foot ledge can be run best on the far left. Around the next bend is a rapid, running some 75 yards, that one should approach cautiously on the right and run on the right. At medium to high levels a giant eddy is formed between this rapid and the next ledge downstream, which is a natural dam. It should be scouted—left or right—and given the same respect one should give any dam. There are breaks that can be run, but hydraulics form at higher levels.

A fine detailed map of the French Broad River from Rosman to Newport, Tennessee, is available for a fee from Land of Sky Regional Council, 25 Heritage Drive, Asheville, NC 28808; (704) 251-2264.

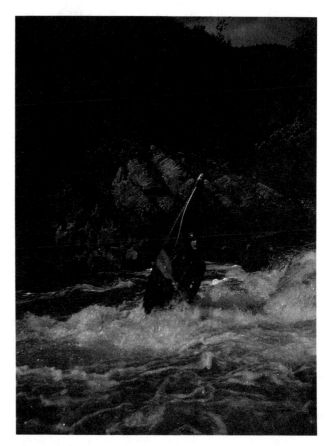

Ender action at Frank Bell's Rapids on the French Broad. Photo by Ed Grove.

North Fork of the Catawba River

The North Fork has its headwaters on Humpback Mountain in McDowell County below the Blue Ridge Parkway. It is a small shallow stream, which US 221 follows down the mountain, until Armstrong Creek comes in and it picks up considerable volume. In the Sevier area it receives some degree of industrial pollution. Below Sevier it enters a small gorge and continues on its way to Lake James. The river runs parallel to and below the western ridge of the Linville Gorge Wilderness Area. With the exception of the Clinchfield Railroad running along the east bank for about half of the way down, this is a relatively uninhabited area. The North Fork remains fairly narrow as it courses over ledges and through small boulder gardens.

There is a gauge on the northwest side of the railroad bridge at the put-in. The minimum level for solo is two inches below zero. With a reading of approximately four inches above the bottom of zero on the gauge, several of the rapids will require scouting. The North Fork can generally be run during wet seasons or immediately after a rain. Runoff will be fast. To reach the put-in, drive north of Marion on US 221 to Woodlawn, then east on Route 1556 to Route 1559 and then 100 yards to the put-in (A) on the river's edge, between the creek bridge and railroad bridge.

Difficulties on this run begin 600 yards below the put-in, where a boulder garden about 100 yards long requires a great deal of maneuvering. The best scouting is on the right bank. There are several interesting rapids before arriving at the railroad bridge about midway through the run, but below it an eight-foot slanting falls should be approached with caution. Three two- to three-foot ledges

Section: Route 1559 to Route 1552
County: McDowell
USGS Quad: Little Switzerland
Difficulty: Class II–III
Gradient: 29 feet per mile
Average Width: 25–120 feet
Velocity: Fast
Rescue Index: Accessible but difficult
Hazards: Difficult rapids, possible deadfalls
Scouting: Scout on right below railroad bridge
Portages: None required
Scenery: Pretty to beautiful
Highlights: Scenery, whitewater, geology
Gauge: Visual only. Gauge on northwest side of railroad bridge at put-in

Runnable Water Level	Minimum	Maximum
	2 inches below 0	Up to flood stage

Months runnable: January through May and after heavy rains
Additional Information: None available

North Fork of the Catawba River • North Carolina

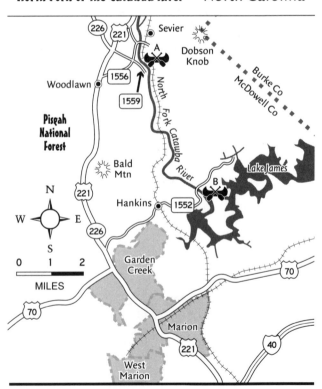

follow it closely. Run these on the right. The river drops about 16 feet within 150 yards through this area. Scout on the right bank again.

The take-out can be reached by driving north of Marion on US 221, then east on Route 1501 (Hankins Road) to Burnett's Landing. Turn left on Route 1552 to the bridge (B). A slightly easier take-out can be made at the Wildlife Access Area a half-mile downstream from the Route 1552 bridge. Look for the sign on the right after passing Burnett's Landing.

Green River

The Green River drops through a great, boulder-strewn gorge after leaving Lake Summit in Henderson County, until it crosses into Polk County. After leaving the deep gorge and entering Polk County, it levels out into a delightful fast-flowing stream cutting between Cove and Chimney Top Mountains on the south and McCraw Mountain to the north. Through this area it is a fairly small stream dropping over small ledges and through small rock gardens. The area is sparsely settled, but evidence of encroaching civilization is growing fast.

Next to the Nantahala, this section of the Green is probably canoed more than any other river in North Carolina. During the summer months hardly a day passes without two or three groups of canoeists from various summer camps holding classes there. It is an excellent stream for teaching the basics of river canoeing. This popularity has created problems for residents. On sum-mer weekends dust hangs in the air as shuttles race up and down the river road, beer bottles and cans are strewn about, and nudity is flaunted. This is a nice place to visit, but not as nice a place to live in as it might be.

Duke Power Company has developed two parking areas—one at the put-in (A) and one at the take-out (B). No parking is allowed on the road between these areas. It is patrolled regularly, especially on weekends, and the rules about parking are rigidly enforced.

The favored whitewater run on the Green River is from Route 1151 (Green Cove Road) to a point six miles downstream where the river leaves the road. The Green is a dam-controlled stream and is runnable only when the plant in Tuxedo is operating. Generally the plant operates

Section: Upstream Duke Power Company parking area to downstream Duke Power Company parking area
County: Polk
USGS Quads: Cliffield Mountain, Lake Lure, Rutherfordton South
Difficulty: Class II
Gradient: 21 feet per mile
Average Width: 20–75 feet
Velocity: Moderate to fast
Rescue Index: Accessible
Hazards: Difficult rapids
Scouting: Little Corky, road on left
Portages: None required
Scenery: Pretty
Highlights : Whitewater
Gauge: Dam-release schedule (800) 829-5253

Runnable Water Level	Minimum	Maximum
	Dam in operation	Up to flood stage

Additional Information: None

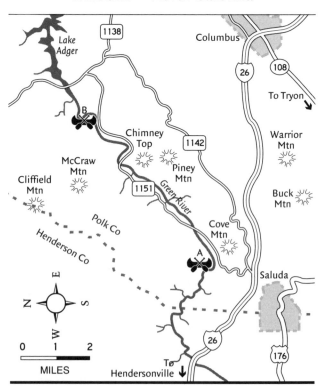

Green River • North Carolina

during the week, in which case water arrives at the put-in each day about 1:00 P.M.

Green Cove Road follows along the river the entire distance, making scouting rather easy. The first rapid of any consequence is Big Corky, 1.3 road miles below the first bridge. It can be recognized by the quiet pool above it and the sandy beach on the left below. When both turbines are running at the dam, it presents a nice standing wave for dousing the bowman.

A second rapid about a quarter mile below Big Corky can present problems to the unwary paddler. It bears to the left and drops over a rock bed for about 75 yards. Farther downstream a series of ledges, called Jacob's Ladder, run for some 200 yards and should be approached cautiously. The road is high above the river at this point.

The approach to Little Corky, a Class II rapid, occurs just beyond a point where the road has dropped down to the river and a sizable island separates the main stream. The more difficult run is on the left of the island. It drops fast, with an apparent straight chute off the right bank. A rock barely under water is the grabber awaiting the straight shooter. A slight movement to the left will shoot the canoe between it and a similar rock on the left. They are little more than one canoe width apart. Scout on the left. Below Little Corky the river continues to drop fast for a half mile; then it slows down somewhat. Primarily fun water follows the last Corky.

To reach the put-in, get off I-26 at the Saluda exit, go east approximately 300 yards to Green Cove Road (Route 1151), and then left down a series of hairpin curves, after which the road straightens. The river is on the left. Turn into the first pull-off on the left. This puts you above a fast-water rapid, requiring some quick maneuvering. Coming from Mill Spring, take NC 9 north about 100 yards, then go west on Route 1138 to Silver Creek Baptist Church. Turn left on Route 1151 to the river. Proceed to the point where the road starts up Cove Mountain and turn right into the parking lot. To reach the take-out drive 6.3 miles toward Lake Adger on Route 1151 to a second parking area, located just beyond a point where one loses sight of the river.

Little Tennessee River

The Little Tennessee first appears to the traveler on US 23-441 south of Franklin in Macon County as a small creek. One wonders how such a small stream can grow to a full-size river between there and Iotla. It flows generally north between the Nantahala Mountain Range on the west and the Cowee Range to the east before emptying into the impoundment at Fontana.

The riverside alternates between farmlands and woodlands above Lost Bridge; below Lost Bridge it becomes heavily forested, except where Route 1114 hits it occasionally. The area near Franklin and around much of Macon County is widely known for its great mineral deposits and is certainly a rock hound's heaven.

The "Little T" is one of the few rivers in North Carolina that lends itself to overnight canoe camping. Generally speaking there is enough water to carry gear; at the same time the rapids aren't so formidable that the paddler is likely to finish the day with it wet. Unfortunately, not many streams remain that can claim both these qualities. The good ones either have been dammed (leaving nothing but flatwater), are too shallow to carry the necessary equipment, or are too rough to maneuver through rapids with the extra weight in the boat.

The best whitewater run on the Little T begins north of Iotla at Lost Bridge off NC 28 (A) and ends where the river joins the sluggish backwaters of Lake Fontana. A gauge is located on the left bank 0.8 mile north of Needmore in Swain County and approximately 6.8 miles below Lost Bridge Road bridge. The Little T is very seldom too low to run, but can become dangerous with high water levels when Lake Fontana is low.

In terms of difficulties several ledges should be approached cautiously at higher levels. When Lake Fontana is quite low (the lake is generally lowered in the fall and winter in preparation for the spring rains) there is a series of ledges that runs for close to 250 yards, following which the entire river (which previously has been up to 300 feet wide) constricts to blast through a sluice no wider than 20 feet! This rapid, appropriately known as the Narrows, should definitely be scouted before attempting a run. In higher waters the rapid can be formidable, with up to five-foot standing waves at the bottom. If the water is high, scout on the right; otherwise the left offers a better view.

Getting off the Little Tennessee is a bit of a problem. You can either climb a nearly vertical "goat path" up to the US 19–NC 28 bridge (C) southwest of Bryson City or paddle about three and a half miles of Lake Fontana to the NC 28 bridge (D).

Section: Lost Bridge to Lake Fontana
Counties: Macon, Swain
USGS Quads: Franklin, Alarka, Wesser
Difficulty: Class I–III (IV)
Gradient: 14 feet per mile
Average Width: 120–300 feet
Velocity: Moderate to fast
Rescue Index: Accessible
Hazards: Difficult rapids
Scouting: The Narrows—river right
Portages: None required
Scenery: Pretty to beautiful
Highlights: Scenery, whitewater, wildlife
Gauge: TVA, (800) 238-2264

Runnable Water Level	Minimum	Maximum
	350 cfs	Up to flood stage

Months runnable: All
Additional Information: None

Little Tennessee River • North Carolina

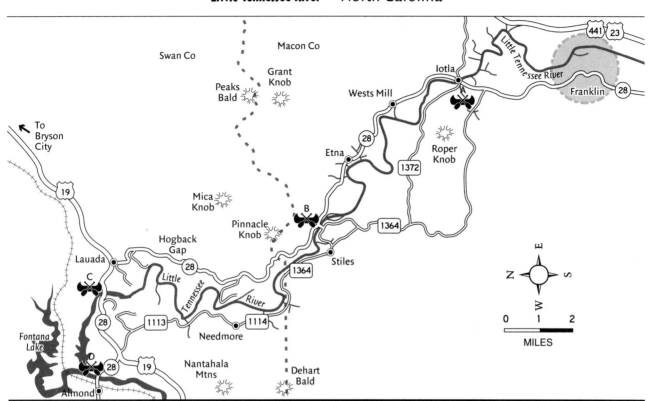

Nantahala River

The Nantahala heads up in Macon County along the edge of Nantahala National Forest before entering Aquone Lake, reportedly the highest lake in North Carolina. From there it is piped and tunneled down the mountain to the power plant a few yards above the put-in point. The water enters the river at a temperature averaging around 45°F. The river then flows down through the beautiful Nantahala Gorge in a mad, shivering dash to Lake Fontana. Nantahala, meaning "Land-of-the-noon-day-sun," was the name given by the Cherokee Indians, because of the deep gorge which shuts out the sun for most of each day.

The cold water can create an unusual phenomenon on a very warm day. A fog rises about three feet above the water, sometimes cutting visibility down to a few feet. Such visibility doesn't leave the newcomer to the river with much margin for error. After one has had some of

the icy water splashed into the boat, it is a rather chilling experience to observe some hardy young souls tubing down the river. This has to be where the "Dead End Kids" got their start.

The course begins at Patton's Pool (A) and runs to the takeout, below Nantahala Falls (C), with continuous whitewater. A bailer—make that a big bailer—is a necessity for the canoeist running the Nantahala. The constant action makes this the most popular canoeing river in the state.

Speaking of which, the exceptional popularity of the Nantahala has in recent years become its most lamentable drawback. Half a dozen commercial outfitters run guided raft trips while a dozen more rent rafts or tubes for

Section: Public launch ramp to Nantahala Outdoor Center

Counties: Macon, Swain

USGS Quads: Hewitt, Wesser

Difficulty: Class II–III

Gradient: 33 feet per mile

Average Width: 20–50 feet

Velocity: Fast

Rescue Index: Accessible

Hazards: Difficult rapids

Scouting: Nantahala Falls, river right

Portages: None required

Scenery: Pretty to beautiful

Highlights: Scenery, whitewater

Gauge: Nantahala Dam Power Plant (704) 369-4556

Runnable Water Level	Minimum	Maximum
	200 cfs	Up to flood stage

Months runnable: All, when water is released from dam

Additional Information: Nantahala Outdoor Center, (704) 488-2175, or during raft season, (704) 488-2176 x426

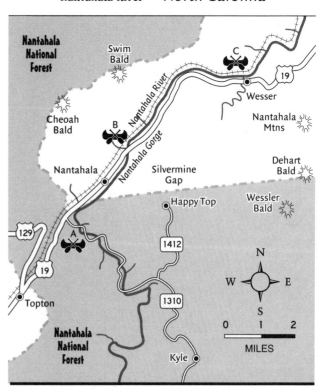

Nantahala River • North Carolina

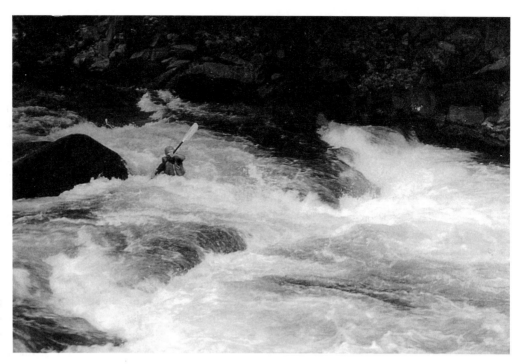

Richard Vest and the last rapid on the Nanty—Nantahala Falls. Photo courtesy Matthew Vest.

self-guided expeditions. Add to this mayhem hundreds (sometimes thousands) of private canoeists and decked boaters and a leisurely day on the river begins to resemble a wet version of rush-hour traffic in Atlanta. Of course, the river isn't the only resource that is strained; campgrounds are packed, long waits develop at the few area restaurants, and parking at the put-in and take-out spots becomes a nightmare. As might be suspected, Saturdays from June through early September are the most crowded days.

If you are determined to paddle the Nantahala on a Saturday you might miss some of the crowd by launching the minute water is released (don't paddle too fast—it is possible to outrun the water), or better yet by making a late afternoon run. Though the gorge is bathed in shadows late in the day, there is plenty of daylight in the summer for runs initiated as late as 4:30 P.M. Sundays are also crowded, but nothing like Saturdays, and the least crowded days are obviously weekdays. A possible alternative if you must go on a summer weekend is to run the nearby Little Tennessee (if water levels permit) on Saturday morning and paddle the Nantahala on Saturday afternoon. The Nantahala, incidentally, does have an intermediate public access point on the north side of where US 19 crosses the river (B). This access essentially allows paddlers to run only half of the river if time is short.

Although the Nantahala can be paddled from the power plant all the way to Lake Fontana (with one mandatory portage), the classic run is from the new pub-

lic parking area just downstream of the power plant to a privately owned take-out a quarter mile below Nantahala Falls made available by the Nantahala Outdoor Center. The river can be run only when the power plant is operating, which is generally the case during the week and quite frequently on weekends.

Cold and fast from start to finish, the Nantahala never stops coming at you. Just below the put-in at the first bend in the river is Patton's Run, the second largest rapid on the run. It's a long Class III, requiring the paddler to stay to the inside of the bend. This is heavy, fast water. Like most of the river, it can be scouted from US 19, which follows the river closely throughout the run. Scout this one from the pull-off on the highway before launching. Patton's Pool and Run were dedicated to the late Charlie Patton of Brevard, an avid paddler of the Nantahala despite the fact that he had practically no use of one arm. He died late one day following a trip down his beloved river.

Action is continuous as the river crashes through the top one-third of the run and crosses under the US 19 bridge. To the right, just past the bridge, is the intermediate take-out/put-in and also a nice spot for lunch and for scouting one of the Nantahala's sneakier rapids, Delabar's Rock. The rapid is located just around a bend to the right, 150 yards downstream of the launch area for the intermediate take-out, and consists of several large rocks, usually awash, on river left, followed by a hole. Paddlers allowing the strong current to pry them to the outside of the bend often do not see the rocks until too late. If a boat dumps here there is a fair possibility it will broach on Delabar's Rock in the middle of the river 30 feet downstream.

The river continues along its fast course with little let-up before approaching the largest rapid on the run, Nantahala Falls. Nantahala Falls, which is about 400 yards above Nantahala Outdoor Center, is a Class III, which at higher levels easily becomes Class IV. There is a short, quiet pool above it where one can pull out easily to scout the falls. There is a concrete pad on the right with a well-marked path. The entrance and approach to the falls are rather difficult and can put a lot of water in the boat before one hits the falls. Be sure to empty the boat before attempting this run. The entrance is generally where the novice or low intermediate skilled paddler gets in trouble, only to be finished off in the falls.

The falls consist of two ledges. The top one doesn't extend all the way across the river, and the passage is just on the left end of it. The paddler then must cut hard back to the right to catch the tongue on the lower drop. With higher water the upper ledge can be run straight through on the right, thereby lining you up for the tongue below. This is about three feet off the large boulder on the right.

In the event you swamp or dump in the falls, get control of the craft immediately. Lesser Falls, which is a quarter mile downstream, will only spew out little pieces.

To reach the put-in, go south on US 19 from Wesser and the Nantahala Outdoor Center to the first paved road on the left (Macon County Route 1310) where the launch and parking areas are immediately identifiable. The take-out can be reached by going north on US 19 to a point just above the Nantahala Outdoor Center Restaurant where an easy take-out drive has been graded—courtesy of the center. Please note: The takeout on the other side is primarily for Nantahala Outdoor Center rentals and groups.

There is now a fee to run the Nantahala. In 1998, the fee was $1 per boat per day or $5 per boat for a season pass. Daily passes can be obtained at the NOC store or, less likely, at the Patton Run parking area. Season passes can be obtained by mail from the USFS, 90 Sloan Road, Franklin, NC, 28734. Just include a note that the check is for a season pass. For more information, call (704) 524-6441.

North Fork of the New River

The head of the North Fork of the New River is located north of Ashe County, just over the Tennessee line. It flows northeast in the shadows of The Peak, Three Top Mountain, and Phoenix Mountain on the south before its confluence with the South Fork and the formation of the New River.

It is primarily a stream of shallow ledges with an occasional gravel bar through its upper reaches. Then it flattens out to where it presents a few riffles and a ledge now and then. River access is quite easy with roads following alongside most of the entire distance. This also gives it a pastoral setting through most of the sections.

It may be of interest to note that Ashe County has

almost 110 miles of water that is canoeable throughout most of the year. The North Fork can be paddled from the community of Maxwell (A) all the way to its confluence with the South Fork. Difficulties include a series of gravel bars which drop about 25 feet per mile one and a half miles below Maxwell; some low-water bridges between Creston (B) and the NC 88 bridge west of Clifton; a 12-foot dam just below Clifton; a rapid below the bridge at Crumpler where the river flows hard right and narrows considerably (scouting from the rocks on the left is quite easy); and another low-water bridge farther downstream that can cause problems at higher water levels.

A gauge is located on the northeast piling of the Route 1644 bridge (Rowie McNeil Road) at Sprague Electric Plant. From Maxwell to Creston, four inches below zero is considered the minimum runnable level, with six inches below zero the minimum from Creston to the confluence with the South Fork.

Section: Maxwell to confluence with South Fork

Counties: Ashe

USGS Quads: Baldwin Gap, Warrensville, Jefferson, Grassy Creek

Difficulty: Class I–II

Gradient: 11 feet per mile

Average Width: 20–100 feet

Velocity: Moderate to fast

Rescue Index: Accessible

Hazards: One dam, low-water bridges, low-hanging branches

Scouting: None required

Portages: Portage dam below Clifton and washed-out bridge below NC 16 on left

Scenery: Fair to beautiful

Highlights: Scenery, whitewater, wildlife, history

Gauge: Visual only. Gauge located on northeast piling of Route 1644 bridge.

Runnable Water Level	Minimum	Maximum
Maxwell to Creston	4 inches below bottom of 0	Up to flood stage
Creston to South Fork	6 inches below 0	Up to flood stage

Additional Information: Zaloos Canoes, (800) 535-4027 or (910) 246-3066

North Fork of the New River • North Carolina

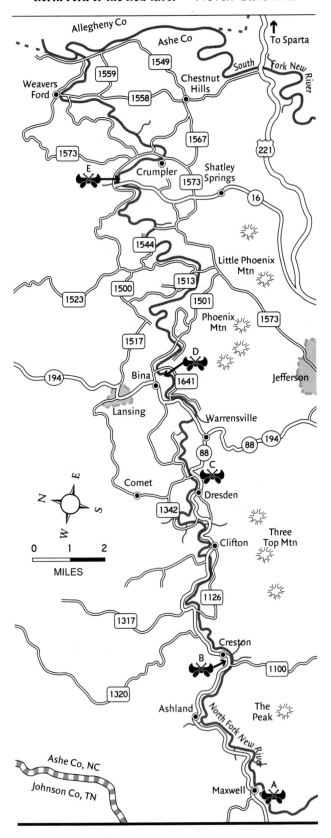

South Fork of the New River

The South Fork of the New River, which begins at the confluence of several small streams southeast of Boone, meanders across the three most northwesterly counties in North Carolina before joining the North Fork and forming the New River just south of the Virginia line. It is primarily an easy-flowing stream over rocky beds, with occasional riffles as it threads its way between mountains on one side and fields on the other. The South Fork is an excellent stream for canoe camping, even though there are low bridges on practically every section that will generally require carrying.

Section: US 421 to Mouth of Wilson, Virginia

Counties: Watauga, Ashe, Alleghany, Grayson (VA)

USGS Quads: Boone, Deep Gap, Todd, Glendale Springs, Jefferson, Laurel Springs, Mouth of Wilson (VA)

Difficulty: Class I–II

Gradient: 7 feet per mile

Average Width: 25–100 feet

Velocity: Moderate to fast

Rescue Index: Accessible

Hazards: Low-water bridges, deadfalls, low-hanging branches

Scouting: None required

Portages: None required

Scenery: Pretty to beautiful

Highlights: Scenery, whitewater, wildlife, history

Gauge: Visual only. Gauge on southwest side of US 221-421 bridge; USGS gauge 200 yards upstream of NC 16/88 near Index

Runnable Water Level	Minimum	Maximum
US 221-421 bridge gauge		
Runs above Todd	5 inches below 0	Up to flood stage
Runs below Todd	5 inches below 0	Up to flood stage
USGS gauge near Index		
Above Watauga Rt 1347	2.50	Up to flood stage
Below Watauga Rt 1347	2.50	Up to flood stage

Additional Information: Zaloos Canoes, (800) 535-4027 or (910) 246-3066

The forks, as well as the New itself, were known as the Teays River on maps showing ancient rivers, and at one time the New River basin was considered the master water system of North America. The New River cuts north and west across Virginia into West Virginia, where it is joined by the Gauley and becomes the Kanawha.

The river, the oldest in the country and second oldest in the world, appeared to be facing its demise when plans for a giant hydroelectric plant were firming up in the early 1970s. Two dams were planned, which would have flooded some 42,000 acres, mostly in North Carolina. After a long, hard battle that gathered national attention, the river was saved when President Gerald Ford signed a bill on September 1, 1976, establishing a 26.5-mile section as a National Wild and Scenic River. This section

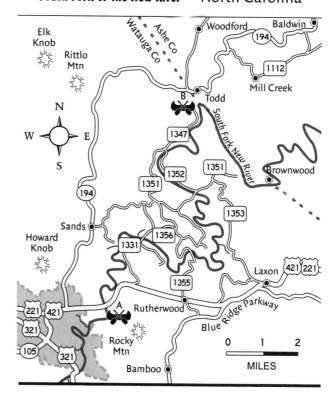

South Fork of the New River • North Carolina

South Fork of the New River • North Carolina

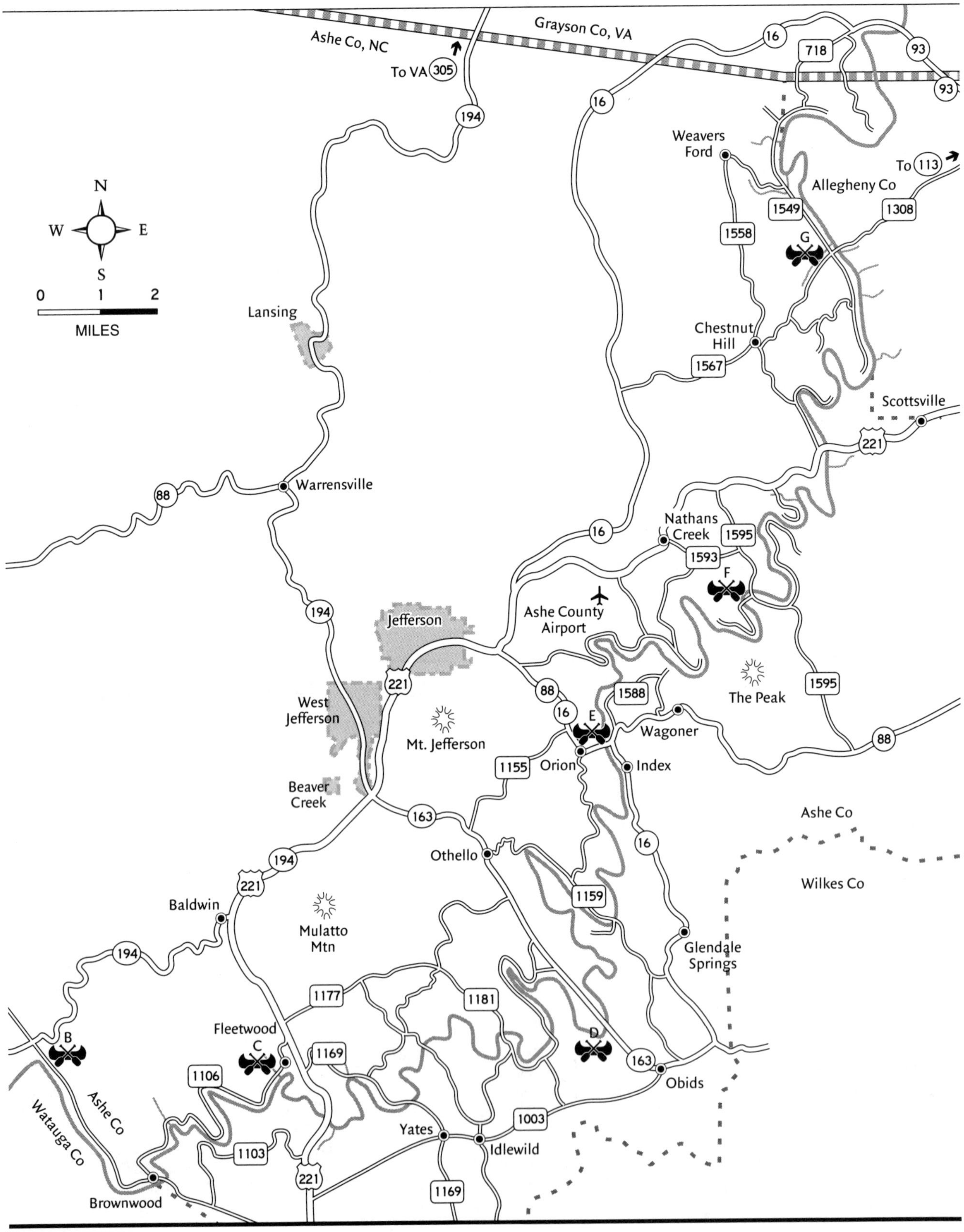

Ashe Co, NC
Grayson Co, VA
To VA (305)
16
718
93
93
194
Weavers Ford
To (113)
Allegheny Co
1549
1558
1308
G
Lansing
Chestnut Hill
1567
Scottsville
221
88
Warrensville
16
Nathans Creek
1595
1593
F
194
Ashe County Airport
Jefferson
1595
221
88
16
The Peak
West Jefferson
Mt. Jefferson
1588
1155
E
Wagoner
Index
88
Orion
Beaver Creek
163
Ashe Co
194
Othello
Wilkes Co
221
Baldwin
1159
16
194
Mulatto Mtn
Glendale Springs
1177
1181
Fleetwood
D
B
C
163
1106
1169
Obids
1103
1003
Ashe Co
Watauga Co
Yates
1169
Brownwood
221
1169
Idlewild

N
W   E
S
0   1   2
MILES

consists of 22 miles of the South Fork plus the first 4.5 miles of the main stem. Naturally this has brought an influx of paddlers to the river, especially on the Wild and Scenic section, which quite often has resulted in property damage and hard feelings on the part of residents. Please keep this in mind when floating here.

Basically Class I with some mild Class II rapids, the South Fork can be run all year except during periods of extreme dryness in the upper sections (above Todd). A USGS gauge is located on the right bank 200 yards upstream of NC 16-88 at the community of Index. Minimum for solo paddling is 2.50 from the US 22-421 bridge to Watauga Route 1347 and 2.40–2.30 down to the confluence with the North Fork. Another gauge can be found at the put-in on the southwest side of the US 221-421 bridge. Minimum for solo paddling is five inches below zero above Todd and six inches below zero for the lower sections.

There are no difficulties other than low-water bridges, low-hanging branches, shallow gravel bars at lower water levels, and some occasional shoals. One series of shoals begins about two miles below the NC 163 bridge and continues to the entrance to the Methodist campground along the right bank. The camp does have an area for family camping, which the paddler passes along the river. It is available for a reasonable fee during the spring and summer. Another series of shoals above the confluence with the North Fork runs for over 200 yards. After entering the New there is still another series of shoals just above the mouth of Big Wilson Creek.

New River

The New River begins with the confluence of the North and South Forks just south of Virginia on the border between Ashe and Alleghany counties. At this point it is already a fairly wide river although still fairly shallow. From the mouth of Big Wilson Creek to Stuart Dam the New is mostly flat; we are therefore not discussing these two and a half miles.

The river flows through forested rolling hills and pastoral lands and generally is a very scenic stream. The favored whitewater run on the Virginia–North Carolina stretch of the New is from Stuart Dam (A) in Grayson County, Virginia, downstream eleven miles to the US 221-21 bridge (B). There is no gauge, but the river can be run all year. During periods of high water, however, extra caution should be taken because the width of the New makes rescue difficult.

The run is generally Class I–II with one Class III. Scenery is pleasant and water quality is good. One mile downstream from the Grayson County 601 bridge in the community of Cox Chapel, as the river bends to the right, there are two rapids. The first, a long Class II, should be scouted from the left in higher water. The second, a couple of hundred yards beyond the first, is a Class III where most of the water flows hard left by a large boulder on the bank. Watch for the drop just beyond the boulder. Attempt to scout on the right. At higher water levels this can be run in the center.

Below the US 221-21 bridge and continuing on to the US 58-221 bridge (C) west of Galax, Virginia, the New is primarily flat with occasional riffles and a few shoals. This is a very scenic section and makes for an excellent overnight run.

Section: Below Stuart Dam to US 58-221 bridge

Counties: Grayson (VA), Alleghany (NC)

USGS Quads: Mouth of Wilson (VA), Sparta West and Sparta East (NC-VA), Briarpatch Mountain (VA), Galax (VA)

Difficulty: Class I–II (III)

Gradient: 6 feet per mile

Average Width: 150–400 feet

Velocity: Moderate to fast

Rescue Index: Accessible to accessible but difficult

Hazards: Difficult rapids, dam, low-water bridges

Scouting: Scout two rapids below Cox Chapel (601 bridge), first left, second right

Portages: If running from Mouth of Wilson, portage Stuart Dam left

Scenery: Pretty to beautiful

Highlights: Scenery, whitewater, wildlife

Gauge: Visual only

Runnable Water Level   Minimum   Maximum

                                    None   Up to flood stage

Additional Information: Zaloos Canoes, (800) 535-4027 or (910) 246-3066

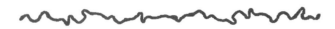

New River • North Carolina and Virginia

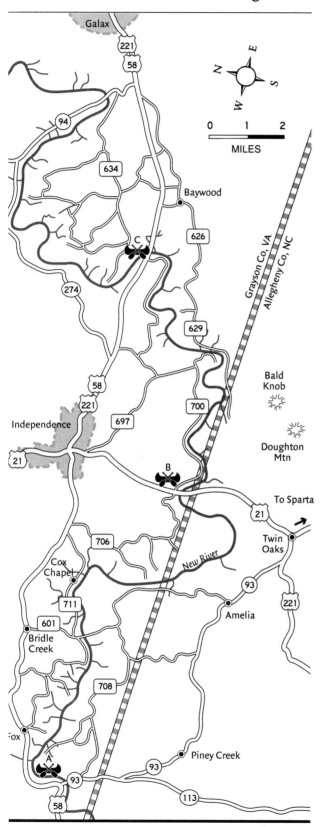

Raven Fork River

Forming in northeastern Swain County, the Raven Fork comes off Breakneck Ridge at what quite often seems to be just that speed. It flows through the Cherokee Indian Reservation to a point just above the town of Cherokee, where it joins the Oconaluftee River. Running through boulder fields and rock gardens the Raven Fork presents one of the most delightful trips the paddler can find anywhere.

The Cherokee have designated the river as "enterprise waters" (see the Oconaluftee), thereby closing the main stretch to paddling except on Wednesdays. The short stretch running from the Great Smoky Mountains National Park boundary just above Crack-in-the-Rock down to the confluence with the Oconaluftee River is runnable on Tuesdays only, as is the Oconaluftee. Trout season on the reservation is open year-round except from the first of March through the last Friday in March.

Section: Confluence with Straight Fork to Job Corps Center
Counties: Swain
USGS Quads: Bunches Bald, Smokemont
Difficulty: Class II–III
Gradient: 51 feet per mile (one mile at 60 feet, 0.5 mile at 75 feet)
Average Width: 15–60 feet
Velocity: Fast
Rescue Index: Accessible
Hazards: Difficult rapids
Scouting: Scout rapids in gorge from right bank
Portages: None required
Scenery: Pretty to beautiful
Highlights: Scenery, whitewater
Gauge: TVA, (800) 238-2264
Runnable Water Level   Minimum   Maximum
                              1.60 feet (700 cfs) 2.5 feet (1000 cfs)
Months runnable: January through June and after rains
Additional Information: None

The run begins at the confluence with the Straight Fork (A) and runs for eight challenging miles to the bridge at the Job Corps Center (B). There is a USGS gauge at Sherries Cove Creek bridge. The minimum for solo is 1.50, while the maximum for a safe trip is 2.50. At a level of 1.50 it is better to cut the trip short and put in at the confluence with Bunches Creek.

Coming at you with incredible speed, the Raven Fork churns down a slalom course of rocks and boulders. A rapid with a large hydraulic just below the put-in may encourage one to start below it (it makes for a rather unpleasant trip to take two strokes and find oneself out of the boat). The river drops at a rate of 75 feet per mile through the first half mile. Fortunately, this stretch, as

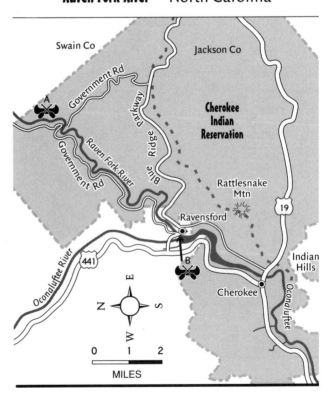

Raven Fork River • North Carolina

well as much of the rest of the trip, can be scouted from the road (highly recommended).

There are numerous Class II rapids before reaching the first Class III, which cannot be seen completely from the road. This rapid is in the bend of the river behind Smith Memorial Pentecostal Holiness Church. At higher water levels it requires a great deal of difficult maneuvering to prevent swamping an open canoe. After passing Sherries Cove Creek bridge the river enters a 900-foot-deep gorge and makes a large bend around River Valley Camp, a private campground. There are three Class IIIs in the gorge, all of which should be scouted, and the gradient increases to over 60 feet per mile. The approach to the first two rapids will vary somewhat with the water level, but both can be scouted from the right. The third, Crack-in-the-Rock, can be scouted on the left and run on the left. It is located just beyond the campground and just above the national park boundary sign. There is fairly heavy water above the rapid so care should be taken in the approach.

To reach the put-in, take the Government Road east of the US 441 bridge over the Oconaluftee in Cherokee for approximately 10 miles. To find the take-out, turn west on the first paved road south of the Government Road bridge crossing the Raven Fork (this road goes to the Job Corps Center).

Oconaluftee River

The Oconaluftee heads up in northern Swain County between Indian Gap (elevation 5,286 feet) and Newfound Gap (elevation 5,048 feet) and generally flows beside US 441 through the Great Smoky Mountains National Park, until its confluence with the Tuckaseigee River east of Bryson City. The run above Cherokee goes through many rock gardens in crystal-clear water. Below Cherokee the water quality diminishes considerably due to sewage being dumped in. A distinct odor may be noticeable below the US 441 bridge, but it doesn't continue for long.

The river enters the Cherokee Indian Reservation a half mile below its confluence with the Raven Fork River, and from this point to the take-out is again designated as "enterprise waters." This stretch can be paddled only on Tuesdays during trout season, when the river is being stocked (trout season is year-round except from first of March through the last Friday of March).

The approximately four-and-a-half-mile stretch above the reservation boundary can be paddled at any time. In order to do so one should check in at the ranger station at park headquarters, located at Pioneer Structures on US 441 north of Cherokee, to inform them of plans to canoe the river. This might save one from being "pulled" off the river by park rangers. This actually happened to Ed Gertler several years ago. It could not only prove embarrassing but could also lead to a rather long hike.

A gauge located on the south bank 200 feet upstream from the Route 1359 bridge below Birdtown should be checked before putting in. Minimum for solo run is 1.70. The river can be run at 1.32 from Ravensford Bridge (above Pioneer Structures), which cuts about four miles

Section: Smokemont Campground to Birdtown
County: Swain
USGS Quads: Smokemont, Whittier
Difficulty: Class II–III
Gradient: 27 feet per mile
Average Width: 25–80 feet
Velocity: Fast
Rescue Index: Accessible
Hazards: Difficult rapids
Scouting: None required
Portages: None required
Scenery: Unattractive to beautiful
Highlights: Scenery, whitewater
Gauge: TVA, (800) 238-2264

Runnable Water Level	Minimum	Maximum
Smokemont to Raven Fork	1.70 (400 cfs)	Up to flood stage
Raven Fork to Birdtown	(200 cfs)	Up to flood stage

Additional Information: None

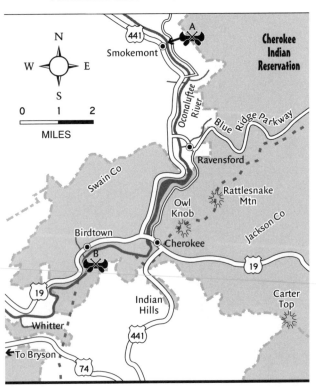

Oconaluftee River • North Carolina

off the total trip. A gauge directly across on the opposite bank (along US 19) will read approximately .05 lower than the opposite gauge, so estimate accordingly.

The most challenging whitewater is in the upper third. Tight runs over ledges and through gravel bars that require fast thinking and faster maneuvering characterize the Oconaluftee, with the first five miles being the toughest part of this Class II–III run. After entering Cherokee, you'll see the remains of an old washed-out dam along US 441. Iron rods protrude from some of the rocks, and it is best to run on the far right directly behind the trailer. This is located about 80 yards above the Cherokee Information Station and picnic area. Other difficulties include low branches and an occasional fallen tree.

For anyone wishing to extend the trip into the Tucka-seigee or on to Bryson City, there is a 30-foot dam three miles below Birdtown. It can be portaged on the right.

To reach the put-in, take US 441 north of Cherokee to the entrance to Smokemont Campground; cross the bridge. To reach the take-out, take US 19 west of Cherokee to Birdtown; cross the Route 1359 bridge (at the Cherokee Recreation Park Campground sign) to the gauge.

Wilson Creek

Tumbling down Calloway Peak off the eastern side of Grandfather Mountain, Wilson Creek starts as a tiny tributary in eastern Avery County. Shortly after crossing into Caldwell County, Wilson Creek and Lost Cove Creek join together at Edgemont and Mortimer. There Wilson Creek doubles its volume. Settled in the 1700s, the communities of Edgemont and Mortimer were supported by the lumber and textile industries. The area was heavily logged and a narrow-gauge railroad was built to haul the wood. Evidence of the old railroad bed is present along the creek. In 1940 the textile plant and logging operation were wiped out by floods. Today the ruins of the old mill can be seen on the way to the put-in for the upper section. Below Mortimer the stream courses through a valley for several miles and contains pleasant Class II water before abruptly entering the two-and-a-half-mile gorge. Running nearly its entire length within Pisgah National Forest, the creek is normally clear enough to allow visibility up to 12 feet.

Due to its ease of access, beauty, and demanding whitewater, Wilson Creek Gorge has long been one of the most popular difficult water runs in the southeast. The paddling season here normally runs from late October to June. Wilson is a classic drop-and-pool creek interspersed with several tight boulder gardens. There are many blind drops that will require scouting for those unfamiliar with this stretch. First run by Bob Benner, Tony Comer, and others back in 1970, the trip was done in 15- and 17-foot

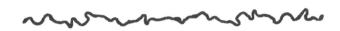

Section: 400 yards upstream of Pisgah National Forest boundary sign to Brown Mountain Beach

County: Caldwell

USGS Quads: Chestnut Mountain, Collettsville

Difficulty: Class IV

Gradient: 92 feet per mile (1.5 miles at 110+ feet)

Average Width: 10–50 feet

Velocity: Moderate to fast

Rescue Index: Accessible but difficult

Hazards: Strainers, pinning spots, numerous hydraulics

Scouting: Ten Foot Falls, Boatbuster, Triple Drop, Razorback, numerous blind drops

Portages: None required

Scenery: Excellent

Highlights: Scenery, geology, whitewater

Gauge: Visual only. Located on the upstream side of the river left pylon of the Route 1337 (Adako Road) bridge.

Runnable Water Level	Minimum	Maximum
	4 inches below 0	6 inches above 0

Additional Information: Brown Mountain Beach Campground, (828) 758-4257

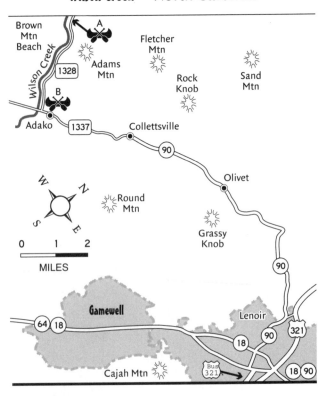

Wilson Creek • North Carolina

Brown Mtn Beach
Fletcher Mtn
Adams Mtn
Rock Knob
Sand Mtn
1328
Wilson Creek
Adako
1337
Collettsville
90
Olivet
Round Mtn
Grassy Knob
0 1 2
MILES
90
Gamewell
Lenoir
64 18
18
90
321
Cajah Mtn
Bus 321
18 90

open boats back when canoes were truly open (i.e., no flotation). The trips, under these circumstances, took close to a full day. Today, with favorable water levels, experts in decked boats have cruised the gorge in less than 25 minutes.

There are five major rapids in the gorge. At minimal levels (up to zero) these drops are a forgiving Class IV; at levels of zero to one foot they progressively increase to hard Class V. Above one foot the drops are quite intimidating with sketchier clean lines and big keeper hydraulics that reel unwilling boaters back in for an extended chat. Everything in the gorge has been run at slightly over one and a half feet. Most of the run has been done up to three feet, but is not recommended at that level. The gauge is located on the upstream side of the river left pylon of the Route 1337 (Adako Road) bridge.

The dirt road (Route 1328) that parallels the gorge makes for ease of scouting, evacuation, and aborted trips, all positive items for paddlers. Due to this accessibility, the area is very popular for people with other interests. Indeed, during warmer months the creek can be quite crowded with tubers, swimmers, sunbathers, and those who like to party. Car break-ins are not unknown to this area and in the past five years paddlers have not been immune. Do not leave valuables at the put-in but rather in vehicles at the less secluded take-out.

Below the put-in, located two and a half miles above Brown Mountain Beach, you'll find several ledges and two tricky boulder mazes prior to the entrance to Ten Foot Falls, the first major rapid. If you have a good run through the entrance rapid, chances are you will exit the falls in good shape. Enter the approach far right and maintain a slight left angle above the falls. A stout diagonal above will surf you to the left. Enter the falls center or left of center with speed. Entry on the right will either plaster you on the slab midway down, surf you in the hole at the bottom, or both.

Below Ten Foot Falls is another interesting rock garden followed by two ledges before the entry to Boatbuster and Thunderhole. The river bends sharply to the left above these drops—that's your cue to get out and scout. Boatbuster is a six-foot ramp that drops into barely buried, sharp boulder calvings. This should be run by angling right to left across the drop so as not to offer your bow wholly unprotected to this nastiness. If you feel unsure here, walk. This is the most potentially lethal rapid on the river, so do not turn over at this point.

Immediately 20 yards) downstream is Thunderhole, a five-foot-wide slot with the whole river pouring down a four-foot drop. Enter left and brace.

Downstream from Thunderhole are several ledges and easy rapids for 0.4 mile before reaching Triple Drop. As seen from above, Triple Drop is a major boulder chokedown with the river disappearing around the far left side. You'll see a series of three drops in succession (each about three feet); run this far left along the rock wall. Be aware of two potential problems: the first drop will invariably throw you far left and the last drop has a sticky hole with a large boulder immediately downstream. This is no place for a swim.

Directly below Triple Drop is another boulder clog with a runnable slot on the far right at water levels above zero. Angle left to avoid bow pinning. Two hundred yards downstream beware of a five-foot ledge with a large undercut boulder on the left. Stay as far right as the water allows here. This drop can be sneaked on the far left at higher water. Below this point the river narrows and runs through some nice Class III and culminates in a large eddy overlooking Razorback. This nine-foot slide can be run far right or far left at levels above zero. At lower levels it's hammer city. Angle hard left and boof if running the right side. The left side does not look runnable but can be accomplished by staying in the trough and clearing the tight slot between the large boulder and the rock forming the roostertail.

Immediately downstream of Razorback is Huntley's Retreat (a.k.a. **S** turn). Without giving away too much, let us say that Dennis Huntley had an interesting run/climb with the creek running three feet. Luckily (since there was snow and ice on the 50-foot sheer "retreat"), Dennis is also an accomplished climber. Huntley's Retreat is a series of ledges in close succession and is run through the only obvious route. Below this rapid is a large pool that denotes the end of the hard stuff, with only two drops of consequence for the next 0.8 mile.

In the past, boaters have been allowed to park across from the Brown Mountain Beach Store and carry boats through the property to reach their cars. This is no longer the case. The owners now charge $2 to either park on or walk across the property. If this is unappetizing to you, take out 0.75 mile upstream, at the first pull-off past the store. The store is open from April 1 to December 1 and can be called at (828) 758-4257 to get a rough idea of the water level.

SOUTH CAROLINA

Chauga River

The Chauga River is a tributary of the Savannah River system. It lies in Oconee County and is mostly within the Sumter National Forest. The Chauga has been described as a miniature version of the Chattooga or the Chattooga alternative. However, these descriptions fail to do it justice. The Chauga can speak for itself.

Although slack areas do appear on the Chauga, the lasting impression is one of plunging in frenzy. The gradient averages 60–80 feet per mile through several small gorges. Numerous tributary creeks cascade periodically into the Chauga from both sides. This is a land of steep, rocky banks, hanging ferns, and rushing water. The scenery is nothing short of splendid.

The Chauga can be divided into three sections for descriptive purposes. The first section is from Blackwell bridge (A), just east of Whetstone, to Cassidy bridge (B),

Section: Blackwell bridge to Cassidy bridge
County: Oconee
USGS Quads: Whetstone, Holly Springs
Difficulty: Class II–IV
Gradient: 51.8 feet per mile
Average Width: 20–35 feet
Velocity: Fast
Rescue Index: Remote
Hazards: Strainers, deadfalls, difficult rapids, undercut rocks, keeper hydraulics, waterfalls
Scouting: At all major rapids
Portages: As needed
Scenery: Exceptionally beautiful
Highlights: Scenery, wildlife, whitewater
Gauge: Visual only at Cassidy bridge

Runnable Water Levels	Minimum	Maximum
	3 inches above 0	2.5 feet

Additional Information: Chattooga Whitewater Shop, (864) 647-9083; Nantahala Outdoor Center, (864) 647-9014; Wildwater, Ltd., (864) 647-9587

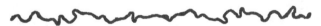

east of Long Creek. Blackwell bridge is on South Carolina secondary road 193 (Whetstone Road). Cassidy bridge is on Cassidy Bridge Road (SC 290). The second section ends at Cobbs bridge (C). The third section encompasses the river from Cobbs bridge to US 123 (H) just north of the Chauga's entry into Hartwell Reservoir.

With favorable high-water conditions (at least 1.7 on the US 76 Chattooga gauge or at least three inches above zero at the gauge painted on the Cassidy bridge pillar), boaters may launch at Blackwell bridge. Be careful not to park on private property near the bridge without asking for permission. A four-wheel-drive dirt road on the western side of the stream provides alternate launch sites. A 45-foot waterfall is encountered within the first half mile. Land and portage on the right bank. You'll find an unusual 20-foot column of rock at the base of the falls. Just below is a 10-foot sliding drop that can sometimes be run. The river drops another 70 feet in the next mile and has some technical Class II and III shoals. Things quiet down a little, but expect plenty of Class II rapids, some downed trees, and one more Class III rapid a little past midrun.

The second section, from Cassidy bridge to Cobbs bridge, known as the Chauga Gorge, is very difficult and should be attempted only by very advanced and expert paddlers. For those who have mastered Section IV of the Chattooga River, this run is a challenge. Frequent scouting, seeing throw ropes, and several portages consume a lot of extra time, so get to the river early and don't plan on running one of the other sections of the Chauga on the same day. A water level of three on the Cassidy bridge gauge is the minimum necessary; one foot is the maximum for a first-time run. Above that, expect heavy and dangerous water. The first mile is in a little valley with only gentle rapids. Recent logging in this area has put a great deal of debris in the stream; watch for possible strainers during and after high water flows. The valley ends abruptly with a waterfall that must be portaged on the left.

Chauga River • South Carolina

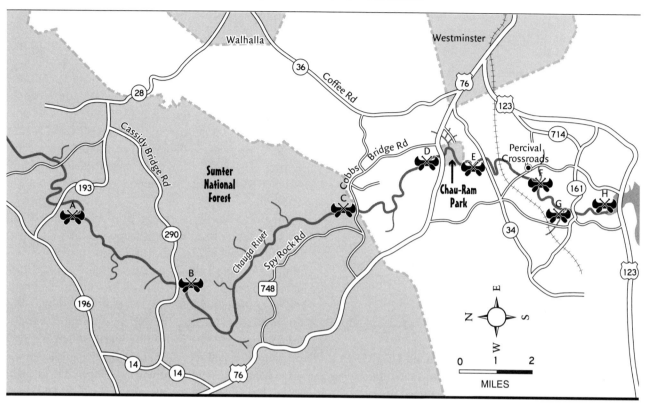

Section: Cassidy bridge to Cobbs bridge
County: Oconee
USGS Quads: Whetstone, Holly Springs
Difficulty: Class III–V
Gradient: 51.8 feet per mile
Average Width: 20–35 feet
Velocity: Fast
Rescue Index: Accessible but difficult to remote
Hazards: Strainers, deadfalls, difficult rapids, undercut rocks, keeper hydraulics, waterfalls
Scouting: At all major rapids
Portages: Falls below Cassidy bridge and falls two miles above Cobbs bridge; elsewhere as needed
Scenery: Spectacular
Highlights: Scenery, wildlife, whitewater
Gauge: Visual only

Runnable Water Level	Minimum	Maximum
	3 inches above 0	1 foot above 0

Additional Information: Chattooga Whitewater Shop, (864) 647-9083; Nantahala Outdoor Center, (864) 647-9014; Wildwater, Ltd., (864) 647-9587

Within the next mile another waterfall is encountered with a strong Class II rapid just above. Get to the left bank promptly to scout or portage. This drop can be run in favorable conditions. At the Spider Valley Creek junction the river turns east and starts dropping in earnest, with the gradient initially exceeding 180 feet per mile. A slanting waterfall that many will choose to portage is followed by almost continuous Class III and IV rapids for the next two miles. Most drops are quite technical and recovery pools are short. Careful scouting along with the use of safety boats and ropes is especially important because you may be the only party on the river and evacuation from the gorge is very difficult.

After a couple of miles the gradient decreases, but several more Class III rapids remain, and about two miles above Cobbs bridge is a sheer fall that must be portaged on the right. Riley Moore Fall has been run on the left but it is not advisable due to the high possibility of ankle damage in kayaks. The flow is relatively placid from the falls to Cobbs bridge. An alternate take-out is off Spy Rock US Forest Service Road 748. USFS Road 748H is the access road.

The most popular run on the lower Chauga is from

Section: Cobbs bridge to US 123

Counties: Oconee

USGS Quads: Holly Springs

Difficulty: Class I–III

Gradient: 14.2 feet per mile

Average Width: 40–50 feet

Velocity: Moderate to fast

Rescue Index: Accessible but difficult

Hazards: Strainers, deadfalls, difficult rapids, undercut rocks

Scouting: At major rapids

Portages: As needed

Scenery: Exceptional

Highlights: Scenery, wildlife, whitewater

Gauge: Visual only

Runnable Water Levels	Minimum	Maximum
	0.3 feet	2.5 feet

Additional Information: Chattooga Whitewater Shop, (864) 647-9083; Nantahala Outdoor Center, (864) 647-9014; Wildwater, Ltd., (864) 647-9587

Cobbs bridge to Horseshoe Bend bridge on US 123. This section is really a piedmont rather than a mountain river, with long stretches of flatwater interrupted occasionally by granite shoals. The high, sandy banks and loblolly pines are also characteristic of the piedmont. Though there are only seven significant rapids, they offer great interest and variety, and portaging back upstream for reruns is unusually easy. This makes the lower Chauga an excellent training ground for intermediates. The most convenient gauge is on the Chattooga at US 76, right on the way for most Georgia paddlers. A reading of 1.8 is the minimum for a decent run, 2.5 is optimum, and, above that, some of the rapids get mean and dangerous. There are private homes at the put-in and take-out, so be extra considerate.

The Class II rapid below Cobbs bridge is run down the right side. Just downriver is a big, slanting ledge that can be scouted from the left bank. At about three and a half miles, cables across the river precede a really interesting Class II rapid that you can scout from a center landing. The right eddy turn after the left-side chute will nearly dislocate your shoulder. This is a good spot for lunch.

Soon after the US 76 bridge is a complex shoal that can be scouted from the left bank. A short pool leads to Pumphouse, a Class III rapid named for the water-pumping facility just below. Land carefully on the rocks just left of center to scout. Chau-Ram County Park is just below on the left, where you can stop to see the falls on Ramsey Creek. This is a convenient take-out if you don't mind missing the last two rapids. Just downstream, get to the right bank and scout the slanting, five-foot ledge with the waterspout. The hole there gets dangerous in higher water. The last rapid is just around the bend and can be scouted from the left. The water pours over a V-shaped slot and past an undercut rock to some smaller drops. The two remaining miles are mostly flat, and deadfalls are the only hazard. Past Horseshoe Bend bridge, there is little gradient, and the river soon reaches the backwaters of Hartwell Reservoir.

TENNESSEE

Doe River

A paddle trip through the infamous Doe River Gorge in Carter County is reminiscent of Jules Verne's Voyage to the Center of the Earth. One moment you are running your shuttle through bustling Elizabethton and fighting traffic up four-lane US 19E on Roan Mountain, and minutes later, on the water, you and your boat have been swallowed up by a mountain wilderness so complete that you can scarcely believe you are still in Tennessee. Traversing a pristine area, only an antique, narrow-gauge railroad unobtrusively accompanies the paddler through the bowels of the hulking gorge. Scenery on the Doe is extremely spectacular with the steep rock and evergreen facade of Fork Mountain on the west and Cedar Moun-

tain on the east scrambling skyward almost 1,100 feet from the water's edge. Indeed, it appears from the shady depths of the gorge that only this narrow ribbon of dancing water keeps the giant mountains apart.

Beginning high on Roan Mountain near the North Carolina state line, the Doe River rumbles through the town of Roan Mountain and along US 19E before disappearing into the gorge. Emerging from the gorge south of Hampton, the stream continues north through Elizabethton before reaching its mouth at the Watauga.

The Doe is runnable from around the town of Roan Mountain to its mouth. Between Roan Mountain (A) and Crabtree (B) the stream is narrow and rocky but fairly straightforward with a Class II difficulty level. Scenery

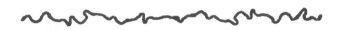

Section: Roan Mountain to Hampton

County: Carter

USGS Quads: White Rocks Mountain, Iron Mountain Gap, Elizabethton

Difficulty: Class II–III (IV); gorge, Class IV–VI

Gradient: 90 feet per mile; (gorge), 115 feet per mile

Average Width: 25–40 feet

Velocity: Fast

Rescue Index: accessible; gorge, remote

Hazards: Strainers, flash flooding, undercut rocks, keeper hydraulics, difficult rapids

Scouting: Frequent and mandatory

Portages: Unrunnable boulder clogs as described in gorge section

Scenery: beautiful in spots to spectacular in the gorge

Highlights: Scenery, wildlife, whitewater, local culture and industry, geology

Gauge: TVA, (423) 632-2264; (800) 238-2264

Runnable Water Levels	Minimum	Maximum
	240 cfs	600 cfs
gorge	300 cfs	600 cfs

Additional Information: USDA Forest Service, Watauga District, (423) 542-2942

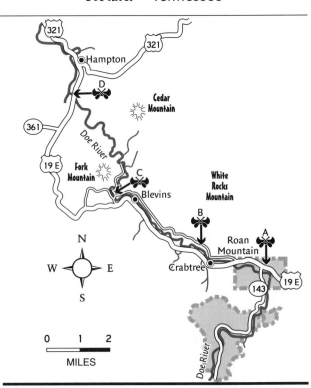

Doe River • Tennessee

here is pleasant with a good cross-sectional view of Tennessee mountain culture. Below Crabtree the Doe becomes challenging, with the gradient reaching 60 feet per mile and two Class III (IV) rapids a half mile downstream of the confluence with Roaring Creek. Both of these rapids are very technical, congested, and have a tendency to catch deadfalls. Under no circumstances should they be run without scouting.

At the tiny town of Blevins (C) the parallel highway (US 19E) cuts sharply west while the Doe continues down and out of sight into the gorge. Civilization follows the stream for a couple of miles with a few small farms at streamside. Several put-ins are available for the gorge run because the road running out of Blevins crosses the Doe in three places.

The gorge section is rated Class III–IV. Narrow, boulder-clogged, and congested with limited visibility (because of rocks in the stream and occlusion of direct sunlight by surrounding mountains), the river's volume accelerates through tight passages and over drops of up to seven feet. Generally, the best advice is to give yourself plenty of time to make the run and be prepared to do a lot of scouting. If nobody in your group is familiar with the river, spend a day scouting from the road and the railroad tracks. Particular spots to watch out for include a sharp turning four-foot drop to the left just above the first railroad bridge, known as Body Snatcher (Class III–IV). You'll find a boulder garden on a river curve to the right approximately one mile downstream from the first railroad bridge where the flow is diverted around and under the obstructing rocks to the extent that no navigable channel remains. Carry on the left. Next comes Tennessee's version of Seven-Foot Falls (at the downstream end of the obstructed channel). Carry left or run right. Man-made rock walls constructed to prevent the river from eroding the base of the railroad tracks are landmarks of the next two danger spots. At the first rock wall is a Class IV series of diagonal drops with some particularly capricious converging currents. At the second wall the flow splits with the main current crunching through a horrendous and unrunnable Class VI rapid on the left. The right, which unfortunately is also unrunnable, consists of a boulder maze that can (with difficulty) be carried or lined through.

From here to the take-out at Hampton (D) you'll run into at least three additional rapids that require scouting and at least that many more where boulders and curves in the river inhibit the paddler's downstream view. The latter are not rated above Class III, but they should be scouted anyway to ensure that the passage is clear of deadfalls or other obstructions. Though the entire gorge run is only six miles or less in length (depending on where you put in), it is incredibly exhausting or depleting and requires, on average, an hour

Section: Hampton to Watauga River

County: Carter

USGS Quads: White Rocks Mountain, Iron Mountain Gap, Elizabethton

Difficulty: Class II (III)

Gradient: 30 feet per mile

Average Width: 25–40 feet

Velocity: Fast

Rescue Index: Accessible but difficult

Hazards: Ledges north of US 19E bridge

Scouting: Scout ledges north of US 19E bridge

Portages: None required

Scenery: Beautiful in spots

Highlights: Scenery, wildlife, whitewater, local culture and industry, geology

Gauge: TVA, (423) 632-2264; (800) 238-2264

Runnable Water Levels	Minimum	Maximum
	300 cfs	NA

Additional Information: USDA Forest Service, Watauga District, (423) 542-2942

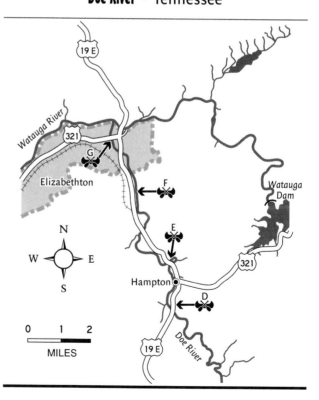

Doe River • Tennessee

and fifteen minutes for a group of four advanced, decked boaters to run each mile. Expressed differently, do not be lulled by the brevity of the run; the Doe Gorge is not the run to catch quickly on Sunday morning before you drive home.

From the US 19E bridge south of Hampton to its mouth at the Watauga in downtown Elizabethton (G), the Doe River widens slightly and calms down a lot. Whitewater is still continuous but primarily Class II in difficulty with one solid Class III area where the river makes a tight loop beneath rock cliffs after passing under the first US 19E bridge north of Hampton. Emerging from the loop, the Doe passes under US 19E again before running over a wide, technical succession of ledges that are somewhat difficult to scout from the bank. At moderate to lower water levels there is usually a route to the right of the center. However, the nature of the rapid is such that perhaps the best approach is to scout from the water by ferrying from eddy to eddy at the top of the rapid. Scenery on this section is not as inspiring because of the population explosion along the stream, but the stretch between North Hampton and Valley Forge is quite beautiful.

The Doe is primarily a wet-weather stream, but it can be run from December to late April in many years. Oddly enough, some of the upper sections (Roan Mountain to Crabtree) can be run into midsummer in years of average rainfall. Hazards to navigation other than rapids and deadfalls mentioned above include a dam in Elizabethton 300 yards downstream from the covered bridge. Access to the river is readily available and good (except, of course, in the gorge).

Tellico River

Upper Tellico River

The upper Tellico River, which originates in the Unicoi Mountains of eastern Monroe County, bears little resemblance to the slow pastoral stream it becomes after it leaves the gorge. The upper Tellico is a raging whitewater river with many Class II, III, and IV rapids. The river is also located in the scenic Cherokee National Forest in and among the same mountain chain that contains the Great Smoky Mountains National Park, farther north. The Tellico River, a trout stream, is noted for its clear woodland drainage with only the indigenous Tellico hogs and bears to muddy the flow (along with an occasional flatlander who might dislodge a riverbed rock or two on his careening trip downstream).

Generally the water level on the upper Tellico is too low to float, but in the winter or early spring this free-flowing little gem jumps up in cfs and eager boaters follow the flow down the 100-foot-per-mile rapids.

Section: Trout Hatchery to bridge at Ranger Station Road
County: Monroe
USGS Quad: Bald River Falls
Difficulty: Class II-IV (V)
Gradient: 71 feet per mile (A–B); 120 feet per mile (B-C); 60 feet per mile (C–D)
Average Width: 30 feet
Velocity: Fast
Rescue Index: Accessible
Hazards: Undercut rocks, difficult rapids, waterfalls
Scouting: At major rapids
Portages: Ledges and fails below North River confluence
Scenery: Beautiful
Highlights: Scenery, whitewater
Gauge: River Flow Rate, (900) 288-8732

Runnable Water Levels	Minimum	Maximum
	200 cfs	1,200 cfs

Months runnable: January through mid-April
Additional Information: TVA, (423) 632-2264; (800) 238-2264

Canoeists look for 250 cfs on TVA's Tellico gauge as optimum for an upper Tellico run. One hundred to 150 cfs is considered low, and, above 500 cfs, good boaters like to take nature hikes to erase the ominous-looking, Class V traps from their minds. A road follows the stream and nerve-shattering scouting is possible all the way to the put-in.

The upper Tellico is somewhat arbitrarily divided into two parts with the bridge below Bald River Falls (C) marking the dividing point. At 350 cfs on the Tellico gauge, the floatable upstream portion, known by the unimaginative name of "Upper, Upper Tellico," begins at the trout hatchery (A) operated by the Tennessee Wildlife Resources Agency. Here up to 140,000 rainbow trout are

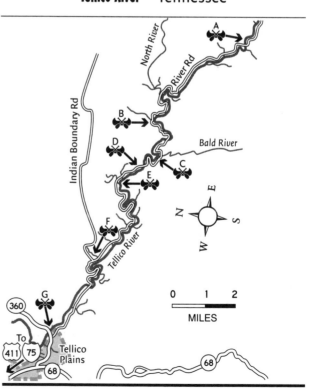

Tellico River • Tennessee

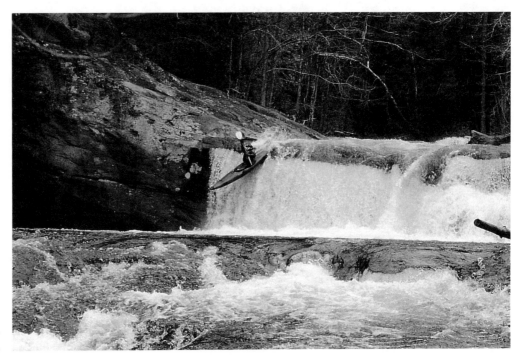

Baby Falls on the Tellico.
Photo by Mayo Gravatt.

penned, fed, and grown to keeper size each year. You may look but not touch.

Action on the river starts quickly with a pair of ledges three feet in height (Class III). For the next 2.5 miles the river presents numerous Class II chutes and a few rock gardens requiring good water-reading skills and a strong pry stroke. Less than a mile below the private Green Cove Campground, visible from the river, there is a four-foot ledge followed by another series of four-foot ledges

Section: Bridge at Ranger Station Road to Tellico Plains
County: Monroe
USGS Quad: Bald River Falls
Difficulty: Class I–II
Gradient: 14 feet per mile
Average Width: 30 feet
Velocity: Moderate to Fast
Rescue Index: Accessible
Hazards: Undercut rocks, difficult rapids
Scouting: At major rapids
Portages: None required
Scenery: Beautiful
Highlights: Scenery, whitewater
Gauge: River Flow Rate, (615) 253-7951 or (615) 253-2520

Runnable Water Level	Minimum	Maximum
	200 cfs	Up to flood
stage		

after 400 yards. All are runnable but scouting is advised. After these ledges the river flows past Panther Branch Picnic Area (USFS) and again becomes an exercise in water reading and Class II chutes. Just below here the North River joins the flow from river right. (Look for 200 cfs for a minimum flow for the rest of the Upper, Upper Tellico.)

Unless you want to run Class IV ledges of four to eight feet each, take out at the next bridge (B, three miles below North River.) For the next 2.5 miles, you will be in the "Ledges" section of the Upper, Upper Tellico. This small section can be a full day's effort to scout and run the technical rapids. Refer to Monte Smith's 1995 edition of Southeastern Whitewater for a good drop-by-drop description of this short section of river (Pahsimeroi Press, Box 190442, Boise, ID 83709). If you're confident and decide to run these drops be aware that the 14-foot, Class V Baby Falls is just around the corner. A paddler who inadvertently encounters this straight-down drop is in for a bruising encounter. Portage Baby Falls on the left and watch for cars. From just below Baby Falls to Bald River the Tellico is nonstop, Class III–IV, expect-no-rest technical paddling. This segment of river has devoured more than its share of plastic boats. The 0.8-mile run from Bald River Falls to the bridge contains the "Jerrods Knee" rapid, which is extremely difficult and hard on equipment. A convenient put-in right in the teeth of a Class III rapid appears at the bridge. This is the common Upper Tellico put-in (C). It's also a convenient place to use four-wheel-drive traction to pull wrapped boats off the rocks 20 feet into the trip (that has been done!). The normal Upper Tellico run at optimum water levels is from this put-in to the Ranger Station Road bridge (F) 5.5 miles downstream. It's short, but there's a lot of bubbling water. This is not a trip for beginners or those who over-rate their abilities or depend on luck. The water remains cold through the springtime, so dry suits and wet suits are an excellent precaution.

Should you complete the Class III, put-in rapid under the bridge intact, you will find a good recovery pool just below which signals another Class III shelf system up ahead. The river is rather wide at this point and an early overturn in this rapid could present rescue prob-lems. We suggest that you not overturn at the begin-ning of this rapid. A half mile from the put-in bridge you will make a straight approach toward an enormous boulder. A powerful right turn is needed. This could be a dangerous place in the event of an upset because the boulder is undercut and can snare partially submerged debris. If you do overturn, get away from your craft and keep your feet on the surface. Avoid that boulder if at all possible.

At 1.5 miles below the put-in bridge you'll come to the Turkey Creek access area. At high water levels, this is a prudent put-in for open craft. The next four miles are rated Class II with occasional Class III drops. Three-foot drops, shelves, and souse holes all enliven the run. The drop in this run averages 60 feet per mile, but it hits 110 feet per mile above the put-in bridge.

As Dick Wooten, a Nashville canoeist, has been known to observe, "The Tellico is a fun run on beautiful water, especially when the mountain laurel is at its height of bloom." He looks at the flowers?!

Lower Tellico River

The Lower Tellico becomes a pastoral stream working its way across the foothills into the heart of the great Tennessee Valley. Below the Ranger Station Road bridge (F) and for the next four miles to Tellico Plains, the river widens, flattens, but still gathers together a few times to provide strong Class II shoals. At lower water levels there are two wide, rocky shoal areas above Tellico Plains that are hard to completely navigate. You'll probably get your feet wet dragging the canoe.

Below Tellico Plains the stream still retains its beauty and appeal but it begins to meander. The Cherokee National Forest is on one bank and agricultural land is on the other. Similar minimum water levels are needed for the Lower Tellico as for the upper whitewater stretches, but optimum flow occurs at about 1,000 cfs. Excessive flow creates trouble typical of pastoral streams. You're advised to stay off when the river is muddy and out of its banks. There are many alternate access points along the Lower Tellico.

The Lower Tellico is a pleasant, pastoral, family float trip through the rural countryside of the historical Little Tennessee valley lands. Unfortunately, most of the time the water level will be too low or marginal.

Tellico River Flow Rate (Conversion from feet to CFS)

Feet .	0	.1	.2	.3	.4	.5	.6	.7	.8	.9
0						12.5	19.5	28	39	51
1	66	83	102	123	147	173	202	234	368	305
2	330	365	403	442	483	526	571	618	667	717
3	770	814	858	904	951	998	1047	1096	1147	1198
4	1250	1301	1354	1407	1461	1515	1571	1627	1684	1742
5	1800	1857	1915	1973	2032	2092	2152	2213	2275	2337
6	2400	2471	2543	2616	2689	2764	2839	2916	2993	3071
7	3150	3239	3330	3422	3515	3610	3705	3802	3900	3999
8	4100	4221	4344	4469	5495	4724	4855	4988	5124	5261
9	5400	5574	5752	5933	6118	6307	6499	6696	6896	7100
10	7308	7519	7735	7955	8179	8406	8638	8874	9115	9359
11	9608	9861	10129	10380	10650	10920	11190	11470	11750	12040
12	12330	12630	12930	13240	12550	13870	14190	14520	14850	15180
13	15520	15870	16220	16570	16930	17300	17670	18040	18420	18810
14	19200	19600	20000							

Nolichucky River

The Nolichucky River erupts at the confluence of the Toe and Cane Rivers on the northeast side of Mount Mitchell, the highest point in North Carolina. Throwing everything it's got at you right at the beginning, the Nolichucky foams and rattles through an awe-inspiring, 900-foot gorge cut through the Bald and Unicoi Mountains below Poplar, North Carolina. Exhausting itself quickly, the Nolichucky enters the gorge like the proverbial lion and exits at Erwin, Tennessee, like a feisty and not-so-proverbial lamb.

Nolichucky Gorge

Excerpts from other descriptions of this spectacular whitewater adventure might give you an idea of what is in store:

> For those who would like to enjoy the rugged grandeur of the gorge and the river to the fullest, hiking is the way. The paddler can only enjoy the river, for it gives one little opportunity to view the magnificent scenery above. (Bob Benner in *Carolina Whitewater*).

> The difficulty of the float trip through the gorge will depend on the water level, however, this trip is difficult at any water level. (Rick Phelps in the *Tennessee Eastman Bulletin*).

> The Nolichucky Gorge is spectacularly wild in spite of the Clinchfield Railroad which follows the river. However, most boaters will be too busy with the challenge of the technical, powerful rapids to see much scenery. (Don Bodley in the *Tennessee Valley Canoe Club Bulletin*).

The Nolichucky Gorge is a respected, challenging piece of whitewater found where this big drainage forces itself through the North Carolina–Tennessee border where the rugged Appalachian mountains make a spine-like boundary. The Clinchfield Railroad is a small connector line across those saw-toothed ridges; but that line is one of the few consistently profitable railroads purely because they had the foresight to note there were almost no passageways across the rugged highlands. Years ago they hacked out a bench along the Nolichucky to lock up that cross-ridge traffic. Heavy (profitable) traffic continues along that track to this day.

The gorge run (for both train and paddler) is 8.5 miles long. The U.S. Forest Service has provided a rustic access and parking area at the village of Poplar, North Carolina (A). Poplar is in a scenic little cove on the North Carolina side of the mountain that doesn't quite qualify as even a crossroads on the map, just a gathering of dwellings. Erwin, Tennessee, at the take-out (B,C), is a healthy railroad town although it is still relatively remote.

Between these two points on the map lie parts of the

Section: Poplar (NC) to Erwin (TN)
Counties: Mitchell (NC), Unicoi (TN)
USGS Quads: Huntdale (NC), Chestoa (TN), Erwin (TN)
Difficulty: Class III–IV
Gradient: 36 feet per mile
Average Width: 50–100 feet
Velocity: Fast
Rescue Index: Accessible but difficult
Hazards: Undercut rocks, keeper hydraulics, difficult rapids
Scouting: At major rapids
Portages: As water level requires
Scenery: Exceptionally beautiful
Highlights: Scenery, whitewater, geology
Gauge: Visual only

Runnable Water Level	Minimum	Maximum
Embreeville gauge	500 cfs	2,000 cfs

Additional Information: Nolichucky Expeditions, (615) 743-3221; US Forest Service, Pisgah National Forest, (704) 682-6146; TVA (423) 632-6065

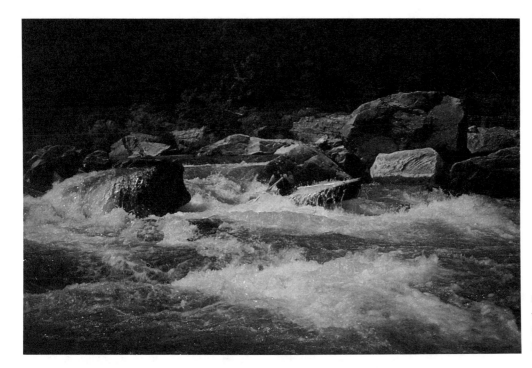

Bill Micks paddling
through On the
Rocks on the Nolichucky.
Photo by Ed Grove

Cherokee National Forest, the border mountains, and the superb Nolichucky whitewater. The TVA-monitored gauge at Embreeville (downstream from the gorge) gives an accurate reference point for the gorge canoeist. Open canoes are advised to outfit with extra flotation at any level. Optimum flow is found at 1,000 cfs. The stream is dangerously difficult and almost too pushy at 1,500 cfs. All knowledgeable local canoe clubs cancel their trips if the flow is above 2,000 cfs. (You ought to take that hint because these people are experienced with this river and know what they are doing.)

The entrance set of rapids is a good test for your particular boating skills for that day. It is a long, technical drop requiring movement from one side of the river to the center, judicious use of eddies, and hole-avoidance maneuvers. Should you experience difficulty maintaining control in this rapid, the long, arduous, brush-beating portage back to the shuttle car can be accomplished (as has been done many times) to avoid an even longer, more difficult, enforced midrun take-out when the going gets considerably harder. You still must face Riverboat Rapids, Big Mother, and other complex drops. The river drops an average of almost 60 feet per mile in the early part of the run, which is a powerful stream in the heavy flow above 1,000 cfs. Rapids rate from II to IV below 1,000 cfs, and from III to V, above.

To summarize, the Nolichucky Gorge begins and ends with a railroad trestle. Most of the heavier-duty rapids are packed into the first third of the run. At higher water

levels multiple routes are available. At moderate to lower levels the gorge can become a technical maze. Specific hazards include On-the-Rocks Rapid in the early part of the run where the main current splits around a large

Nolichucky River • Tennessee, North Carolina

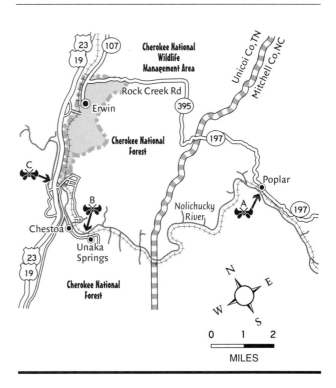

Nolichucky River • Tennessee

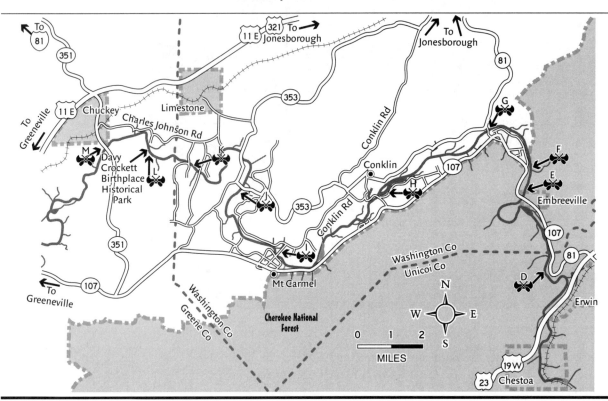

boulder that has eaten its share of boats. Quarter Mile Rapid (because it is a quarter of a mile long) sports large,

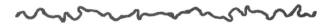

Section: Erwin to Chuckey
Counties: Unicoi, Washington, Greene
USGS Quads: Erwin, Telford, Chuckey
Difficulty: Class I–II
Gradient: 12 feet per mile
Average Width: 70 feet
Velocity: Moderate to fast
Rescue Index: Accessible
Hazards: Moderate Class II (III) rapid above Embreeville
Scouting: None required
Portages: None required
Scenery: Beautiful
Highlights: Scenery, wildlife, whitewater, camping, local culture and industry, history (Davy Crockett Birthplace)
Gauge: Visual only

Runnable Water Level	Minimum	Maximum
Embreeville gauge	550 cfs	Up to flood stage

Additional Information: Nolichucky Expeditions, (615) 743-3221; TVA, (423) 632-6065

jagged fragments of old iron railroad canisters. Immediately below Quarter Mile Rapid, just when you think the worst is over, a riverwide hydraulic that tends to be a keeper materializes to grab the complacent boater. This should be run far right. Several more of these riverwide holes crop up throughout the run. At practically all levels these holes should be run to the extreme left or right.

Commercial rafting companies use this section of the river heavily. The water quality suffers from heavy, sandy/silty loads derived from mining higher in the North Carolina watershed. Newly formed sandbars are evident wherever the water slows down. But the scenery and excitement of the whitewater are spectacular.

Below the Nolichucky Gorge

After the Nolichucky Gorge, between Erwin (C) and Embreeville (E), the river assumes the characteristics of the typical Great Smoky Mountain valley stream; it has a broad, rocky bottom, frequent ripples, small waves, and an occasional big surprise. Scenery is beautiful in spite of parallel highways and considerable industrial development. Exposed rock bluffs rise and recede from the river's

Nolichucky River • Tennessee

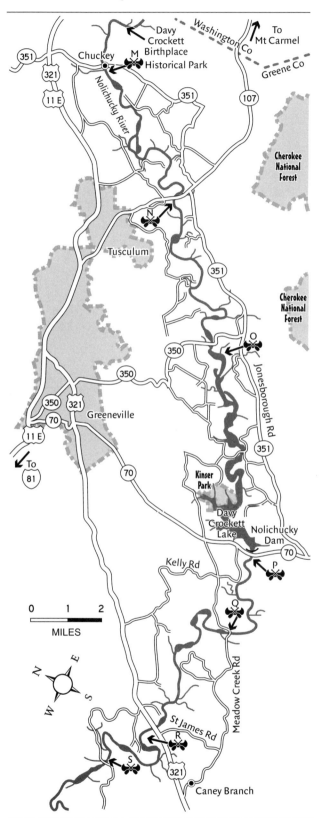

edge. The level of difficulty of this section is Class II with one borderline Class III rapid a half mile downstream from the TN 81 bridge as the river loops around a mammoth rocky pinnacle just upstream from Embreeville. Access is fair to good and navigational dangers are essentially limited to the one large rapid mentioned above. Runnable from late November through early June in most years, this section makes a good practice run for the novice whitewater paddler. River width varies from 65 to over 90 feet.

Below Embreeville, the Nolichucky continues to flow through mountainous terrain for five miles and then exits into the rolling hills of Washington, Greene, and Hamblen counties before emptying into the French Broad River at the headwaters of Douglas Lake south of Morristown. This section offers numerous paddle trip opportunities because it has plentiful access, lively Class I+ water, and pleasant scenery. Upstream from Davy Crockett Lake in Greene County the Nolichucky is characterized by high banks and some exposed rock walls rising from the river. Hardwoods shade the stream, which averages 70 feet in width.

While almost all property along the river is privately owned, an exception is the Davy Crockett Birthplace Historical Park (L) just downstream of the Washington-Greene county line. Camping is allowed here, making canoe camping practical on this section.

Four hundred yards below Davy Crockett Birthplace

Section: Chuckey to Douglas Lake
Counties: Greene, Cocke
USGS Quads: Chuckey, Greeneville, Davy Crockett Lake, Cedar Creek, Parrottsville, Springvale, Rankin
Difficulty: Class I+
Average Width: 70 feet
Gradient: 5.65 feet per mile
Velocity: Moderate
Rescue Index: Accessible to accessible but difficult
Hazards: Deadfalls
Scouting: None required
Portages: Greeneville Dam
Scenery: Pretty to beautiful in spots
Highlights: Scenery, camping, wildlife, local culture and industry
Gauge: Visual only

Runnable Water Levels	Minimum	Maximum
Embreeville gauge	500 cfs	Up to flood stage

Months runnable: All except during dry weather
Additional Information: TVA, (423) 632-6065

Nolichucky River • Tennessee

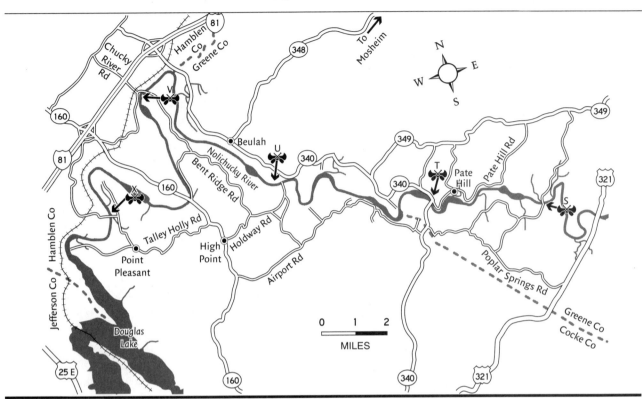

Historical Park watch for a 50-yard-long series of Class II ledges. This rapid can easily be run on the far right or portaged on the right bank. Hazards to navigation for the remainder of the section are limited primarily to deadfalls. The Nolichucky from Embreeville to Davy Crockett Lake can be run from mid-November through mid-July in most years. Though certainly not a wilderness stream, the farms bordering the river are usually not visible from the water, and the atmosphere of natural solitude remains largely intact.

Below Greeneville Dam on Davy Crockett Lake the Nolichucky River meanders through rolling, rich farmland and is guarded by sharply inclined banks 15 feet high. Small shoals and ripples keep the paddler busy as the stream threads through bottomland at the base of tall, curving hills, and islands appear frequently in midstream. As the Nolichucky approaches its confluence with the French Broad River on Douglas Lake, it widens perceptibly from 80 to 100 and finally to almost 300 feet. The dense hardwoods of the upstream reaches are replaced by intermittent foliage and short, scrub vegetation. The level of difficulty is Class I+, with few or no dangers to navigation. Access is fair and signs of human habitation are frequent. The Nolichucky can be run from Davy Crockett Lake to its mouth whenever the Greeneville Dam is releasing.

Little River of Sevier and Blount Counties

The Little River originates high on the northwest side of Clingmans Dome in the Great Smoky Mountains and cascades precipitously down the mountainside to become, between Elkmont and Townsend, one of the most difficult whitewater runs in Tennessee. Firing off the mountain at a furious pace, the Little River squeezes through a continuously narrowing, boulder-infested bed with an average gradient of 70 feet per mile and higher. Technical to the extreme and almost devoid of eddies for long stretches, the Little River is stuffed mile after mile with successive Class III and IV rapids disguised by exploding foam and mined with boat-crunching rocks. To say the least, this is a run for experts only.

For most of us, catching the Little with sufficient water for a run is almost as tricky as getting home with boat and limbs in one piece. Definitely a wet-weather stream with tremendously quick runoff in the upper sections, the Little River draws most of its following from the Knoxville/Oak Ridge/Maryville area, where local paddlers are within striking distance when the water is up. For the rest of us this run is catch-as-catch-can. The Little is usually considered to be runnable downstream from the Millsap Picnic Grounds near Elkmont (A). Right from the put-in the rapids are continuous and come at the paddler with alarming speed; pools just do not exist. Drops are frequent and often severe (three feet and higher); rapids are long and technical. As the river passes under the Little River Road (TN 73) bridge near the mouth of the Poplar Branch, three Class

Section: Elkmont to Townsend

Counties: Sevier, Count

USGS Quads: Gatlinburg, Wear Cove

Difficulty: Class III–IV

Gradient: 65 feet per mile; 76 feet per mile (A-D)

Average Width: 20–35 feet

Velocity: Fast

Rescue Index: Accessible

Hazards: Deadfalls, strainers, flash flooding, undercut rocks, difficult rapids

Scouting: Complete run

Portages: Sinks rapid, Elbow rapid, and other rapids as levels dictate

Scenery: Beautiful to exceptionally beautiful

Highlights: Scenery, whitewater

Gauge: Visual only

Runnable Water Level	Minimum	Maximum
Maryville gauge	400	2,000

Additional Information: TVA, (423) 632-2264 or (800) 238-2264; National Park Service, Great Smoky Mountains National Parks, (423) 436-1200

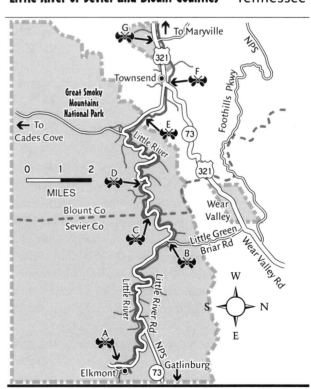

Little River of Sevier and Blount Counties • Tennessee

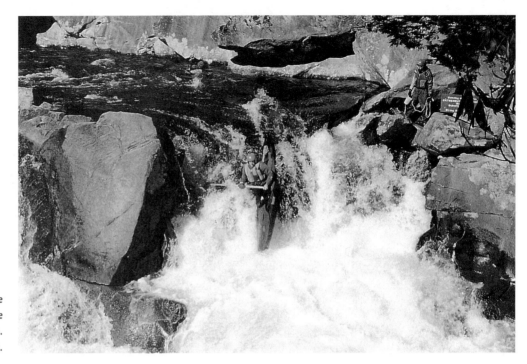

A cold day on the Little River. Bill Hay running the Sinks of the Little. Photo by Mayo Gravatt.

IV rapids occur within 200 yards; scout from the left bank.

After the Little River passes under the bridge leading to Little Greenbrier School, it calms down somewhat (Class II–III) as it parallels Little River Road (TN 73) along the left bank. Following a half-loop to the left, the river curves right and flows relatively straight for about a third of a mile before beginning a large loop to the left. This loop, containing some particularly fierce water, forms the entrance rapids for the 10-foot vertical drop of the Sinks of the Little at the end of the loop, just under the Little River Road bridge crossing (C). This entire segment should be scouted carefully before running. The Sinks probably should be portaged.

Below the Sinks, to the next downstream crossing of Little River Road, the Little River continues true to form with several long, technical, Class IV rapids interspersed with lots of challenging Class III and long Class II rapids. Past the Little River Road bridge (D), the Little calms down somewhat in what is sometimes called the Elbow section. Unlike the Sinks section, normally regarded as suitable for decked-boat experts only, the Elbow section is considered a good run for open- and decked-boat intermediates. The rapids persist in being long and technical, but pools are more frequently encountered here and the gradient flattens out to a mere 50 feet per mile.

Don't relax prematurely, however. One of the most dangerous rapids on the Little River rears its seething head right in the middle of the run. It is the namesake of this section, Elbow Rapid. Elbow is Class IV at moderate levels when there's a good collection pool below. It consists of a tricky approach on the right, followed by a drop, and a sharp left turn in a crashing boil of falling, converging currents. An alternate route down the middle is possible at certain water levels but carries the paddler into and sometimes under a head-crunching overhanging rock at the bottom of the drop. Except at lower levels, we

Section: Townsend to Tennessee River
County: Blount
USGS Quads: Wear Cove, Kinzel Springs, Wildwood, Maryville
Difficulty: Class I–II
Gradient: 7.94 feet per mile
Average Width: 30–35 feet
Velocity: Moderate
Rescue Index: Accessible
Hazards: Deadfalls, dams, flash flooding
Scouting: As water level requires
Portages: Dams
Scenery: Beautiful in spots
Highlights: Scenery, wildlife, whitewater, local culture, geology
Gauge: Visual only

Runnable Water Level	Minimum	Maximum
Maryville gauge	230 cfs	Up to flood stage

Additional Information: TVA, (423) 632-2264 or (800) 238-2264

Little River of Sevier and Blount Counties • Tennessee

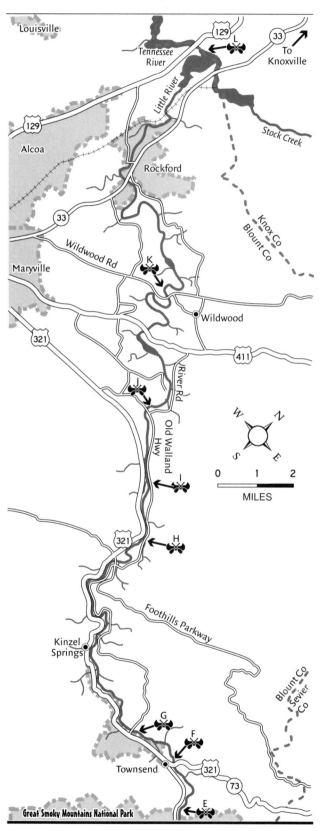

heartily recommended that you portage this rapid. It is reported that this rapid was formerly known as the 90 Percent Rapid—that is, no matter how good the paddler or what technique was used in the run, he or she would be chewed to pieces about 90 percent of the time. Enough said.

A good take-out for this section is the tourist parking area just inside the boundary of Great Smoky Mountains National Park, two miles upstream from Townsend. Because the characteristics of the Little River from Elkmont to the park boundary vary considerably with changing water levels, paddlers should avail themselves of the parallel road network and carefully scout their proposed run in its entirety before putting in. Due to the narrow, rocky nature of the Little River and the distinct absence of alternate routes in some of the more difficult rapids, deadfalls lodged across the stream can be lethal. Paddlers, therefore, should take extra pains while scouting to ensure that the channel is clear of obstructions.

From the park boundary to Melrose (I) the river increases in width and long pools separate the playful Class II rapids and rock gardens. This section is appropriate for well-schooled beginners in both decked and open boats. This section also marks the descent of the river into a gorge with tall cliffs alternately rising up beside the water and receding from its edge. Signs of civilization are common in this area, with resort properties dotting the water's edge wherever the precipitous terrain permits.

Downstream from Melrose the Little River flows almost tranquilly through foothills and farm country before emptying into the Tennessee River near Singleton (L). Here the Little drifts quietly beneath tree-shaded mud banks. Fishing is not bad and anglers in johnboats are encountered frequently. The level of difficulty is Class I with deadfalls and dams at Melrose being the only navigational hazards. Access to this lower section is adequate.

Ocoee River

For years, paddlers traveling the Old Copper Road (US 64) in southeastern Polk County would marvel at the dry, rocky Ocoee riverbed beside the highway. They couldn't help but conjecture about the potential souse holes and rapids. But high on the mountainside, across the river, a leaky 65-year-old wooden flume carried the river's entire flow to a powerhouse seven miles downstream. Many years ago, the old flume began to leak, and 17 megawatts of river-generated power was transformed back into 1,000 cfs of river flow. The paddlers would conjecture no more. Double Trouble, Diamond Splitter, Table Saw, and Hell's Hole were exciting manifestations of the newly found, 57-foot-drop-per-mile water. Instant notoriety came as river runners tried to learn how various flow levels might affect their craft on this new whitewater. Commercial raft outfitters sprang up. National decked-boat championship races appeared.

Despite the Ocoee's growing popularity and its contribution to southeastern Tennessee's economy, the TVA was determined to reconstruct the flume and once again drain the river. The TVA's inflexible position precipitated an opposing coalition of private boaters and commercial rafters, joined later by conservationists, local businesspeople, commercial raft customers, concerned citizens, country singers, members of Congress, governors, and ultimately the state of Tennessee. As the controversy heated up, the TVA continued to rebuild the flume and placed "temporary bridges" and other construction equipment amidst several of the rapids in the middle of the run. Finally, an agreement was reached whereby TVA would be reimbursed for the power it didn't create on the days when water was released down the natural riverbed.

The agreement mandates releases on all weekends in March, April, May, September, October, and the first weekend of November. During June, July, and August, water is released every day except Tuesday and Wednesday. In addition to these scheduled releases, water is also released during the annual 7- to 14-day powerhouse maintenance period in the fall.

The Ocoee outfitters have done all they can to educate TVA to the true values of this river as a nationally significant whitewater flow. But TVA remains hidebound to their traditions from the 1930s. Still, each year, a release schedule gets negotiated and the information posted.

You probably realize that the 1996 Olympic kayaking events were held on the Ocoee. And that now adds to the management difficulties for water releases. The Olympic course is upstream of the normal, flume-diverted Ocoee whitewater run. Releases through the course can affect water availability for the normal whitewater run. Similar negotiations are currently under way to allow posted times of water release through the upstream Olympic course.

For the time being, one of the most taxing whitewater streams in the southeast exists along seven miles of the Old Copper Road from Ocoee No. 2 dam to Ocoee No. 2 powerhouse. The Ocoee whitewater is not general recreational canoeing. It is solid Class III and IV; however, the road is nearby along the entire run, so you can walk out. Only whitewater canoes rigged with extra flotation should attempt the run, and the paddler should be a confident expert with advanced paddling techniques. Damage reports from the Ocoee are legendary. Know what you are doing or stay off.

The Ocoee is Tennessee's portion of Georgia's Toccoa River, an attractive mountain stream skirting the southern reaches of the Smokies. Unfortunately, at the Georgia-Tennessee border the Copperhill mining basin fouls the water quality. Sulfuric acid leached from 40 years of mining and smelting has completely sterilized the Ocoee tributaries coming out of the great copper basin. Years of airborne acid have also denuded the forested hillsides in the basin. (This red space amid the sea of Great Smoky Mountain green, along with the Great Wall of China, was one of the few man-made earth

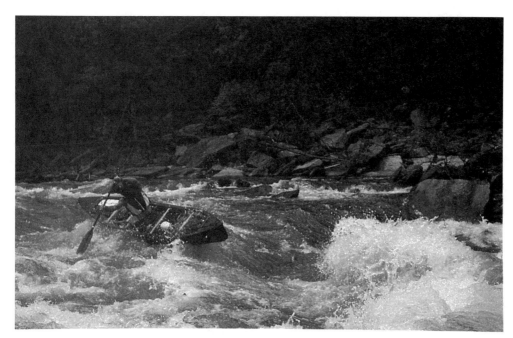

An open boater in Double Trouble. Photo by Ed Grove.

modifications visible to orbiting astronauts.) The bare hillsides of the basin also choke the same tributaries with fine-grained red silt. Water quality coming down this premier whitewater run is somewhere between repulsive and lethal. Keep your mouth closed!

Hazards on this run begin before you even get your boat in the water. The only safe loading and parking area is upstream of the put-in on the lake side of the Ocoee No. 2 dam. It is here that the release levels for the day are reported on a bulletin board—they are usually around 1,200 cfs. This parking area above the raft unloading area is preferred to the challenge of unloading amid the dizzying fumes of speeding diesels and the careening autos of rubbernecking tourists on US 64. Downstream of that parking area, with nothing more at risk than your life, you could park on a constricted ribbon of road shoulder next to the put-in (just below the boat-swamping "Entrance" rapid) and feverishly attempt to unload your gear, a little at a time, when breaks in the traffic allow. However, this type of river access for private boaters is not encouraged. Your vehicle must be completely off the road, with no tolerance offered by the enforcers. It is a dangerous place, and they are correct in their concerns.

Once in the water, the paddler will find the Ocoee to be synonymous with continuous action. The pace is intense and the eddies are not always where you want them. The action starts as soon as you put in. Entrance Rapid can hammer unwary paddlers. The best run is to ferry to river left and paddle down the left side. Below

this, Class II and III rapids follow one upon the other and consist primarily of big waves and some respectable holes. These rapids are agreeably straightforward for the most part, and have recognizable routes. Following this

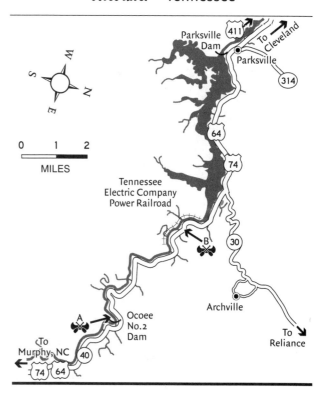

Ocoee River • Tennessee

stretch of warm-up rapids, however, the river broadens and runs shallow over a long series of ledges known as Gonzo Shoals. Route selection is anything but obvious and the going (particularly at minimal flow) gets extremely technical.

Below this shallow stretch, the river begins to narrow slightly and bend to the right. This is the approach to Broken Nose (alternately known as Veg-O-Matic), a potentially lethal series of three drops in rapid succession. The drops are near the right bank. Powerful crosscurrents surge between each of the drops; the last two hydraulics can be very sticky. There is a cheat route along the far left for those who prefer not to encounter the main activity in Broken Nose Rapid.

Action continues and bears back to the left on through a Class II–III series including Second Helping and Moon Shoot. When the river begins to turn back toward the right, prepare for Double Suck. Double Suck gets its name from two closely spaced souse holes. You will recognize the rapid by the large granite boulders thrusting up and blocking the center third of the stream. Go just to the right of these boulders and over a four-foot drop into the first hole. Don't relax after this one, however, because the second hole follows immediately and it will eat the unwary. Eddy out behind the large boulders in the center if you need time to recover your composure or bail the water from your boat.

Continuing downstream, the river swings away from parallel US 64. The paddler should move to the far right

for Double Trouble, a double set of holes and waves. Below Double Trouble, a number of smaller rapids lead into a long pool known as the Doldrums. This, the longest pool on the river, signals the presence of Class IV Table Saw rapid about three-fourths of a mile ahead. At the end of the Doldrums the stream broadens conspicuously and laps playfully over the shallows with little riffles and waves. Protruding from the right bank, a large rock shelf or boulder beach funnels the water to the left.

The river narrows and the current deepens and picks up speed as it enters the most formidable rapid on the Ocoee. Table Saw was named for a large rock situated in the middle of a chute that split the current, sending up an impressive rooster tail. Past floods have removed the rock and rooster tail. Toward the end of the rapid is a violent diagonal hole that fortunately is not a keeper. Table Saw can be scouted from the boulder beach on the right or from eddies on the left. Rescue can be set on river right just below the hole where there is a nice, if not overly spacious eddy. Speedy rescue of people and equipment is important here because of the proximity of Diamond Splitter just downstream.

Consisting of yet another river-dividing boulder, Diamond Splitter rises ponderously out of the water offering a potential for broaching or entrapment. The generally preferred route is to the right of the boulder. From here Class II and III rapids rampage more or less continuously with only one significant pool as the Ocoee approaches the powerhouse. A quarter mile upstream of the power-

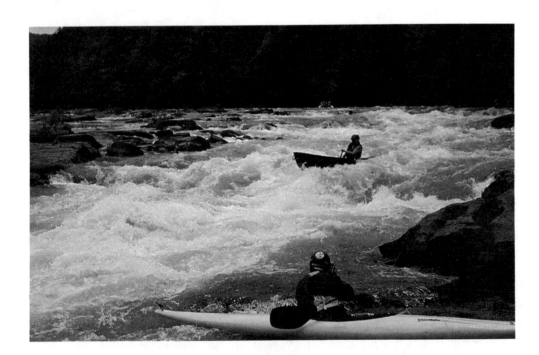

Running through
Table Saw Rapid (before
the "saw" disappeared).
Photo by Ed Grove.

Section: Ocoee No. 2 dam to Ocoee No. 2 powerhouse

County: Polk

USGS Quads: Ducktown, Caney Creek

Difficulty: Class III–IV

Gradient: 57 feet per mile

Average Width: 40–60 feet

Velocity: Fast

Rescue Index: Very accessible

Hazards: Keeper hydraulics, difficult rapids

Scouting: At major rapids

Portages: None required

Scenery: Beautiful

Highlights: Scenery, whitewater, history

Gauge: TVA Hotline, (800) 362-9250; in Southeastern states (800) 251-9242, outside the Southeast (423) 632-4100. Instantaneous flow report available from powerhouse for Ocoee No. 3 (when No. 2 is spilling). Recording gives 24-hour average that is too low for the 8-hour generating period.

Runnable Water Level	Minimum	Maximum
	700 cfs	4000 cfs

Months runnable: Variable dam releases. Generally everyday except Tuesdays and Wednesdays during rafting season.

Additional Information: Ocoee Outdoors, (423) 338-2438; US Forest Service, Cherokee National Forest, (423) 338-5201

house is Torpedo (a.k.a. Cat's Pajamas), a long, confusing, technical rapid with several powerful holes. Frequently omitted in descriptions of the Ocoee, this rapid can be very rough on a boater who chooses the wrong route. Most easily scouted from the road while running the shuttle, Torpedo should be of particular interest to first-timers.

Torpedo is separated from Hell's Hole, an enormous, deep, aerated, river-dominating hole by a pool just upstream of the powerhouse and bridge. Situated toward the right bank of the river at the new powerhouse bridge, Hell's Hole can be played, surfed, or punched with the happy prospect of being flushed out in case of an upset.

Hell's Hole monopolizes the channel, but a technical run skirting the hole on the left is possible (and generally advisable for open boats). Hell's Hole, however, is only the first part of a double rapid. Not twenty yards beyond the fearsome hole itself is the drop known as Powerhouse Rapid. Powerhouse consists of a four-foot vertical ledge and nasty hydraulic spanning the left two-thirds of the stream, with a more manageable tongue spilling down on the right.

Arriving safely at the bottom of all this requires making it through or around Hell's Hole, fighting the current at the bottom, which tries to carry you left, and working hard to the right to line up for the tongue through Powerhouse. Have a good roll if you try to play Hell's Hole, and anticipate the current kicking you left as you wash out. When the water is high (1,800+ cfs) Hell's Hole washes out while the Powerhouse hydraulic becomes lethal. In this situation, run close to the right bank to avoid being carried too far left as you approach the bridge. Scout this complex stretch either while running the shuttle or from the TVA plant bridge.

If you make it this far you can drift for awhile (a quarter mile) to the raft take-out shortly downstream. Continuing past this study in (un)organized human activity and milling about, the stream flows through some shoals to the new, private boater take-out another half mile downstream.

Once the basic route down the river is learned, competent paddlers will find endless variations for running different rapids. Some can add considerably to the difficulty of the river. Though the house-sized eddies of some drop-and-pool rivers are not common, you can find countless eddies large enough for at least one skillful boater in even the most technical rapids. The majority of the river consists of sizable waves, rocks, and scattered holes (some large enough to turn unsuspecting paddlers into fish counters in a heartbeat). Generally the rocks are not undercut (provided you're going downstream), but they are plentiful and tend to pop up in front of your boat at inopportune moments.

Hiwassee River

Cold water, fast current, rock ledges—an ideal habitat for whitewater canoeing or put-and-take fly fishing. You'll find both on the Hiwassee, a Tennessee State Scenic River. The trout supply is stocked and the canoeists seem to be, too, when the water rises. In northeastern Polk County, near the North Carolina border, the Appalachia Dam impounds this major drainage of the southern Blue Ridge Mountains. The Hiwassee begins on a ridge near the Appalachian Trail high above Helen, Georgia, and meanders northward through some highland patch-farm, north Georgia country. It rests in an impoundment or two, masquerades under the more Indian "Hiawassee" spelling, and then cuts across the forested foot of several North Carolina peaks and plunges into Tennessee via the Appalachia powerhouse release. It's a big water-

shed and an equally large riverbed for this Tennessee portion of the river.

For a different experience on the Hiwassee, take a look at the interesting and scenic 15-mile section of the river between the dam and the powerhouse. This bed is now mostly dry and carries water only during periods of extremely high natural flow from heavy rainfall. Hiking access is via the railroad tracks (still in regular use) on river right or the John Muir trail on river left. The scenery is beautiful, with mountains on both sides and unusual rock formations. High trestles cross over brooks and at one point the track crosses over itself, which is famous in railroad circles. The railroad makes more than a complete circle, known as the Hiwassee Loop, to gain elevation. Nearer the powerhouse is the abandoned town site

Section: Powerhouse to Reliance
County: Polk
USGS Quads: McFarland, Oswald Dome
Difficulty: Class I–II
Gradient: 14.54 feet per mile
Average Width: 100–150 feet
Velocity: Fast
Rescue Index: Accessible
Hazards: Undercut rocks
Scouting: None required
Portages: None required
Scenery: Beautiful
Highlights: Scenery, whitewater
Gauge: TVA Hotline in Tennessee, (800) 362-9250; in other Southeastern states (800) 251-9242; outside of the Southeast call (615) 632-4100. Gives release from Appalachia Dam as well as natural flow.

Runnable Water Level	Minimum	Maximum
	1,000 cfs	10,000 cfs

Additional Information: Hiwassee Outfitters, (423) 338-8115; US Forest Service, Cherokee National Forest, (423) 338-5201

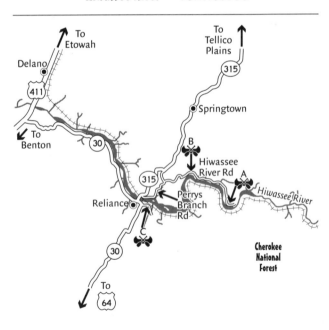

Hiwassee River • Tennessee

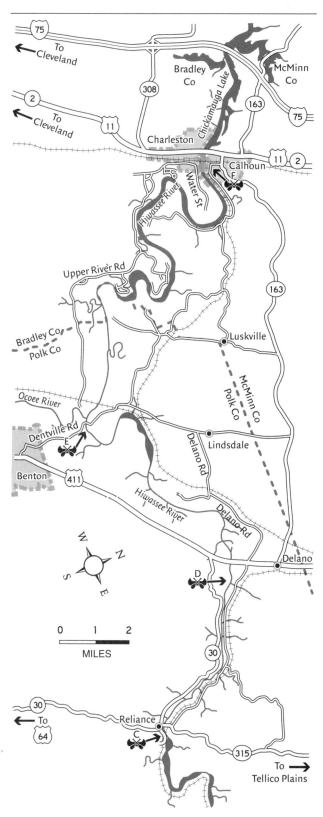

Hiwassee River • Tennessee

(Map labels:)

75
To Cleveland

Bradley Co

McMinn Co

308

2

11
To Cleveland

163

75

Charleston

Chickamauga Lake

11 2

Calhoun
F

Water St

Hiwassee River

163

Upper River Rd

Bradley Co
Polk Co

Luskville

McMinn Co
Polk Co

Ocoee River

Dentville Rd
E

Benton

411

Delano Rd

Lindsdale

Hiwassee River

Delano Rd

Delano

D

N
W   E
S

0   1   2
MILES

30

30
To
64

Reliance
C

315

To
Tellico Plains

Section: Reliance to Calhoun

Counties: Polk, Bradley, McMinn

USGS Quads: Oswald Dome, Benton, Calhoun, Charleston

Difficulty: Class I (II)

Gradient: 4.62 feet per mile

Average Width: 300–450 feet

Velocity: Moderate to fast

Rescue Index: Accessible

Hazards: Strainers, powerboats

Scouting: None required

Portages: None required

Scenery: Beautiful

Highlights: Scenery, history, camping

Gauge: TVA Hotline in Tennessee, (800) 362-9250; in other Southeastern states (800) 251-9242; outside of the Southeast call (615) 632-4100

Runnable Water Level	Minimum	Maximum
	500 cfs	Up to flood stage

Months runnable: All (dam-controlled)

Additional Information: Hiwassee Outfitters, (423) 338-8115; US Forest Service, Cherokee National Forest, (423) 338-5201

of McFarland and the Narrows, where the river is constricted between the tracks and high rocks of unusual formation.

Downstream from the powerhouse, where the river is again canoeable, the water is cold. Releases come from deep in the impoundment. It is rather unusual to find such cold water in a wide, shallow stream. Trout thrive; dunked canoeists shiver.

After all its mountain meandering, this river still has one ridge left to clear in its surge toward the Tennessee River. And it is a beautiful, scenic setting as the clear, bouncing river makes a dramatic horseshoe bend at the foot of Tennessee's Hood Mountain. It is truly a worthy member of the state's scenic river system.

Fishermen and canoeists have almost learned to coexist on this stretch of rockbound water. When there's no dam release, the waders line the rocky outcroppings in the riverbed hunting the pooled-up fish. When the 1,500-cfs dam release comes along, tubers, rafters, and paddlers of all types come with it, plunging over those same rock ledges and recovering in those same fished-out pools.

The first five miles of the Hiwassee below the powerhouse (A) is Class I and II with a couple of rapids rating a strong Class II. It's a fun ride—the Hiwassee is a forgiving stream—but one that accelerates a desire to hone your skills. The swift current and the wide reach across the river can often make recovery a difficult, chilly experience. The put-in is at the powerhouse access ramp (about a quarter mile below the powerhouse). Two miles downstream is the Big Bend parking lot (B) hidden in the trees at the foot of a series of ledges. If rain, cold, or mishap creates a need to take out early, you should know how to find that access—there isn't another one until the ramp at Reliance (C).

Between the powerhouse and Reliance, you'll encounter a mixed bag of paddling possibilities: swift current and bouncy waves at Cabin Bend (there's no cabin there anymore, but there's still a bend); big, unstable drops at No. 2 Rapids and Oblique Falls; tricky crosscurrents at Bigneys Rock; follow-the-flow, water-reading exercises at the Ledges and the Stairsteps; peel-off and eddy-turn practice at the Needles; and big swamper waves at Devils Shoals.

As of 1998, the US Forest Service began charging parking fees. The fee is $2 per vehicle, $30 for a season pass. For more information or to get a pass, write to Hiwassee Ranger Station, P.O. Box D, Etowah, TN 37331.

Below Reliance, the river flattens out as it makes it's final run out of the mountains to Calhoun (F). Six miles downstream you'll find the US Forest Service Quinn Springs fee campground across TN 30 from the fishing access on river left and the Tennessee State Park's Gee Creek campground along the right just below. The Gee Creek ramp is up the creek a few yards and its entrance is marked by an old Indian-built fishtrap of V-shaped shallow rock shoals just below the mouth of Gee creek in the Hiwassee.

Conasauga River

A cold, clear scenic river, a Tennessee State Scenic River, and Georgia claims it! The Conasauga River is born deep in Georgia's Cohutta Wilderness, where it falls off the slopes of those north Georgia mountains. The waters drain only national forestlands as they gather together as a streamway. The upper Conasauga, this little, crystal-clear gem of the woodlands, then flows north through steep, almost inaccessible terrain until the highland Alaculsy Valley is reached near the Georgia-Tennessee border. It is there that Jacks River joins the Conasauga and doubles its flow.

In high-water periods, experienced boaters may begin their trip as high as Chicken Coop Gap (A) off Forest Service Road 17 at the edge of the Cohutta Wilderness Area. Putting in at this point requires map-reading skills, determination, and a high skill level. Map-reading skills are required to locate Chicken Coop Gap. Determination is required to get your boat and equipment approximately one quarter mile straight down into the gorge. Above all,

a high skill level is required to successfully navigate down to Alaculsy Valley (B). This is rugged and wild terrain. In some areas the river drops over 100 feet per mile, creating intense, lengthy rapids (Class IV+). It can only be run in high water, and when the water is high all conditions combine to create a potentially lethal situation. It is no place for beginners.

For those with the above-mentioned qualities, however, the rewards are great. The scenery is pristine and stunningly beautiful. The water is crystalline and contains native trout. Rapids range in difficulty to Class IV+ and the quick rate of descent keeps the adrenaline level high. Scouting is frequently necessary around blind drops and turns. All rapids on this section have been run, but

Section: Chicken Coop Gap (GA) to Jacks River (GA)
Counties: Murray (GA); Polk, Bradley (TN)
USGS Quads: Tennga (GA), Parksville (TN)
Difficulty: Class I–IV+
Gradient: 125 feet per mile
Average Width: 15–40 feet
Velocity: Moderate to fast
Rescue Index: Accessible to extremely remote
Hazards: Strainers, deadfalls, difficult rapids, keeper hydraulics
Scouting: All rapids in section A-B, falls in B-C section
Portages: Rapids, as necessary
Scenery: Beautiful to spectacular
Highlights: Scenery, wildlife, whitewater
Gauge: Visual only

Runnable Water Level	Minimum	Maximum
	NA	NA

Additional Information: None

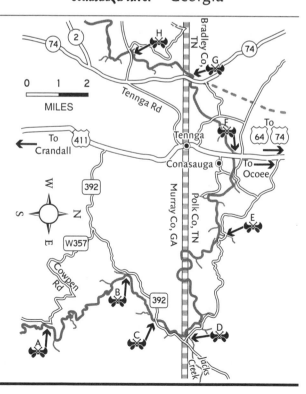

Conasauga River • Georgia

Section: Jacks River confluence to upstream of US 411 bridge
County: Polk
USGS Quad: Parksville
Difficulty: Class II (III)
Gradient: 14.54 feet per mile
Average Width: 15–40 feet
Velocity: Fast
Rescue Index: Accessible
Hazards: Strainers
Scouting: The Falls
Portages: None required
Scenery: Beautiful
Highlights: Scenery, whitewater
Gauge: Visual only

Runnable Water Level	Minimum	Maximum
	NA	NA

Additional Information: None

Section: US 411 (TN) to Browns Bridge Road
Counties: Polk, Bradley (TN); Murray, Whitefield (GA)
USGS Quads: Beaverdale, Chatsworth, Calhoun NE
Difficulty: Class I
Gradient: 1.5 feet per mile
Average Width: 25–45 feet
Velocity: Slack to slow
Rescue Index: Accessible to accessible but difficult
Hazards: Strainers, deadfalls
Scouting: None required
Portages: None required
Scenery: Fair
Highlights: Scenery, Camping
Gauge: Visual only

Runnable Water Level	Minimum	Maximum
	NA	NA

Additional Information: None

portages are prudent at certain times.

Below the second access point the river remains in the Alaculsy Valley until the Jacks River junction. The valley is pretty, but in comparison to the upper section, it might produce either ennui or welcome relief to the paddler. At the Jacks River confluence (D) the stream becomes canoeable to mere mortals. Here, the newly combined flow enters Tennessee. But natural boundaries and political boundaries don't always agree. Twice in the next five miles of flow, the Conasauga, a Tennessee State Scenic River, leaves Tennessee and drops back into Georgia only to reenter soon after. Eventually it makes a permanent southern plunge into Georgia about 15 miles from where it first enters Tennessee. But your float will remain uninterrupted by those political boundaries. No matter where you are, your concern will be only with the rocks and rapids, the flowers, trees, and trout. This naturally flowing stream drains mostly forestlands in southeastern Polk County. The only sustained season of floatable water is during winter and early spring; during this time of year, however, the water is cold—cold enough, in fact, to support native trout. Even at the high levels needed for floating, the water remains clear and clean; even clean enough to drink.

This is an absolutely superb river run. As Don Hixson of Chattanooga once observed in a past newsletter of the Tennessee Scenic Rivers Association: "The Conasauga is among the most beautiful rivers you will ever paddle." Many of the rapids require intricate Class II maneuvering—excellent waters for skill sharpening. But the river

isn't pushy or threatening. Put in near the Jacks River confluence for a 10-mile run. This gives you a half-mile warm-up for the Class II+ shoal, Taylor Branch Rapid. There's good primitive camping and river access just above the rapid if you think warm-ups are superfluous. A mile and a half downstream, you'll find The Falls, a Class III, three-foot drop following a difficult, technical approach. This is the most difficult rapid on the river, but there's a convenient recovery pool below. A fishing camp on the right is often used for lunch while dunked boaters drag their canoes back up to run this approach and drop over and over again until success smiles on their grim, wet, cold, and determined faces. This usually happens soon after the boater realizes that there is a tricky, strategic crosscurrent that has a tendency to push the bow of the otherwise perfectly aligned canoe to the right just before entering the drop.

About four miles downriver, in deceptively swift shoals stands the infamous Fiberglass Covered Rock. Beware this innocent, rounded menace. You're lulled to inattention by the scenery and your past rapid-running successes. You see the river valley opening up and know the whitewater is playing out. Yet this final kiss good-bye from the river has claimed more canoes than any of the upper rapids yet encountered. It's simple—all the recently accelerated river currents converge on this rock. By the time you realize your impending impact, the shallow, swift shoals allow no purchase no matter how hard you stab the slick rock riverbed with your paddle. You'll regain your normal river-running alertness at the sound

Conasauga River • Georgia

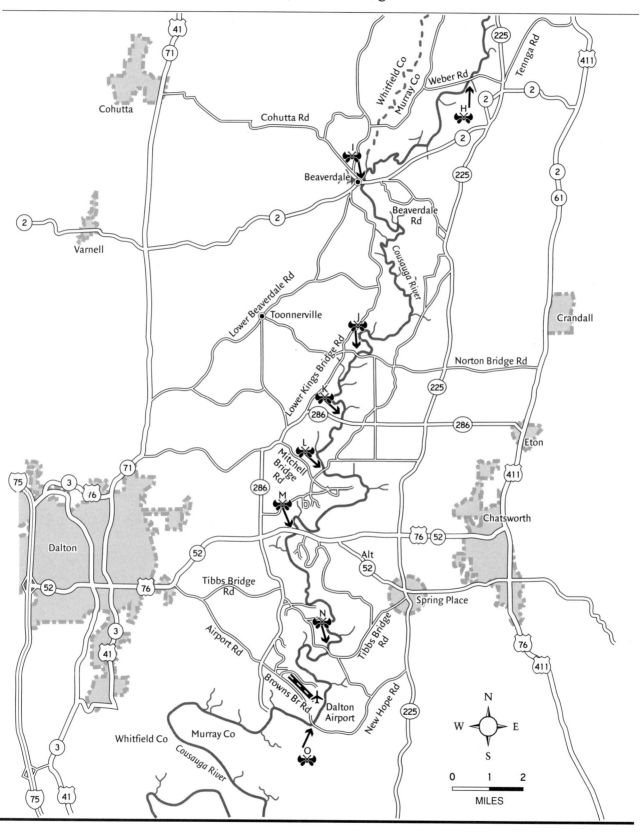

of a crunching canoe and the feel of a chilling dunking. Beyond "Fiberglass Rock" (named in the days before Royalex canoes), the river settles into an agricultural valley and the float becomes more leisurely. The current remains helpful until the take-out on river right about a half mile upstream of the US 411 bridge (F).

It should be noted that an old logging road, now a 6.5-mile hiking trail, exists along the river from Taylor Branch Camp until the river leaves the mountains for the agricultural valley. The trail starts on river right and crosses the river twice. (Canoe assists for the hikers might be needed.) One crossing is near the Georgia-Tennessee border where the river again reenters Tennessee below Taylor Branch Camp, about two miles below The Falls. The second crossing is near where the trail terminates. It crosses back from the river's left to its right, then shortly heads away from the river to intersect the shuttle road 4.3 miles west of Taylor Branch Camp.

Whether canoeing the whitewater or hiking through the well-watered forest, the clean and clear Conasauga is a beautiful springtime expression of Mother Nature's bounty. From US 411 on down to the Coosawattee River junction near Calhoun, the Conasauga is definitely a pastoral stream. Rapids have disappeared and the presence of man becomes more prevalent. Some attractive wooded sections remain, but all pale in comparison to the delights of the mountainous region.

Clear Fork River

Clear Fork River, as its name implies, is a fresh, crisp, clean-water run. It begins on the border between Fentress and Morgan counties and ends in Scott County. After 26 canoeable miles, Clear Fork finally joins with Tennessee's often muddy New River to form the better-known Big South Fork of the Cumberland River. The lower part of this Clear Fork run is also included (as a tributary) in the 125,000-acre Big South Fork National River and Recreation Area. Hence, you should begin to suspect some excellent canoeing potential for this major Cumberland Plateau streamway.

Clear Fork is free-flowing, clear water through wild country and gorgeous scenery. Clear Fork is a remote, scenic experience, a rural escape from familiar urban pressures. But, you should know that Clear Fork is not a wild, crashing, hair-raising mountainside cascade. Rather it is a remarkably well-behaved cruising waterway, cut-

Section: Gatewood Bridge to Burnt Mill Bridge
Counties: Morgan, Scott
USGS Quads: Burrville, Rugby, Honey Creek
Difficulty: Class I–II (III)
Gradient: 18.3 feet per mile
Average Width: 30–40 feet
Velocity: Moderate to fast
Rescue Index: Remote
Hazards: Deadfalls, flash flooding, undercut rocks
Scouting: Decapitation Rock rapid below Brewster bridge
Portages: None required
Scenery: Beautiful
Highlights: Scenery, wildlife, whitewater, history, geology
Gauge: TVA, (800) 362-9250

Runnable Water Level	Minimum	Maximum
Stearns Gauge	1,000 cfs	10,000 cfs

Months runnable: November to June
Additional Information: None

ting deeper and deeper into the old sandstone plateau as it completes the descending river miles heading toward its confluence with the New River.

From Gatewood bridge (A) to Burnt Mill bridge (D), Clear Fork is a Class I and II stream with only one rapid of significant note: Decapitation Rock. Here, on the run below Brewster bridge, you'll remember this Class III brainbuster if you don't note the whole stream swinging under an overhanging rock. If prepared, you can maneuver along the outer edge of this undercut so as to keep your skull intact, but—surprise!—you also maneuvered into a certain line-up for the swamper hole below a sudden three-foot drop just beyond the head-knocker. You can't seem to win—hence the definition of Class III whitewater.

Clear Fork is favored for canoe camping as well as for day floats. Starting at Gatewood bridge, the placid stream immediately sets forth its streamside greenery of thick-set laurel and rhododendron to screen you from any non-river concerns. Shoals and occasional boulders start to hint at a deeper penetration into the plateau. By the time you get to about a mile above Peters Ford bridge (B), you'll be right at the foot of sheer, massive, rock-face sidewall bluffs, but you'll be engrossed in maneuvering through the solid Class II whitewater caused by the resultant bluff-cut rockfalls. It's an exciting end to a short, scenic, six-mile run.

The next six miles to Brewster bridge (C) contain more shoals, small drops, and enjoyable scenery. Large indentations under the riverside bluffs (called "rockhouses") contain remnants of Indian encampments and still provide shelter for knowledgeable people who know how to seek water and comfort in these primitive conditions. From Brewster bridge to Burnt Mill bridge, conditions keep improving.

Just before you pass the mouth of White Oak Creek, you'll pass through a couple of still-water, rock-bottomed pools known locally as The Gentlemen's Swimming Hole. This is where the English residents of Rugby frol-

Clear Fork River • Tennessee

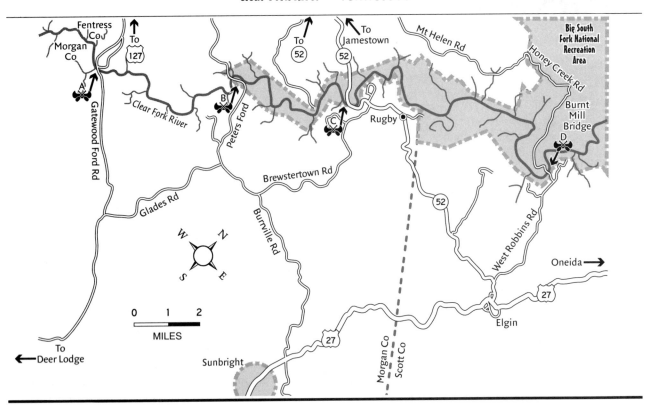

icked (and probably bathed) during an interesting late-nineteenth-century European community experiment. It's worth your time to visit restored Rugby while in the area.

Beyond Rugby at "The Meeting of the Waters," White Oak Creek adds considerably to the flow and the stream becomes bigger and slightly more placid. Twenty-two miles downstream from Gatewood is the quiet pool (and old gauging station) at Burnt Mill bridge, which is an old, one-lane steel truss. This is the final take-out for the enjoyable and scenic Clear Fork float. No novices or campers should plan to float below this bridge.

Clear Fork changes considerably below Burnt Mill. It uses its final three and a half miles to whip the whitewater wanderer into shape for tackling the Big South

Fork Gorge of the Cumberland River just below the confluence with the New River. It is serious, technical whitewater below Burnt Mill bridge and should only be attempted by experienced teams of experts who know what they are doing, have all the proper equipment, and know and understand exactly what the present river flow reading will mean to their trip. External rescue is next to impossible below Burnt Mill bridge. Any party should be able to handle any condition or emergency as a self-contained unit. Knowledge, equipment, skill, and endurance are all necessary for those who will float below this bridge. No reason for alarm, but Clear Fork paddlers should definitely realize that Burnt Mill bridge marks the boundary for casual floating experiences.

Big South Fork of the Cumberland River

The Big South Fork Gorge

The Big South Fork Gorge is part of the headwaters of the Big South Fork of the Cumberland River. Consisting of almost continuous Class III and IV whitewater, the run begins at the confluence of the Clear Fork and New Rivers about 12 miles southwest of Oneida and ends at Leatherwood Ford west of Oneida. In all there are 13 major rapids and several dozen smaller ones. Since there are no roads to the confluence, you might choose to put in on Clear Creek or run the New River.

The New River forms the primary drainage for Scott County in northern Tennessee as it flows west to join the Clear Fork River to form the Big South Fork of the Cumberland River. Runnable below the US 27 bridge (A') to late May, the New River winds placidly through a deep, wooded valley, working its way around rocks or over small ledges and shoals for the first five and a half miles. Then, as the New begins to drop down to its confluence with the Clear Fork, the gradient picks up and several Class II and III ledges are encountered in quick succession. The kicker for this run is that it is part of a package deal; when you run the New River, you get the Class III and IV Big South Fork Gorge thrown in at no extra charge. When you reach the mouth of the New, there is no place to go except down the gorge. This turns the reasonably friendly little eight-mile zip down the New into a rowdy, 16-mile expedition on one of the toughest stretches of whitewater in Tennessee.

If your interest is primarily in the Big South Fork Gorge, an alternative way of getting there is down the Clear Fork River from the Burnt Mill bridge put-in (A). Many veterans of both routes prefer the Clear Fork since they wish to avoid the silt and the acid-mine drainage that pollute the New.

The Big South Fork was once considered by many to be a decked-boat-only river, but the Gorge is now run successfully by both solo and tandem open boaters. The nature of the run varies widely with water level. It is extremely technical at lower water and big and pushy (much like the New River Gorge in West Virginia) when flowing high. At moderate levels the paddler gets a taste of both worlds with quick, technical water on the Clear Fork and bigger, less technical water below the confluence of the Clear Fork and the New River.

Scenery is magnificent, when you have time to notice it. Boulders line the banks and canyon walls rise on both sides. For a Class III (IV) river, the Big South Fork Gorge is surprisingly free of dangers; deadfalls and logjams are infrequent and the holes are washouts at almost all levels. The drops, however, are huge (several exceeding four feet), and helmets are a must for all paddlers. Also, some of the rapids are extremely long, making rescue difficult (especially at higher water levels). Extra flotation is essential for open canoes and a good roll is definitely recommended for decked boaters. Access at the

Section: Burnt Mill bridge (on Clear Fork River) to Leatherwood Ford
County: Scott
USGS Quads: Oneida South, Honey Creek
Difficulty: Class III–IV
Gradient: 19.44 feet per mile
Average Width: 35–70 feet
Velocity: Moderate to fast
Rescue Index: Remote to extremely remote
Hazards: Undercut rocks, difficult rapids
Scouting: At major rapids
Portages: Routes around major rapids are extremely difficult
Scenery: Exceptionally beautiful to spectacular
Highlights: Scenery, wildlife, whitewater, geology
Gauge: US Army Corps of Engineers, (800) 261-5033

Runnable Water Level	Minimum	Maximum
(intermediates)	400 cfs	2,000 cfs
(advanced)		6,000+ cfs

Additional Information: TVA Hotline in Tennessee, (800) 362-9250; in other Southeastern states (800) 251-9242; outside of the Southeast, (615) 632-4100

Big South Fork Gorge of the Cumberland River • Tennessee & Kentucky

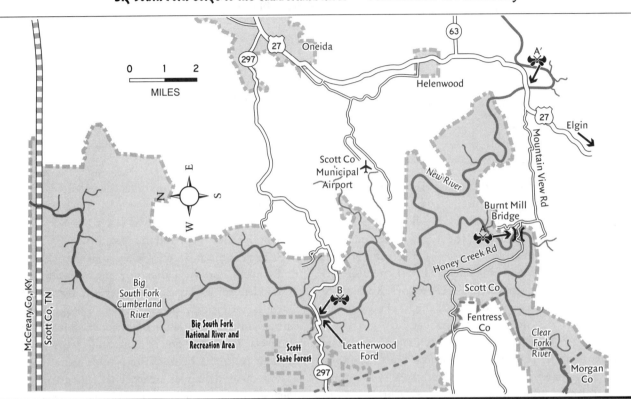

river is good at both put-in and take-out (B), but connecting roads are sometimes muddy and slippery. The Big South Fork Gorge is runnable from late Fall to mid-May in years of average rainfall.

Leatherwood Ford to Lake Cumberland

Flowing out of Scott County (Tennessee), the Big South Fork of the Cumberland River flows north from Leatherwood Ford (B) through McCreary County (Kentucky) before emptying into Lake Cumberland (E). One of the most popular canoe-camping runs in the southeastern United States, the Big South Fork winds through the heart of the Big South Fork National River and Recreation Area in Tennessee. An exceptionally beautiful river flowing swiftly below exposed rock pinnacles, the Big South Fork is dotted with huge boulders both midstream and along the banks, and is padded along either side by steep hillsides of hardwoods and evergreens. Wildflowers brighten the vista in the spring and wildlife is plentiful.

Paddling is interesting with as many as five legitimate (and six borderline) Class II rapids (some of them quite long) consisting primarily of nontechnical small ledges and standing waves. The main channel is easily dis-

cerned in these rapids and scouting is normally not required. At moderate to low water all the Class IIs can be run with a loaded boat. At higher water, loaded, open boats can avail themselves of sneak routes to avoid swamping.

Two Class III–IV rapids are encountered on this section of the Big South Fork. Both are technical, complex, high-velocity chutes that are dangerous at certain water levels. First is Angel Falls, 1.5 miles into the run, where the river takes an eight-foot drop in closely spaced one- and two-foot increments with the main flow forced between two large rocks toward the right of the river. After the first two ledges (normally run from the left), converging smaller chutes of water join the main flow from the right, further aerating the water and causing the current to impact a large boulder to the left. A smaller boulder at the bottom of the rapid, in conjunction with the converging currents from the right, causes the current to turn left at the end of the rapid before pooling out. This rapid must be scouted and different strategies are appropriate at different water levels (though Angel Falls is usually run far left to left center to right center). Regardless of water level, boats should be emptied of all gear before attempting the run. Portage is possible via a

Big South Fork of the Cumberland River • Tennessee and Kentucky

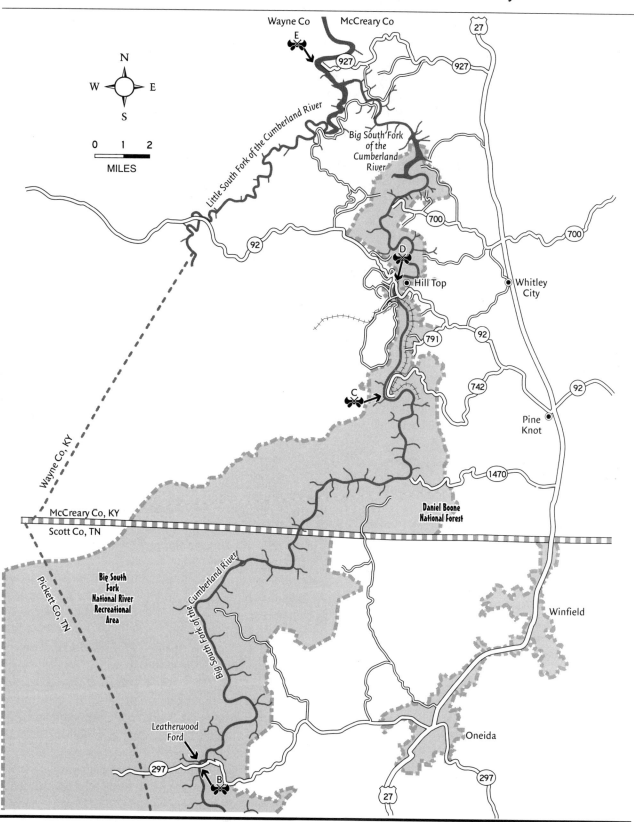

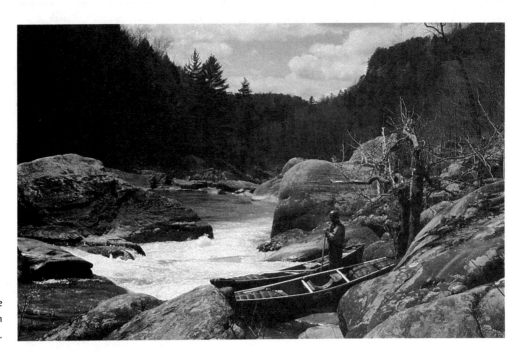

A beautiful clear day above Double Falls on the Big South Fork. Photo by Ed Grove.

trail on the right 50 yards upstream of the rapid and is highly recommended at all water levels except for competent, experienced boaters. (Why trash your boat in the first two miles of a weekend canoe-camping trip?) Canoes have been wedged for weeks at that 90-degree left turn in

Section: Leatherwood Ford to Lake Cumberland (KY)
Counties: Scott (TN), McCreary (KY)
USGS Quads: Oneida South, Oneida North (TN); Earthen, Nevelsville, Burnside (KY)
Difficulty: Class II (III–IV)
Gradient: 6.82 feet per mile
Average Width: 55–80 feet (A–C); 100–150 feet (C–D)
Velocity: Moderate to fast
Rescue Index: Extremely remote
Hazards: Flash flooding, undercut rocks, keeper hydraulics, difficult rapids, concrete ford
Scouting: At Angel Falls and Devils Jump
Portages: Angel Falls and Devils Jump, except for advanced paddlers; concrete ford between Blue Heron and Yamacraw
Scenery: Beautiful to exceptionally beautiful
Highlights: Scenery, wildlife, whitewater
Gauge: U.S. Army Corps of Engineers, (800) 261-5033

Runnable Level	Minimum	Maximum
	350 cfs	Up to flood stage

Additional Information: TVA Water Resources, (423) 632-6065; National Park Service, (423) 879-4890

the Angel Falls chute due to small miscalculations by even expert canoeists. Most of the other expert canoeists choose to portage.

Devils Jump, a difficult Class IV rapid, is closer to the end of the run, upstream from the Blue Heron Mine. Here, current flows into a house-sized boulder and is diverted at an angle through a high-velocity chute. The trick is to align your boat for the chute by riding the pillow off the left of that boulder. This is done at low to moderate water levels by practically setting your bow on a collision course for the giant boulder and then allowing the pillow to divert your bow into the top of the chute. The route to the right of the giant boulder is usually avoided because of a mean hydraulic at the bottom. Once again, all boats should be run without gear and after careful scouting (if you do not understand the dynamics of converging currents, leave this rapid alone). Portage is possible and is recommended at all water levels except for competent, experienced boaters.

The Big South Fork is runnable from late fall through early June in this section. Because of the scouting required, and so on, it is not recommended that the Big South Fork from Leatherwood Ford downstream be attempted in one day. Several nice camping locations are available along the run (which can be lengthened to three or more days by continuing on down into Lake Cumberland). Between Leatherwood and Devils Jump, the river averages eighty to 100 feet and settles down conspicuously with fewer rapids in evidence. Downstream from

Yamacraw the current comes to a halt as it reaches the lake pool. Dangers to navigation are as described above plus a damaged concrete ford between Blue Heron and Yamacraw that must be portaged on the right, and the potential of the river to rise at an alarming rate after heavy rains (remember this when you set up camp). Because of the remoteness of the Big South Fork, access points are few and far between with connecting roads often unpaved and rugged (but generally passable in a passenger car).

The Obed-Emory River System

Tennessee's only National Wild and Scenic River—but a river that does the national system proud! With the type of cascading, clean, clear water almost nonexistent in the populated eastern United States, this deeply cut, free-flowing river system is a statewide favorite for whitewater canoeing in season. Through a quirk of political boundaries, only half of the Obed-Emory system is nationally designated, but of that half, a full 42 of the 44 protected miles qualify as "wild," the highest wilderness classification. And wilderness canoeing it is!

The Obed-Emory, in Cumberland and Morgan Counties, is a major drainage of the northern half of Tennessee's Cumberland Plateau, a wear-resistant sandstone remnant of prehistoric marine geology. Over the eons, the streams in the area have only cut narrow defiles in the hard sandstone caprock. These waterways are now noted for their steep-sided "gorge" topography. As the streams carved their narrow ways, large boulders tumbled off the undercut gorge walls, often landing in the water's flow. The natural pool–drop, descending-elevation whitewater became even more interesting as blind passages, undercut rocks, and tricky crosscurrents were added.

The Obed-Emory is technical whitewater—not of the pushy variety where enough cresting waves will finally swamp your canoe, but rather of the water-reading-required variety where a lack of skillful, multidirectional maneuvering will leave your canoe plastered all over the front of some stream-splitting sandstone. But do not despair. On your (long) hike out, while climbing through some hard-found break in the nearly continuous gorge-wall rimrock, if you pause and look back at the view, you'll note the incredible beauty of this undisturbed natural wilderness. The combination of high rainfall, sheltered canyons, and general inaccessibility has produced a lush forest with excellent second growth and possibly some virgin forest. Huge hemlocks and white pines vie with the ever-present streamside rhododendron and mountain laurel to command your attention.

The same riverway boulders that alter the canoeist's downstream run also support lush lichens, mosses, and ferns. With such abundant and fertile flora comes a similar abundance of fauna. In fact, a large part of the Obed-Emory system lies within a state game preserve, the Catoosa Wildlife Management Area. Deer, turkeys, hawks, bobcats, rattlesnakes, and copperheads all inhabit the area. Undoubtedly, you'll see one of the above on your sojourn in the area. Just remember, this river system is free-flowing! A rainfall pushes the flow rates up within hours, but within days of a sudden storm, the water has completely passed by. Check the water's flow at put-in and take note of incipient weather. Don't expect much canoeing opportunity in the long, dry months late in the season, but if you hit it right, you've got it all going for you: exciting whitewater, beautiful scenery, and a taste of the primeval wilderness.

Clear Creek

Clear Creek (US 127, A to Obed River, F) is probably the most favored whitewater in the Obed-Emory system. It forms the boundary between Cumberland and Fentress Counties before entering Morgan County and its confluence with the Obed River. The creek begins narrow and intimate for floaters who put in at the US 127 bridge. Blow-down obstructions and other pastoral hazards might be found in the early stages of this high-on-the-watershed float.

Sharp-eyed canoeists will note that the farther they float, the deeper the stream cuts into the terrain. Creek-side banks become bluffs. The meandering stream gains a stronger, swifter character, and outside intrusions cease. It's 20 miles to the next bridge, with numerous Class II drops along the way. Twenty miles is too far for a single-day whitewater trip, so you are challenged to direct a camping gear–laden canoe through the shoals and rapids.

Two Class III rapids are found in this upper section, but they are easy to portage. By the time you reach the

Clear Creek • Tennessee

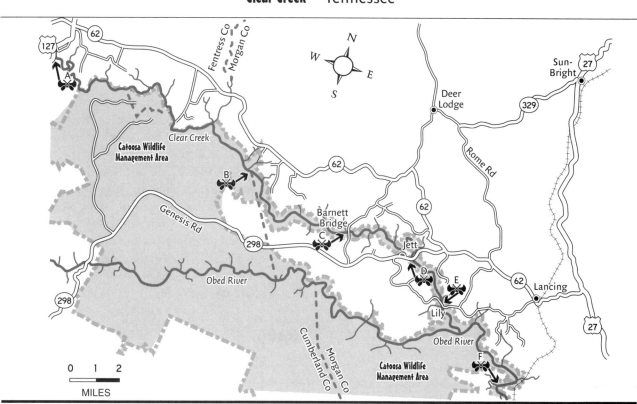

site where Burkhardt's concrete cabin stood in a previous decade (downstream left at river mile 15), you'll be within the boundaries of the national system. Along the big pool at the cabin site, an old logging road (B) can be found on the left bank flood plain. This road connects to the ancient Norris Ford Road (just downstream), which is now a four-wheel-drive-plus, washed-out creekway that offers the first (emergency) vehicular access since the US 127 bridge.

Down at about mile nine you come to a major access, Barnett bridge (C, also called Waltman Ford bridge), but before you get there you have to get past Double Drop Falls. This Class III rapid is commonly portaged when you're loaded with camping gear. At the Barnett bridge access area, White Creek enters the stream from river left and almost doubles the flow. Shed your camping gear and enjoy the brisk five-mile run to Jett bridge. This particular segment of Clear Creek has the longest paddling season; it can still be run when the rest is too low. It's also the best introduction to the Obed-Emory system in the entire watershed. It's got beautiful scenery, solid Class II rapids, and reasonable access to the bridges.

If you've piloted your craft without mishap to Jett (D), then you're ready for the short, snappy, renowned Jett-to-Lilly (E) run. Probably more canoes float this short, two-and-a-half-mile run than any other section in the system. It's a delightful hour in your life. The clean waters of Clear Creek (the best water quality in the entire river system) playfully jump, funnel, and splash while your canoe bounces, rocks, and rolls on down the 20-foot-per-mile gradient. An obvious discontinuity in the river gives notice that you're approaching The Grunch, named after the sound the aft end of your canoe makes after the rest of your craft clears that pushy, three-foot waterfall. Around the bend is the Washing Machine, always operating on its spin-dry cycle. And those are just preludes for Lilly Rapids just upstream of the take-out at Lilly bridge.

Lilly is the longest rapid on this section and allows the canoeist opportunity to show off for the spectators on the bridge. There is no more access below Lilly bridge, but there are still one and a half miles of Clear Creek before its confluence with the Obed. But those one and a half miles drop at 67.3 feet per mile—dangerous by anyone's ratings. Jacks Rock Falls, Camel Rock, and Wootens Folly are three mean Class IVs in rapid succession. Good, high-quality, whitewater canoes have been torn to shreds by this trio. And still there's more. In fact, you can see the waters of the Obed and still be eaten alive by the last big,

Section: US 127 Bridge to Obed River

Counties: Fentress, Morgan, Cumberland

USGS Quads: Herbertsburg, Lancing, Clarkrange, Jones Knob, Pilot Mountain

Difficulty: Class II (III, IV)

Gradient: 18 feet per mile (A–E); 67 feet per mile (E–F)

Average Width: 20 feet

Velocity: Moderate to fast

Rescue Index: Remote

Hazards: Deadfalls, strainers, flash flooding, undercut rocks, difficult rapids

Scouting: As water level requires

Portages: As water level requires; at Double Drop above Barnett; below Lilly at major rapids

Scenery: Spectacular

Highlights: Scenery, wildlife, whitewater, geology

Gauge: TVA, (423) 632-2264 or (800) 238-2264

Runnable Water Level	Minimum	Maximum
A–C	1,500 cfs	6,000 cfs
C–D	800 cfs	4,000 cfs
D–E	1,000 cfs	5,000 cfs
E–F	1,200 cfs	4,000 cfs

Months runnable: December through April

Additional Information: TVA Water Resources, (423) 632-6065; Obed Wild and Scenic River National Park Office, (423) 346-6295

offset double drop in an unnamed rapid just above the confluence. Canoeing below Lilly is for well-experienced paddlers following normal safety procedures and paddling in groups with a minimum of three craft.

The next convenient take-out (and the next bridge crossing) is at Nemo bridge (F) on the Emory River (just past the Obed-Emory confluence), 7.1 miles downstream from Lilly. So don't set off lightly to view the Clear Creek confluence or you just might end your float with a hike. At the Obed–Clear Creek confluence a trail scales the end of the point of land that separates the two rivers; on Clear Creek look to the right just before the confluence. Start climbing the talus slope on the end of the point and you'll intersect the trail at the base of the bluff caprock. It's a tough chug as you steeply ascend 450 feet, but the trail does wind up through the caprock and onto a ridgeway dirt road heading toward the rural settlements. Take care of your own problems if possible; the people out there are hard-pressed enough with their own survival.

Daddys Creek

This creek has no middle ground. Starting in northeastern Cumberland County and flowing into Morgan County, you'll find pastoral, easy floating in the upper reaches and terrifying, dangerous whitewater below. If there is plenty of water in the system, you might have enough flow for the meandering float from Big Lick (A) to

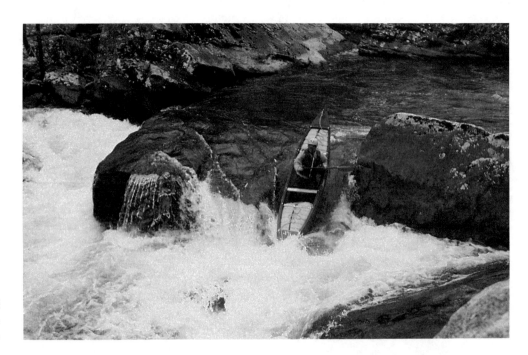

Running Fang Falls on Daddys Creek. Photo by Ed Grove.

Section: Big Lick to Antioch Bridge

County: Cumberland

USGS Quads: Dorton, Herbertsburg, Ozone, Grassy Cove,
Vandever

Difficulty: Class I–II

Gradient: 11 feet per mile

Average Width: 20 feet

Velocity: Moderate to fast

Rescue Index: Remote

Hazards: Strainers, dam at Linary

Scouting: None required

Portages: Dam at Linary

Scenery: Beautiful in spots

Highlights: Scenery, wildlife, local culture and industry

Gauge: TVA Water Resources, (423) 632-6065

Runnable Water Level	Minimum	Maximum
Oakdale gauge	1,000 cfs	4,000 cfs

Months Runnable: November through March

Additional Information: Obed Wild and Scenic River National
Park Office, (423) 346-6295

Linary (B). Portage the dam at Linary (just above TN 28) and continue your placid way to Meridian (C), US 70 (D), and Center bridges (E). You'll see evidences of mining and farming all along the way. At times the land forms close in and you penetrate some shallow canyons.

Below Center bridge the gradient picks up and your canoeing becomes more serious. Take out at the Antioch bridge (F). Don't boat below this bridge until you've hiked the three miles of Daddys Creek below the Yellow Creek confluence to scout the action. Here you'll see the distorted piles of massive boulders that torture the streamway (not to mention the boater), and Class IV and V rapids set in a drop of 100 feet per mile amid the pounding and crashing water. Not only are there dangerous undercut rocks in this section, but in one place you'll find an undercut bluff that's probably the single most dangerous spot in the entire Obed-Emory system. Portage in many cases is difficult to impossible. (It's hard to climb a house-sized boulder with a boat on your back). This is the most difficult and hazardous section of the entire system, but the scenery is outstanding.

About a mile below this "Daddys Creek Canyon" is the Devils Breakfast Table bridge (G) and the boundary for the national system. This bridge is a put-in for the lower Obed run with the last two and a half miles of Daddys Creek being extremely scenic and the water a solid Class II. You then come to Obed Junction and will probably

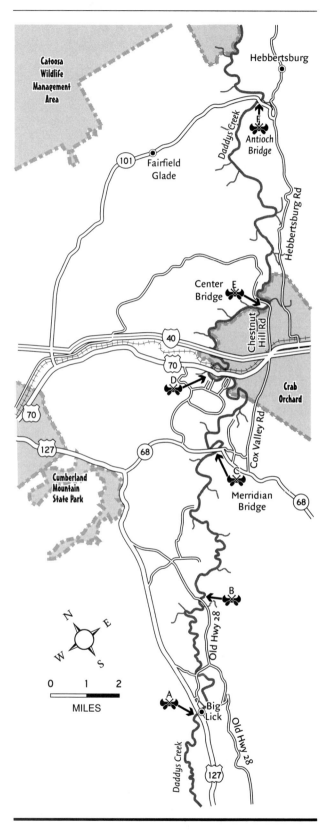

Daddys Creek • Tennessee

Section: Antioch Bridge to Devils Breakfast Table Bridge

Counties: Cumberland, Morgan

USGS Quad: Herbertsburg

Difficulty: Class III–V

Gradient: 46 feet per mile (one mile of 100 feet per mile)

Average Width: 20 feet

Velocity: Fast

Rescue Index: Remote

Hazards: Undercut rocks, keeper hydraulics, difficult rapids

Scouting: Frequent, as needed

Portages: At undercut bluff a half-mile below Yellow Creek; as
   water level requires

Scenery: Spectacular

Highlights: Scenery, wildlife, whitewater, geology

Gauge: TVA Water Resources, (423) 632-6065

Runnable Water Level	Minimum	Maximum
	1,200 cfs	10,000 cfs

Months runnable: November through March

Additional Information: Obed Wild and Scenic River National
   Park Office, (423) 346-6295

continue on to more taxing paddling on the Obed, or you
can carry out on the four-wheel-drive access road on the
Obed River's left, across from the confluence.

Obed River

The city of Crossville in Cumberland County com-
mands the headwaters of the Obed River. Tributary lakes
and a necessary water plant push canoeists down to the
last available highway access before the river heads off
cross-country towards the Catoosa Wildlife Management
Area. US 127 (A) is a tough, steep put-in, but maybe that's
good, because this upper, upper stretch of the Obed River
features tough, steep rapids. It's a narrow stream up here
and high water readings are required before the run is feasible.

This section of the Obed is called the Goulds Bend
run, and it starts easily and ends placidly, but in the
middle the bottom drops out at 80 feet per mile!
Knucklebuster and Hellhole are Class IV rapids, but the
Esses should be portaged. You can tell the Esses because
the stream makes two sharp, 90-degree turns in opposite
directions, and it looks for all the world as if a 16-foot
canoe couldn't swing that far in those tight spaces. Many
canoeists walk out from this spot in the river. Landowners have posted much of the access at Adams bridge (B),
so be particularly careful during take-out or when parking shuttle cars here.

Daddys Creek • Tennessee

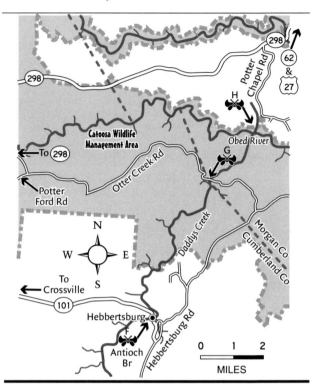

A mile below the bridge the river enters the Catoosa
Wildlife Management Area and simultaneously crosses
the boundary for national designation. Automobiles cannot reach Potters Ford bridge during turkey or deer hunts
(or when the Catoosa is closed for winter road care), so it
is best to check with the Catoosa managers before planning a trip below Adams bridge.

Many solid Class II rapids, with a couple of surprising
Class IIIs thrown in, characterize this extremely scenic
and wild float between Adams bridge and Obed Junction
(D). At 16 miles, this trip is too long for a day trip, and
consequently is probably the least-run section in the system. Obed Junction is actually the confluence of Daddys
Creek and the Obed River and was named at the turn of
the century when an old narrow-gauge logging railroad
used to come down Daddys Creek and turn down the
Obed. The old bridge pilings are still visible at the confluence. There's a four-wheel-drive access road out on the
Obed River's left here. Actually, you can find a trail out
on the river's right just down from the confluence, but it
only leads to a road in the middle of Catoosa that may
not be of much help. Your best bet when forced to leave
the Obed past this point is to try to scale the bluffs on
river's left.

Below Obed Junction you'll enter the wild and woolly
Obed that most floaters talk about. This run usually

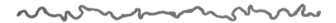

Section: US 127 Bridge to Adams Bridge

County: Cumberland

USGS Quads: Fox Creek, Isoline, Crossville

Difficulty: Class II–III (IV+)

Gradient: 32 feet per mile with 1 mile at 80 feet per mile

Average Width: 25 feet

Velocity: Moderate to fast

Rescue Index: Remote

Hazards: Strainers, undercut rocks, keeper hydraulics, difficult rapids

Scouting: At major rapids

Portages: At Esses rapid

Scenery: Beautiful

Highlights: Scenery, wildlife, whitewater

Gauge: TVA Water Resources, (423) 632-6065

Runnable Water Level	Minimum	Maximum
Emory gauge at Oakdale	3,000 cfs	10,000 cfs

Additional Information: Obed Wild and Scenic River National Park Office, (423) 346-6295

Obed River • Tennessee

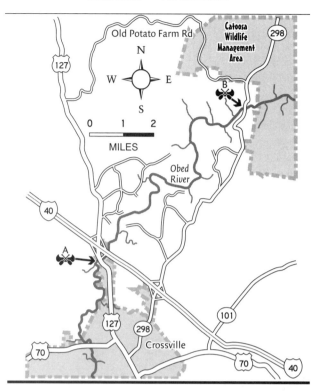

starts either from the four-wheel-drive Obed Junction road or from two miles up Daddys Creek (above the junction) at the Devils Breakfast Table bridge. The run ends 10 miles below the junction, at Nemo bridge (F) on the Emory. The water from Daddys Creek doubles the flow of the Obed, and the river gets pushy as the gorge gets deeper. A rapid called 90-Right/90-Left kind of lets you know what to expect. The next one, Ohmigod!, is very similar but is entered via a blind approach. Sturdy white-water canoes have been ripped to pieces under the rocks

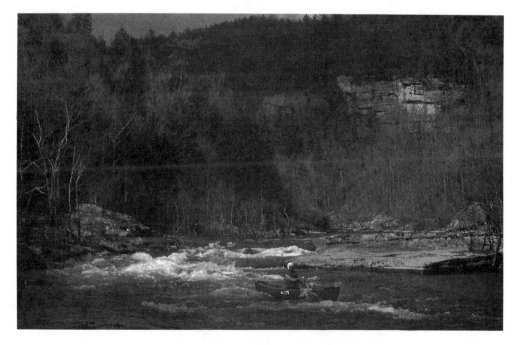

View of the cliffs above the Obed River. Photo by Ed Grove.

Section: Adams bridge to Emory River

Counties: Cumberland, Morgan

USGS Quads: Herbertsburg, Lancing

Difficulty: Class II-III (IV)

Gradient: 14 feet per mile

Average Width: 40 feet

Velocity: Moderate to fast

Rescue Index: Remote

Hazards: Strainers, flash flooding, undercut rocks, difficult rapids

Scouting: At major rapids below Daddys Creek

Portages: At Rockgarden Rapid (mile 5.5)

Scenery: Spectacular

Highlights: Scenery, wildlife, whitewater, geology

Gauge: TVA Water Resources, (615) 632-6065

Runnable Water Level	Minimum	Maximum
Section B–D	1,300 cfs	4,000
Section D–F	600 cfs	5,000

Additional Information: Obed Wild and Scenic River National Park Office, (423) 346-6295

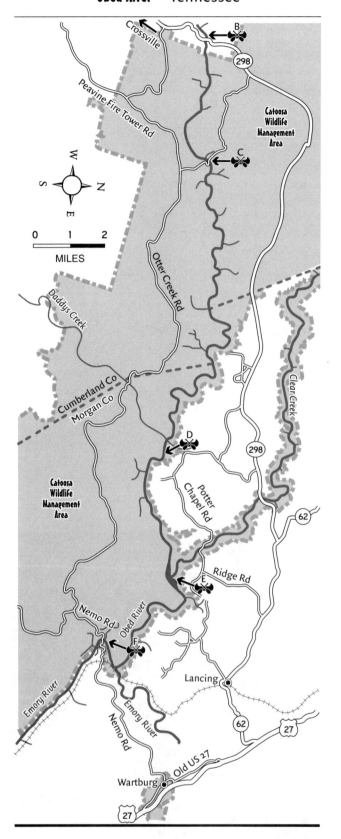

Obed River • Tennessee

during high-water attempts at this rapid. Shortly thereafter, the Class IV Rockgarden rapid has spilled many an expert and has taken a life. Many excellent, experienced canoeists portage Rockgarden.

There follow more narrow drops, more chances for pinned canoes, more opportunities to walk out (remember, to the left). Then you reach Clear Creek junction. A long cascading delta rapid propels you on into Canoe Hole, where an old logging road provides four-wheel-drive-plus access to the river (most people park at the top and portage the quarter mile up or down the bluff).

Beyond this point the canoeing settles down to three great Class II+ rapids in a row followed by the added excitement of The Widowmaker, making a fourth rapid. The river slows down, letting the canoeist marvel at the scenery. A slow pool or two allows time for some relaxing before a large side-wall cut ahead signals the railroad tunnel and tracks running along the Emory. The oversized pool found here is actually the confluence of the Obed with the Emory. The name changes because the river turns 90 degrees; but 90 percent of the water comes down the Obed. Look off to your left in the bend of the river and you'll see a small tributary sneaking in under the ever-present foliage. That's the Emory River and you are now on it.

A frolicking mile of a wider river and some interesting shoals bring you to the take-out and the old iron bridge at

Emory River • Tennessee

Nemo. In May 1973, when Barnett and Lilly bridges washed out on Clear Creek, and Antioch and Devils Breakfast Table bridges washed out on Daddys Creek, the water lapped over the deck on Nemo bridge. It's interesting to think about as you wind up your long, eventful whitewater run.

Emory River

By a quirk of geology, the Emory River retains its name after joining its overgrown "tributary," the Obed River, and continues toward the Clinch River and the big Tennessee River. Upstream, in northeastern Morgan County, the little Emory drains a lovely, covelike valley amid the towering peaks of the Cumberland Mountains. Scenic farmlands on the valley floor are offset by the hardwood flanks of the adjacent mountains. The stream is slow and pastoral near Gobey. You'll also see many traces of past and current strip-mining all along the Emory as this stream penetrates deep into a coal-bearing region of this part of the Appalachians. The Emory is second only to its neighbor the New River (of Tennessee) in the extent of strip-mining in its watershed. You'll note the murky water quality as you float the Emory. You'll also note the active strip mines and the ineffective silt

traps on the more poorly situated ones just before you reach the Obed.

The upper part of the Emory is a pleasant, easy float from under the new US 27 bridge (B) and on to Montgomery bridge (C), where John Muir stayed overnight on his "thousand-mile walk to the sea." Below Montgomery bridge the stream continues its Class I flow for three more miles to where the solid rock riverbed finally begins to break up. At this point the Emory River falls off the Cumberland Plateau.

For two miles, the canoeist drops at 62 feet per mile, crashing between boulders as the narrow stream bounces back and forth in the steep-sided terrain. It is best to run this section at marginal water flows; too much water can push even expert canoeists beyond their skills. Portages are not difficult and are feasible alternatives to some of the dead-end drops, especially at the higher water levels. Interesting abandoned railroad tunnels are visible on both sides of the river toward the end of this canyon. Finally, the railroad bridge over the Emory signals the upcoming confluence with the Obed—a whole different river. It's big and wide and has much more water, and the water quality improves. After a mile of cascading joyrides, the iron bridge of Nemo comes into view. Only this short section of the Emory between the Obed con-

Section: Gobey Bridge to Oakdale

County: Morgan

USGS Quads: Gobey, Camp Austin, Lancing, Harriman

Difficulty: Class I–III (IV)

Gradient: 13.21 feet per mile

Average Width: 20–50 feet

Velocity: Slack to slow

Rescue Index: Accessible but difficult

Hazards: Undercut rocks, difficult rapids

Scouting: At major rapids (above Nemo)

Portages: As water level requires (above Nemo)

Scenery: Beautiful in spots

Highlights: Scenery, wildlife, whitewater, local culture, coal industry, history, geology

Gauge: Oakdale gauge; TVA Water Resources, (615) 632-6065

Runnable Water Level	Minimum	Maximum
Section A–C	10,000+ cfs	NA
Section C–D	300+ cfs	4,000+ cfs

Additional Information: Obed Wild and Scenic River National Park Office, (423) 346-6295

fluence and the Nemo bridge (D) is included in the national system.

Just below the bridge and out of sight around a bend, a Class III rapid awaits. Nemo Rapid is a bouncy double-dip into a plunge-pool recovery basin. This signals the beginning of a nine-mile run to Oakdale, rated Class I and II. You're floating on the combined waters of the entire Obed-Emory system, so the season lasts longer. The river is wider but it channels up as the flow decreases. This section is ideal for the beginning canoeist to try the Obed-Emory experience. The Catoosa Wildlife Management Area is still on the river's right, but a railroad track runs on the river's left (it can be a trail out in emergencies).

The scenery and water remain attractive. Midway, you'll pass under the Camp Austin bridge (E). Several long pools make you complacent before the Class II+ rapids below Camp Austin and Oakdale bridges wake you up again. Take out at the Oakdale bridge. The park-like area around the bend is private property, belonging to one of Oakdale's law enforcement officers; permission to use the area is difficult to obtain. This run is a pleasant, drifting, mountain-scenery run and is almost a relief from the crashing whitewater of the upper Obed stretches. There are about five more free-flowing miles left, then the Emory feeds the clean mountain waters to the tailwaters of Watts Bar Lake on the Clinch and Tennessee Rivers.

Piney Creek

Until popular whitewater canoes got shorter than 14 feet in length, few canoeists had ever floated the narrow, tight Piney Creek in Rhea county. Located on Cumberland Plateau's Walden Ridge escarpment overlooking the great Tennessee River Valley in east Tennessee, this little stream is in rugged, wild, remote terrain—land not suited for human habitation. It's not even fair to request any rescue aid in land like this, and a paddler trying to walk out is just as apt to fall off a 20-foot bluff as to get woefully trapped in the omnipresent rhododendron and laurel thickets. The put-in is on the dead-end, gravel Wash-Pelfrey Road creek crossing and the take-out is 10 miles downstream at Shut-in Gap Road. There is nothing between these two backwoods roads anywhere near this stream except boulders, bluffs, ledges, hemlock, white pine, rhododendron, laurel, and clean, clear water.

Wash-Pelfrey Road is the right fork after Mountain Road out of Evensville, Tennessee, climbs the Walden Ridge escarpment and splits to head off, on the left side, towards Liberty Hill. Shut-in Gap Road is a road climbing that same escarpment directly out of Spring City, Tennessee (not TN 68). Piney Creek runs through a narrow, deep gorge on the ridge above the escarpment. It is a narrow stream with scenic side branches tumbling in as waterfalls all along the way. The float down this creek is rated Class IV and V, mostly suitable for closed craft. You'll find numerous strainers, keepers, and undercut rocks. The portages are difficult and numerous. The run is too long to dally during any of the many scoutings and portages required. Nightfall can easily overtake a large, slow-moving group. High water levels are needed. The only gauge nearby is over on the Tellico River (not in the same watershed, or even in the same mountains), and where it has been found that a Tellico reading of 800 to 1,200 cfs generally provides the level needed to float the Piney.

VIRGINIA

South Fork of the Shenandoah River

The Shenandoah River is legendary throughout the world. In song, story, and among canoeists it is part of the vocabulary of the English-speaking world. The valley through which it flows is synonymous with agricultural richness, and the very name conjures images of pastoral serenity and farm living. For the paddler the Shenandoah offers little in the way of whitewater but provides a beautiful river experience running through a combination of scenic farmland and steep mountain forest. This section of the South Fork from Bixler Bridge to Karo Landing has probably been paddled by more beginning paddlers, as well as veterans, than any other stream. Boy Scouts have baptized their paddles in the South Fork for generations and outing groups of all varieties continue to do so in droves. For any Virginia paddler, a trip down the South Fork of the Shenandoah continues to be an essential part of the Old Dominion experience.

The Shenandoah Valley was beloved by the Native Americans who lived and traveled here before the coming of the Europeans. The valley seems to have been largely used as a hunting ground in the years immediately preceding the arrival of colonists, although remains of pre-colonial villages continue to be found along the South Fork. These villages were very small and tended to revolve around cave dwellings in the limestone cliffs of the valley. The inhabitants of these villages greatly predated the Susquehannock and Catawba tribes of popular legend and were apparently not related culturally or racially to these later Native American groups.

The identity of the first European to see the Shenandoah Valley is a matter of controversy. There is evidence that French Jesuits visited the area before 1632. John Lederer, the early geographer, was certainly there in 1669. The most entertaining account of the early explorations of the valley, however, is that of Virginia Governor Alexander Spotswood and friends in 1716. History records that Spotswood was not much of a geographer or explorer but he certainly knew how to have a good time in the Virginia mountains, a skill still pursued by pad-

dlers. Accompanying Spotswood was the young John Fontaine, ancestor of Matthew Fontaine Maury. His diary records the particulars of the journey. The expedition consisted of many gentlemen of Virginia, along with servants, slaves, women, drovers, and so on, and the party carried with them "Virginia red wine and white wine, Irish uisgebaugh [whiskey], brandy shrub, two sorts of rum, canary punch, cider, etc." (Blair Niles, *The James*, Rivers of America Series, Farrar, Straus & Giroux, 1940). Crossing the Blue Ridge at Swift Run Gap (the present site of US 33), Fontaine says they "all drank the King's health in champagne, and fired a volley . . . the Princess' health in Burgundy, and fired a volley . . . all the rest of

Section: Bixler Bridge to Karo Landing
Counties: Page, Warren
USGS Quads: Luray, Rileyville, Bentonville
Difficulty: Class I-II with one solid Class II (Compton's Rapids)
Gradient: 5 feet per mile
Average Width: 80–150 feet
Velocity: Moderate
Rescue Index: Accessible
Hazards: None
Scouting: Compton's Rapid
Portages: Low-water bridge at Bentonville Landing, three-fourths through the trip
Scenery: Beautiful
Highlights: Scenery, wildlife, history
Gauge: National Weather Service gauge recording, (703) 260-0305

Runnable Water Levels	Minimum	Maximum
	1.2 feet	3.5 feet

Months Runnable: Year-round except for unusually dry summers
Additional Information: There are a number of canoe outfitters active in the area; one is Shenandoah River Outfitters, (540) 743-4159

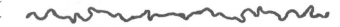

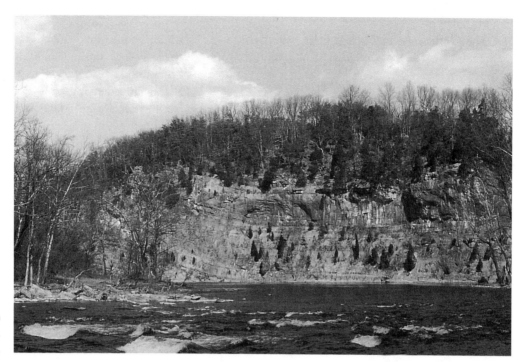

Cliffs overlooking Compton Rapid on the Shenandoah. Photo by Ed Grove.

the Royal Family in Claret, and fired a volley . . . then the Governor's health, and fired a volley." Thus was established the honorable tradition of guns and booze at Appalachian mountain parties, which continues to this day. The Governor's expedition did little to further the cartographic knowledge of the valley but it did draw attention to it as a site of future development. After his expedition, German, Dutch, and Scottish immigrants from Pennsylvania began settling in the valley of the Shenandoah. The names of their descendants are still evident on the mailboxes along Route 11 and other roads in the valley.

During the Civil War the Shenandoah Valley was of critical importance to both sides. The farms of the valley provided a large portion of the food necessary to keep the Confederate troops operating, and the strategic location of the valley meant that an army could easily threaten Washington, DC. As a result, the valley was the site of constant fighting throughout the war. The most famous of the campaigns fought there was Stonewall Jackson's campaign in the spring of 1862. Jackson tied up Federal armies of several times his own strength, weakening the Union attempt to take Richmond and keeping the federal leadership in constant anxiety for the safety of the northern capital. Later in the war, when Confederate fortunes began to sink, Union General Philip Sheridan was charged with reducing the valley to such an extent that "a crow flying over the valley would have to carry his own rations" (Mark M. Boatner, *The Civil War Dic-*

tionary, David McKay, 1959). Following a scorched-earth policy, Sheridan destroyed every barn, burned every crop, and killed animals throughout the length and breadth of the valley, causing great hardship among the inhabitants. When, as predicted by Stonewall Jackson, the valley was destroyed, so went the Confederacy.

The present-day paddler on the Shenandoah will see things much as they might have been before the Civil War, with the addition of the occasional concrete bridge, power line, and tractor. The business of the land—farming—takes place in much the same area it did in earlier years. Some of the fields have been plowed within the same fencerows for generations. The river contains numerous fish dams built by Native Americans. These structures, only visible at low water, are V-shaped arrangements of rocks pointing downstream. Some paddlers grumble about running man-made rapids, but who can be offended by a ripple produced by a thousand-year-old pile of cobbles? It is interesting to think that the stones placed so laboriously by hand long ago now bear the multicolor streaks scraped off the aluminum and plastic pleasure craft of today.

This trip on the magnificent Shenandoah is generally not a whitewater trip. Paddlers can pick which put-in and take-out they want in order to shorten or lengthen a trip. The only rapid of any significance is Compton's Rapids, encountered 17 miles from the put-in at Bixler Bridge. This drop is a Class II drop with nice standing waves at the bottom, the height of which increases with higher

South Fork of the Shenandoah River • Virginia

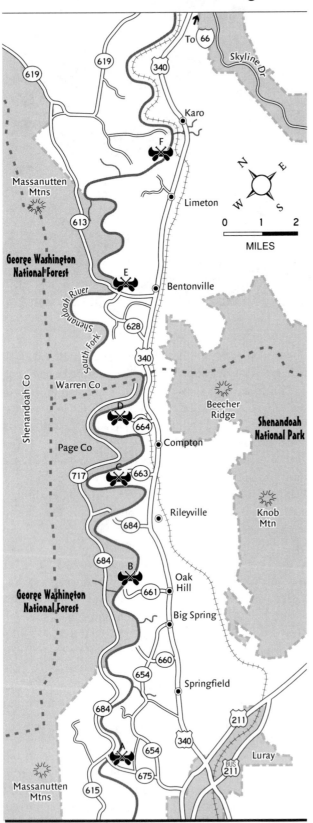

water levels. Compton's is recognized from upstream by a high, golden rock wall that appears to block the stream ahead and by the unusually loud rumble of the rapids. Compton's is not dangerous at reasonable levels but it has swamped many open canoes and soaked a lot of clothing and gear. Make sure everything is battened down before running this drop.

The balance of this stretch of the South Fork consists of widely spaced tiny ledges and ancient fish dams, beautiful vistas of the Blue Ridge and Massanutten Mountains, and relaxed paddling. The river is a sterling example of a geologically mature stream and it meanders back and forth between the above-named ridges. As a result, the view and the orientation of the light is constantly changing, and the paddler is presented with a feast of visual entertainment alternating between steep forested slopes, limestone cliffs, cow pastures, and shady bowers between sandy islands.

Camping is possible in many places along the river, although the "No Trespassing" signs proliferate more and more each year. If there is any doubt as to whether camping is permitted in a particular spot it would be wise to locate the nearest farmhouse and inquire. The river is heavily used in this area and littering is a severe problem for some of the landowners; therefore, protect the relationship between paddlers and landowners by utilizing courtesy, discretion, and a large trash bag.

Ten miles below Compton's Rapids a low-water bridge appears that will probably require a short portage. This bridge at Bentonville Landing signals the final quarter of the trip, as Karo Landing is just nine miles below. Karo Landing, on Gooney Run, is not marked by bridge or other unmistakable landmark so be sure to study it while running the shuttle to ensure that it will be recognized from the river.

Passage Creek

The southern part of the Shenandoah Valley is bisected by the intimidating massif of the Massanutten Mountains. From Harrisonburg to Strasburg the Massanutten holds apart the respective valleys of the North and South Forks of the Shenandoah until Strasburg, where the North Fork abandons its northeasterly course and turns east to join the South Fork near Front Royal. From the floor of either valley the Massanutten appears as an abrupt, even-topped wall separating the lowlands surrounding it. A look at a map, however, reveals that the Massanutten is itself cleaved throughout its northern half by the defile of Passage Creek. As Passage Creek tumbles from its high repose in the Fort Valley to join the North Fork of the Shenandoah it briefly becomes a cascading torrent that will delight the whitewater paddler.

Only slightly over an hour from Washington, DC, Passage Creek rewards the paddler with clear water, easy access, towering cliffs and rock formations, rhododendron thickets, and tight, intricate rapids. There is a price, however, and that price is an ever-changing maze of fallen trees in the lower part of the run. Fortunately the worst part of this labyrinth is in relatively calm water so it is more of an inconvenience than a death trap, as it might be otherwise. Route 678 follows the creek throughout the length of the trip (although it occasionally wanders some distance from the stream), so rescue or a walk-out will not be a disaster.

Section: Elizabeth Furnace Picnic Area to Route 55

Counties: Shenandoah, Warren

USGS Quad: Strasburg

Difficulty: Class II–III at moderate levels; Class III–IV at high levels

Gradient: 40 feet per mile average; 60 feet per mile in steepest section

Average Width: 20–45 feet

Velocity: Fast

Rescue Index: Accessible

Hazards: Possible logjams, strainers, fishermen, dam

Scouting: Scouting from road possible for most rapids except Out-of-Sight Rapids need scouting

Portages: Dam at fish hatchery, probably some logjams to carry around

Scenery: Beautiful

Highlights: Whitewater, scenery

Gauge: National Weather Service gauge recording, (703) 260-0305

Runnable Water Levels	Minimum	Maximum
Route 55 gauge	0.5 feet	3.5 feet
Cootes Store Gauge	3.3 feet	6 feet

Additional Information: None

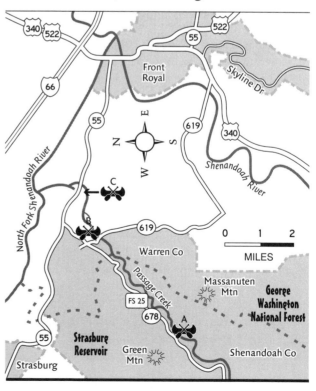

Passage Creek • Virginia

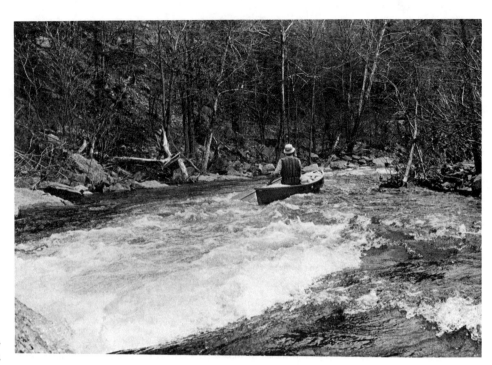

Ed Grove on Passage Creek.
Photo by Bill Kirby.

Passage Creek meanders along peacefully over a sandy bottom in the miles above the Elizabeth Furnace Recreation Area. Upon reaching the picnic area (A), however, the mountain closes in on both sides and the creek begins to head downhill. If putting in at the picnic area, the paddler is treated to a swift current and occasional Class I–II gravel bars and rock gardens for a mile or so. Soon the good stuff begins, with a Class II–III ledge series where the creek closely approaches the road. The stream continues dropping at a rapid pace through ledges for a few hundred yards. When it turns away from the road to the right and a high rock wall appears on the right bank, Out-of-Sight Rapids is fast approaching. A scout from the bank will be in order here, especially if you are not following a paddler familiar with the route through this rather complicated drop.

At higher levels some good surfing waves appear part way through the series. The eddies are small, however, and a flip could put the boat against some angry rocks, as the distance between the individual ledges is very short. Out-of-Sight is followed by another Class II–III ledge series and then the creek turns back against the road. Against a masonry wall supporting the road on the left is a series of entertaining ledges. Soon the fish hatchery dam is reached, a six-foot-high weir. The right side of the dam looks like the proper portage route but this is not the case! Years of paddlers walking over this area have severely eroded the soil there and portaging on the right

side of the dam is prohibited. Carry on the left side with care. Very experienced boaters have run the left side at moderate levels and using appropriate safety precautions. In high water beware of the flow going over the dam.

Below the hatchery dam the stream begins to flow with a decreased gradient and the load of rock rubble and timber carried by the creek through the steep section above is deposited. Passage Creek divides around numerous small islands and between these islands there may be tangles of fallen trees, debris, and branches. Use extreme care when choosing which route to run between the islands and always be prepared to get to shore quickly. The route through this maze can change after high water, so the paddler must use care in negotiating the puzzle. However, there currently is a way to miss most of this maze. Near its beginning, look for a small channel to the left. If you take this channel, it will slowly grow larger until the creek fully collects itself at the end of this puzzle. Don't try to run this tangle on the right; if you do, the channel will get smaller and smaller until you are enmeshed in a maze of small channels.

Below the jackstraw pile the creek flows swiftly between wooded banks until the Route 55 bridge (C) at Waterlick heaves into view. Just above Route 55 is a man-made ledge that forms a grabby hole at certain levels. Between the ledge and Route 55 bridge is the river right take-out on a secondary road. Route 55 is a heavily used truck route so be cautious if you walk on it. The paddling gauge is on the left upstream abutment of the Route 55 bridge.

Passage Creek is a heavily fished trout stream, stocked, as one would expect, from the hatchery at the exit from the steep section. Trout fishing is allowed for the entire season, and we highly recommend prudence in paddling during early spring because of the many fishermen using Passage Creek then. A high-speed collision with a wading fisherman could be a disaster in both the physical and public relations areas especially because there could be many fishermen standing by in the event of a mishap.

For those with a propensity for hiking, a trip to Signal Knob via the Signal Knob Trail will certainly be worthwhile. The trail begins at a small parking area off the road on the west side of the canyon near the Elizabeth Furnace campground and leads to a prominent peak used as an observation post by both sides during the Civil War. The Massanutten Trail heads south from the fish hatchery and follows the crest of Massanutten Mountain all the way to Route 33 east of Harrisonburg. This entire area lies within the George Washington National Forest, which is a public hunting area, so wear bright clothing when hiking during hunting season and don't have a white handkerchief hanging out of your back pocket.

Passage Creek is located between Front Royal and Strasburg on State Route 55. From I-66, go south on Route 340 toward Front Royal and go right (west) on Route 55 for about five miles. The creek is crossed a half mile before the left turn onto Route 678.

Other streams in the area include Cedar Creek, flowing into the North Fork from the north nearby; the South Fork of the Shenandoah to the south; and the Lost River just over the West Virginia line to the west.

Potomac River

The Potomac River forms the northern border of Virginia, separating the Old Dominion from Maryland and the District of Columbia. Throughout the history of the United States the Potomac has functioned as an important waterway for communication and commerce as well as a barrier to the many foreign and domestic military forces that have campaigned in this area. In recent years the Potomac has found new duties as a premier recreational area for the millions that live in the region. Whitewater paddling is the most recent of these activities, but the old river has proven to be a superlative location for the enjoyment of this sport.

The Potomac and its tributaries provide whitewater of all degrees of difficulty throughout its length, from the small headwater streams of West Virginia and western Maryland, through the Blue Ridge at Harpers Ferry, and across the piedmont between the mountains and the coast. The most heavily used section, however, is the stretch between Great Falls and the tidal estuary at Washington, DC, discussed below. This area has access to the river in many spots. The C & O Canal follows the river on the Maryland shore between Washington and Cumberland, Maryland, and provides public access and parking at many locations. The Virginia side of the river is almost entirely in private ownership and public access is rare.

Between Great Falls and Washington the most important access points are Great Falls, Maryland, and Old Anglers Inn (B and C, respectively; both on MacArthur Boulevard), Carderock (D), and Lockhouse number 10 and Lockhouse number 6 (E and F, respectively; both on the Clara Barton Parkway). All of these points are accessible via the Capital Beltway (I-495) at the Clara Barton Parkway exit. The comparable road on the Virginia side of the river is the George Washington Memorial Parkway, but that provides no access to the river. The original plan called for the parkways to be joined by a bridge at Great Falls but fortunately this plan was scrapped, due in large part to the efforts of the late Supreme Court Chief Justice William O. Douglas.

Along the northern border of Virginia lies the largest rapid in the state and one of the largest runnable rapids anywhere. This drop was named by the earliest colonists and through the centuries has retained the designation given to it by them: the Great Falls of the Potomac.

The Falls are created where the Potomac, like all other rivers that flow eastward into the Atlantic, drops over the edge of the continental bedrock onto the sedimentary soil of the Coastal Plain. The fall line proper is actually located farther downstream, at Roosevelt Island in the estuary between Rosslyn, Virginia, and the District of Columbia. The entire section of the river between this spot and the Great Falls, a distance of some nine miles, is a result of the headward (i.e., upstream) erosion of the riverbed by the stream. The present location of the falls represents the latest manifestation of this unending process. All of the downstream rapids (Observation Deck Rapids, S-Turn Rapids, Rocky Island Rapids, Wet Bottom Chute, Difficult Run Rapids, Yellow Falls, Stubblefield Falls, and Little Falls) are the locations of particularly resistant strata of rock, where the falls may have once paused in their slow but inexorable upstream migration. The present-day Great Falls of the Potomac display the steepest and most spectacular fall-line rapid of any on the eastern rivers.

Before beginning a description of the Great Falls section it must be pointed out most emphatically that this area is extremely hazardous. The dangers are high. The most advanced paddlers in the country examined these drops for years before the first attempt was made. Although the passage of many years since has increased the number of paddlers completing the run, it has not decreased the objective hazards presented by these falls, as proven by the hundreds of documented deaths that have occurred here. No one should attempt such a run without the highest degree of skill and confidence, particularly a very fast and sure roll and previous experience in vertical waterfall running. Most important, a newcomer should only paddle the falls with someone who has previously completed a successful run; the choice of the wrong route would almost certainly be fatal.

Finally, the park rangers who administer the land on both shores request that runs be made before 9 A.M. and preferably on weekdays to avoid a public spectacle and the encouragement of unqualified individuals to emulate the paddlers they see but don't understand. A run that turns into a circus or results in a death or costly rescue operation by the National Park Service would almost surely cause the law- and rule-makers to close this incredible resource to those who are best able to appreciate it.

The Potomac flows along lazily all of the way from Harpers Ferry, some 35 miles upstream, across the piedmont with only the lightest riffles disturbing its placid, green surface. Seneca Breaks, five miles upstream from the falls, marks briefly the new sentiment of the river but the Potomac resumes its pastoral quality below Seneca. Only four miles from the Capital Beltway and without further prelude the river drops over the Great Falls Dam, a six-foot stone structure built in the 1850s to provide drinking water for the District of Columbia. The structure still serves in its original capacity, the water thus stored is pumped by gravity through the aqueduct running under the equally aged MacArthur Boulevard into the city. The Potomac pools briefly below the dam and then begins its rush to the estuary in earnest.

The area below the dam for a quarter of a mile, generally lumped together under the designation of Great Falls, begins with gentle rapids. Immediately the chan-

nel, which is 2,500 feet wide at the dam, is split by the long, narrow Falls Island, which separates the main part of the Falls from the so-called Fish Ladder, adjacent to the Maryland shore. Just downstream, the Fish Ladder channel is split again by Olmsted Island, which separates the Fish Ladder from an equally steep but unnamed channel between Olmsted and Falls Islands.

In past years Olmsted and Falls Islands have been linked with the Maryland shore by footbridges, allowing visitors to Great Falls Park, Maryland (known officially as a unit of the C & O Canal National Historic Park) the opportunity to walk across the Fish Ladder channel and the unnamed defile to Falls Island to view the main section of the falls. In June 1972 the flood caused by Hurricane Agnes destroyed these sturdy steel and reinforced-concrete bridges, located 25 to 40 feet above normal water level, and made the islands and their spectacular views of the falls the exclusive preserve of the wildlife and whitewater boaters in all but the lowest water levels. Reconstruction of the bridges was completed by the end of 1992, but they were damaged again by two floods in 1996. The bridges are once again open. Both the Fish Ladder and the unnamed channel were altered by the U.S. Army Corps of Engineers around the turn of the century in an attempt to allow fish to migrate upstream of the falls. The resulting channels have concrete ramps that have weathered to expose the aggregate rock, creating knife-edged boulders in midchannel and impossibly tight turns. These hazards, combined with the extreme gradi-

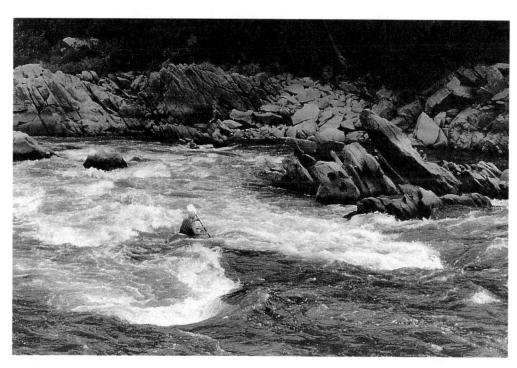

Little Falls on the Potomac River. Photo by Ed Grove.

ent, make both channels horrifyingly dangerous.

The main channel, separated from the Fish Ladder channel immediately below the dam, falls over unnamed drops of increasing severity for a few hundred yards. These drops, reaching Class IV in difficulty, would be significant enough to be named and paddled often anywhere else, but here they are mere prelude to and warning of the main event that awaits just below.

The Falls proper begins on a front approximately 600 feet wide. The Maryland Falls, running alongside Falls Island, reach their full development first, running swiftly to the brink of a convex, 20-foot vertical drop known as Tumblehome. The river immediately regathers its strength and within a few boat lengths drops over a straight-lipped, 10-foot drop called Charlie's Hole that is not quite vertical. The river again "pools" while moving at a rapid pace and turns sharply right and drops over a concave-edged 10-footer named Horseshoe Falls that has a wicked hydraulic at the bottom amid many broken boulders. This hydraulic has held onto boats and boaters for uncomfortably long periods of time. Indeed, while there had been no boater fatalities here at the time of this writing, the hole had kept a couple of pilot-less boats on a permanent basis, tearing them to pieces in lieu of releasing them to their bedraggled owners.

To the right of Maryland Falls the channel known since George Washington's time as the Streamers extends its flat section a few dozen feet farther downstream of the Maryland Falls and then proceeds to drop through a chaos of boulders, narrow chutes, and vertical falls that defies description. At the top of this channel you'll find a very interesting phenomenon: a small chute drops a distance of several feet and apparently runs onto a sharply sloped rock at the base, causing the flow to bubble straight upward in a natural water fountain fully as high as the height from which the water originally fell. This entire section of the river is ridiculously dangerous-looking and has only been run by deranged experts. The name of this section apparently comes from the last drop in the sequence. A relatively small amount of water, at summertime levels, falls over a rocky lip that is fairly regularly notched at the top, creating dozens of tiny waterfalls at intervals of one foot or so, falling a vertical distance of about 10 feet.

Even farther to the right, against the Virginia shore, is the section known as the Spout, possibly named by George Washington (or at least by the time he wrote his diaries). The Spout is separated from the Streamers by a 100-yard-long rock island locally called The Flake, but named officially Kirby Island in USGS records. This channel extends even farther downstream than the

Streamers before becoming unruly, but it makes up for its tardiness with an extra effort at being horrendous, awesome, and downright bodacious. After the initial pool the channel flows over a drop of seven or eight feet, called U-Hole, from a semicircular lip; the paddler drops from the outside to the inside of the circle. The concentration of the resulting hydraulic makes it extremely strong and it tends to back-pop or back-end the paddler, thoroughly frustrating carefully constructed plans for surviving the following drops. Most paddlers of this falls avoid the entire left side of the drop and enter on the far right, even though this necessitates a very sharp right turn at the bottom.

The channel runs straight downhill to the next drop, called Z-Turn, which splits at the top. The right two-thirds consists of another conclave lip and a nasty-looking hydraulic at the bottom. The far left side is a rightward-slanting slide and is actually easier than it looks. Immediately the channels converge and crash together violently against a rock wall straight ahead. The paddler must make a 90-degree turn to the left, proceed over a five-foot drop, make an immediate 90-degree turn to the right, and then drop a couple of feet. The whole sequence of Z-Turn from the slanting drop through the two sharp turns, usually lumped together as the second of three major drops in the Spout, occupies the linear space of only about three boat lengths and drops some 10 to 12 feet. A flip here, even with the quickest and surest of rolls, could be disastrous, particularly in view of what lies downstream.

After twisting through the described second drop the Spout forms a moving pool of 60 feet in length before delivering the coup de grace. The third and final drop consists of a single vertical falls of about 20 to 25 feet. The right two-thirds of the falls drop onto a slanting ledge halfway down and then strike a flat boulder or ledge at the bottom. The exact configuration of the slanting ledge and flat ledge at the bottom are unknown but the surrounding rock is heavily fissured and potholed, suggesting the presence of many nooks and crannies where the bow of a boat might become wedged, trapping the paddler under an enormous weight of water pouring over his boat and body. Rescue from such a situation would appear to be quite impossible due to the steepness of the shoreline and the tremendous power of a large amount of water flowing over a lip only about 12 feet wide.

Only the farthest left portion of the falls drops into clear water. Reaching this clear slot requires a turn at the top of nearly 90 degrees, virtually in midair. In addition, the paddler must simultaneously raise the bow of the boat to avoid a tiny, almost invisible rock at the bottom that's hidden by the curtain of water at all but the lowest levels. This small rock has taken a heavy toll in sterns from those who failed to notice it and achieve some degree of arch in their fall from the lip. Fortunately, within the very narrow range of water levels in which runs of the falls are possible, the hydraulic at the base of the last drop is not a safety problem. The long fall, however, results in a deep penetration of the pool at the base and the water pressure at these depths has popped the seams of some fiberglass boats.

After this frenetic descent the river pools very briefly and runs down to the heavy but more normal rapids of Observation Deck or "O-Deck" as it is known locally. Viewed from Observation Deck, the Spout clearly deserves its name. Survivors of such a run will certainly know that they have really accomplished something. We must again emphasize that for anyone but those who just can't sleep nights without having run Great Falls once in their lives the best advice is to forget it. Or to repeat a phrase heard repeatedly on many rivers, "Let's not, and say we did."

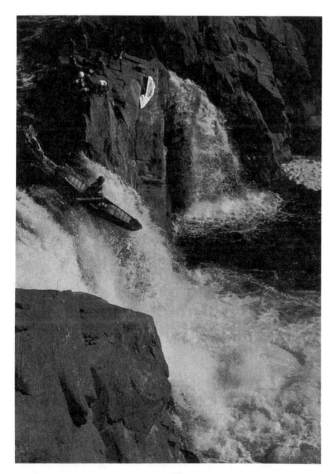

David Simpson running Great Falls. Photo by Ed Grove.

For years the myriad of paddlers who played in the rapids below the Falls gazed up from Observation Deck and wondered about the possibility of a successful run through some section of the very complex drops of the Falls. Many hours were spent discussing the merits of the almost infinite possible routes through the maelstrom. Most paddlers considered any attempt to verify these hotly debated theoretical runs to be tantamount to suicide, a notion reinforced by the steady incidence of fatalities incurred by ill-advised swimmers and rock scramblers. Each year several unfortunates were swept accidentally into the Falls and without exception met death in the foamy green chaos of the two-hundred-yard-long stretch of whitewater. For many years it seemed that the Great Falls of the Potomac would forever remain outside the ken of whitewater paddlers, unexplored and unknown. In 1976 this situation changed.

Two internationally known local paddlers, Wick Walker and Tom McEwan, studied the Falls with others and wondered whether a run was possible and if so, which route would be the most feasible. These two men, one a C-1 paddler and the other a kayaker, chose a route down the Spout section and decided to attempt it based upon their experience running smaller waterfalls during the development of waterfall running in the early 1970s. An additional factor in this decision was their plan to run a steep river in the Himalayas in the near future and their feeling that the Great Falls bore a resemblance to the 300-foot-per-mile gradients they would encounter in the canyons of Asia. Thus, the first successful run of one of the most feared drops in the region was, in point of fact, a mere training run for more severe rapids in Nepal!

After the initial run, it was two years before another attempt was made, in 1978. In late August of that year Bill Kirby and Steve McConaughy, both rangers at Great Falls National Park, successfully ran the Spout. The following year the Maryland Falls was successfully run for the first time. Since that time the number of paddlers completing the run and the variations of route and water level have multiplied. No one has been killed purposefully running the falls so far, but there have been an increasing number of close calls and many destroyed boats. As mentioned above, the first fatal run could be the last legal run of all, so let's be careful out there.

Below the Falls, the Potomac drops over Observation Deck Rapids, named for the tourist overlooks on both sides of the river. At levels of around three to four feet on the Little Falls gauge, this rapids provides large waves for the delight of the paddler. The sure presence of hundreds of amused, awed, and puzzled spectators on sunny weekends provides the hot-dog paddler with an unparalleled

Potomac River • Virginia, Maryland, District of Columbia

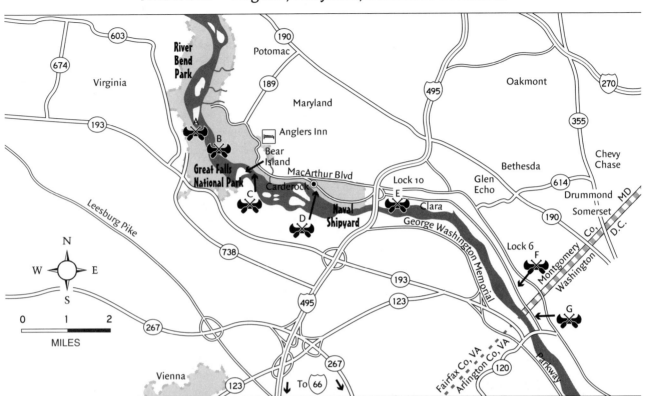

Section: Great Falls to the estuary below Little Falls

Counties: Fairfax (VA), Arlington (VA), Montgomery (MD), Washington DC

USGS Quads: Falls Church, Washington West

Difficulty: Great Falls proper, Class VI; Below Great Falls to Little Falls, Class II–IV; Little Falls proper, Class III–VI

Gradient: 14 feet per mile average

Average Width: 60–2,000 feet

Velocity: Fast

Rescue Index: Accessible except for Mather Gorge section

Hazards: Large rapids, wide river, difficult to swim out of, vertical walls in some sections, waterfalls

Scouting: S-Turn, Yellow Falls, Little Falls

Portages: Great Falls, Brookmont Dam

Scenery: Good to beautiful

Highlights: Scenery, wildlife, geology, whitewater, history

Gauge: National Weather Service, (703) 260-0305

Runnable Water Levels	Minimum	Maximum
Little Falls Gauge	2.5 feet	5 to 7 feet depending on section

Additional Information: None

forum for displaying skills. One such kayaker, a few years ago, apparently in search of female companionship, painted in large letters on the stern deck of his boat his name and phone number, preceded by the message "For a date call . . ." The effectiveness of this technique is unknown to the writers.

Below O-Deck the river turns 90 degrees left and runs toward the reentry of the Fish Ladder on the left. Just before the Fish Ladder drops into the mainstream, the river drops over a three-foot ledge that produces fun surfing waves at lower water levels. Where the Fish Ladder enters, bizarre currents are created in the deep water, which can be fun or frightening depending on the skill level of the paddler. Immediately after receiving the Fish Ladder's flow the river enters the S-Turn, a back-to-back set of right and left turns. At higher levels the Potomac splits again just below the Fish Ladder, with the left fork running hard up against the Maryland shore for a quarter mile before reentering below Rocky Island Rapids. The upper portion of this Maryland channel is called the Catfish Hole and is a popular put-in spot accessible via the C & O Canal towpath from Great Falls, Maryland.

S-Turn Rapids is a strange little place. The rapids are created not so much from a high gradient as from the concentration of the entire Potomac River into a channel only 60 feet wide. At levels between 3.2 and 4.0 feet on the Little Falls gauge a nasty hole forms behind a boulder on river right at the beginning of **S-Turn**. At lower levels this boulder, known as Judy's Rock after the late Judy Waddell (a local paddler and Great Falls Park ranger), becomes exposed. At any level all of the **S-Turn** sequence is full of moving waves, whirlpools, and crosscurrents. After straightening out of **S-Turn** the river flows more or less quietly for 200 yards to Rocky Island Rapids.

Rocky Island Rapids is probably the most heavily paddled rapids on the river. When the gauge reads between 3.8 and 4.6 feet, paddlers flock here to surf the wide, smooth, five-foot waves created here. Shortly below Rocky Island Rapids the Maryland channel from Catfish Hole reenters and the reunited river runs through Wet Bottom Chute, a four-foot ledge offering surfing waves and a nice bouncy ride. For the next mile the Potomac flows placidly between vertical rock walls 50 to 200 feet high on both sides with spectacular scenery and abundant wildlife. It is difficult to believe in this section that you are only a few miles from the Washington, DC, city limits and right in the middle of a suburban community. The land on both banks is part of national park areas and is thus preserved for recreational enjoyment.

As the vertical rock walls recede, the paddler approaches the confluence with Difficult Run, a creek entering from the Virginia (right) side of the river. Just upstream from the mouth of Difficult Run is the rapid named for that creek. Difficult Run Rapids consists of three chutes, separated from one another by rock islands. The left channel, called the Maryland Chute, is a three-foot ledge offering a small hydraulic and two- to three-foot waves. The center channel, appropriately named the Middle Chute, is a longer, gentler rapid with boulders and small ledges scattered over 100 yards. The Virginia Chute, on river right, is a narrow two- to three-foot ledge with a very smooth surfing wave at the top. All three of the chutes are heavily used as a training area by Washington-region paddlers.

Below Difficult Run the river flattens and runs placidly between wooded shores. A half-mile below the rapids the Anglers Inn put-in appears on the left shore. A parking area on MacArthur Boulevard across from a restaurant called the Old Anglers Inn provides access to the river. Paddlers park here for trips both upstream and downstream on the river and on the C & O Canal. Hikers, bicyclers, birdwatchers, and other outdoor types park here also, so in anything approaching good weather arrive early to secure a parking spot. Be certain not to block the emergency gates in the lot because the rescue squad and park rangers use these accesses regularly on busy weekends. Also, forget getting a drink or a bite to eat at the Anglers Inn in paddling clothes. The place is strictly for yuppies; gnarly-looking river rats will be shown the door immediately.

Below Anglers Inn the river continues flowing calmly for about a mile until the Yellow Falls–Calico Falls area is reached. The river is now being split by high rock islands with vertical walls. When a modern-design home is seen on the Virginia (right) shore a choice must be made as to which channel to run. Yellow Falls on the right is the steeper, more entertaining of the two. Calico Falls to the left is a longer, cobble-strewn sequence with no distinct drops. Yellow Falls should be scouted by first-timers because of the nasty hidden boulder located at the bottom that has wrapped and destroyed many canoes.

Below Yellow Falls and Calico Falls the river channels merge once again and soon the Carderock Picnic Area appears on the left, another access point. On the Virginia shore opposite Carderock, Scott Run enters, creating a picturesque little waterfall. Bathing in the cascade is done often, but one must be careful and not swallow any water because the Scott Run watershed is entirely urban and suburban. Immediately below Carderock, Stubblefield Falls is encountered. This is a gradually steepening cobble rapid with entertaining standing waves and whirlpools.

The Cabin John Bridge carrying the Capital Beltway (I-495) is now in sight and without this reminder you might think you were still in some remote mountain location. Below the bridge the Potomac flows tranquilly through a maze of low wooded islands for some three miles until Little Falls is approached. On river left below Cabin John Bridge, access to the river is gained from the Clara Barton Parkway at Lock 10 on the C & O Canal. The take-out spot is hidden among small channels along the Maryland shore, so the paddler new to the area should seek guidance from a local paddler before attempting to take out here. The river between Lock 10 and Little Falls is interesting and scenic but contains no fast water; most whitewater aficionados seldom paddle it.

The Little Falls section of the river is a blessing to local whitewater paddlers but it can be an extremely hazardous place under the wrong conditions. The beginning of this section is marked by the Little Falls dam, a low concrete dam that is deceptively simple looking. The smooth flow over this three-foot barrage creates an absolutely lethal hydraulic at the base that has killed dozens of people over the years. The river is nearly a half mile wide at the dam so rescue from shore or boats in the event of a mishap is virtually impossible. From upstream the dam is not easily seen but can be inferred by the concrete pump building on the left. If one is paddling down the river and this structure becomes visible, start moving left to exit the river well above this dangerous construction.

Immediately below the concrete dam is the old Little Falls dam, a rock-fill structure built to provide water for the canal on the Maryland shore. This dam has no hydraulic but at reasonable levels the rocks are thinly covered in most places and iron bars poke dangerously through the rubble in some areas. Choosing the proper channel is difficult but crucial.

Below the two dams the river narrows rapidly and drops over one long rock garden and several wave trains before reaching Little Falls proper. This rapid is a straightforward ledge at the lowest levels but even the slightest change in water height can alter Little Falls into a thundering, boiling monster. At high levels the normally short Class III drop stretches into a Class VI killer with 15-foot exploding waves stretching for half a mile. No detailed explanation of Little Falls is attempted here because it is essential to attempt this stretch only in the company of paddlers who have experience with this rapid and to scout it from the left bank of the river. It is interesting to note that the highest water velocity ever recorded in nature was seen at Little Falls during the massive flood of 1936.

Aquia Creek

Aquia Creek is one of those little-known gems that delight the heart of the whitewater paddler. Located only 30 miles south of Washington, Aquia Creek promises little based on the land surrounding it. The environs of the creek are mostly agricultural land to the south and the Quantico Marine Base to the north. However, once on the river the jaded paddler is in for a day of surprise and delight. Aquia Creek is one of the most scenic and enjoyable small streams east of the Alleghenies.

The stream at the put-in does not arouse particular hope. Aquia Creek at Route 610 (A) is a tiny, sand- and mud-banked creek. The flow moves along swiftly over a sandy bottom, but the only drops are where the stream flows over fallen logs. Fallen logs of the nonsubmerged

variety are something of a problem for the first couple of miles, but at most water levels one should be able to lift over them or pass underneath with little trouble.

A few miles into the trip a concrete bridge is approached with three large culverts running through it. Barring any accumulation of debris in the pipes, and sufficient clearance depending on water level, any of these passages may be run safely. Be very sure of clearance before entering because, although the current through the bridge is not particularly swift, a broach in the pipe could be very serious. The idea of being wedged with your boat in a debris jam in a culvert is the stuff of paddling nightmares. After passing under the bridge, Aquia Creek begins to gradually steepen. This process

Section: Route 610 to Route 1

County: Stafford

USGS Quad: Stafford

Difficulty: Class I–II (III)

Gradient: 15 feet per mile

Average Width: 15–50 feet

Velocity: Fast

Rescue Index: Accessible

Hazards: Occasional strainers, Smith Lake Dam Spillway

Scouting: None

Portages: None except around downed trees where necessary

Scenery: Beautiful

Highlights: Scenery, wildlife, whitewater

Gauge: Visual only

Runnable Water Levels	Minimum	Maximum
	Riffles runnable below Route 610 and 641	Nearing flood stage

Additional Information: None really. This is a hard stream to catch up. If in the area check out the creek. If it looks runnable at the put-ins on Rt. 610 or Rt. 641, it's runnable all the way. National Weather Service, (703) 260-0305.

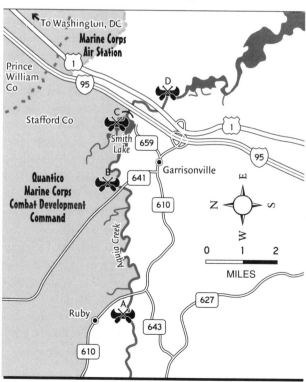

Aquia Creek • Virginia

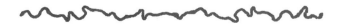

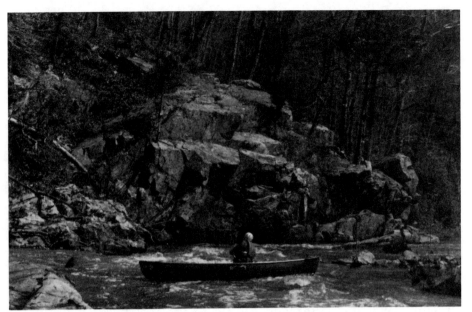

Bill Gordon enjoying one
of the many fall-line
rapids on Aquia Creek.
Photo by Ed Grove.

continues all of the way to Smith Lake near the take-out. Also, in the vicinity of the bridge several tributaries enter and the stream doubles in width, becoming a more respectable size.

Soon the paddler begins to notice that the banks are showing some rock mixed in with the sand and clay and eventually the rock begins to dominate. The slopes on the left bank rise high above the stream and rhododendrons begin to populate the stream's edge, serving notice that the geological environment has changed significantly. Aquia Creek has entered the fall-line area, where all of the eastward-flowing streams drop off the bedrock of the continent onto the sedimentary soils of the coastal plain. Some of the small streams in this area pack all of their drop into a small area, like Accotink and Pohick creeks, creating rapids with four- and five-foot drops. Aquia Creek, however, distributes its gradient more evenly, creating a stream more suitable to the intermediate paddler. As the creek passes downstream the slopes rise higher and higher on both sides, spectacular rock formations appear, and hemlocks tower over the stream, jutting dramatically from the rock. Rapids become steeper, but not nasty, and the relaxed paddler will find his or her adrenal glands beginning to stir into activity. The drops consist mostly of ledges up to three feet in height, some with rather complicated routes, many dropping over tight turns into picturesque little pools at the bases of high rock cliffs. Except for one Class III, none is tougher than a stiff Class II. On the inside of bends, white sandy beaches invite the paddler to linger and soak up sun.

Approximately six miles into the trip the Route 641 bridge (B) is reached. While this bridge would make a convenient take-out, doing so here would deprive the paddler of the best part of the trip. In the three miles between this bridge and the lake, Aquia Creek has all pluses and no minuses. The downed trees of the upper section are gone, the gradient continues to steepen, and the cliffs, hemlocks, and rhododendrons are at their most spectacular. The wildlife in this area is equally pleasing—on one trip we saw beavers, deer, kingfishers, ospreys, hawks, great blue herons, and various waterfowl. The scenery is reminiscent of some of the upper Cheat tributaries in West Virginia, such as Red Creek, subtracting the high mountains in the far distance. The action builds to a crescendo in the 1.5 miles below the Route 641 bridge, until the Aquia drops into Smith Lake. Now the paddler must pay for his enjoyment upstream with a 1.5-mile paddle across the lake.

The route across the lake is not immediately obvious because the dam is earthfill and has the same look as the rest of the shoreline. Just keep paddling straight ahead and look for the take-out (C) at the right end of the lake. There is a concrete spillway on the left edge of the dam. Give the entrance to the spillway a wide berth, as there are no warning signs or buoys.

The dam itself is about 100 feet high and rather impressive. The lake is relatively small for such a large dam, indicating that the gradient of the creek under the reservoir must be quite large. Doubtless some fine rapids were sacrificed to create the water supply for Stafford

County. The upstream end of the reservoir is silting in very heavily, so whitewater paddlers may look forward to the distant day when the lake will be filled by sediment and the creek will reassert its authority over its own destiny.

Below the dam Aquia Creek is rather unattractive and the remaining 1.5 miles to Route 1 (D) are not recommended paddling. Although it still drops at a good rate the creek passes by some dismal scenery and the odor of sewage as one passes a trailer court on the left is depressing.

The land on the left bank for most of the trip is part of the Marine base and is posted against trespassing. It would seem best, then, to arrange lunch or tanning spots on the right bank to avoid any possible federal entanglements. Just as with Aquia's neighbor to the north, Quantico Creek, the Marines will occasionally entertain the paddler with low level jet or helicopter flights over the creek. What you thought was the blood pounding in your ears may turn out to be the sound of huge helicopter blades.

You need a heavy spring rain to paddle Aquia Creek. The upper section requires more water than the lower section; if the upper, six-mile section looks runnable at the Route 610 put-in, Aquia is runnable the entire nine miles to Smith Lake. The lower, three-mile section has enough water if you can paddle the riffles below the Route 641 bridge.

Rappahannock River

The Rappahannock River shares the distinction with the James and the Potomac Rivers of being inextricably intertwined with the history of the state and the nation. Some of the earliest settlements on the continent were founded on the banks of the Rappahannock estuary. President George Washington warned Congress that if measures were not taken to improve the navigation of the Rappahannock below the falls at Fredericksburg then the day might come when that city would be overshadowed as a seaport by the upstart village of New York. According to legend, Washington threw a silver dollar over the Rappahannock in his youth.

Throughout most of the Civil War the Rappahannock and Rapidan formed the de facto border between the Union and the Confederacy. Today many Virginians who live on both sides of the river feel that the state legislature in Richmond still views the Rappahannock as the border between the "real Virginia" south of the Rappahannock and the Yankee country north of that stream, and that they appropriate state monies for roads and other services accordingly. Along the banks of the Rappahannock four major battles were fought during the war. The battles of Fredericksburg, Chancellorsville, the Wilderness, and Spotsylvania Court House resulted in the deaths of over 100,000 Americans between December 1862 and May 1864. John Wilkes Booth, having murdered President Lincoln, ran south through Maryland, crossed the Potomac near what is now the Route 301 bridge and entered Virginia. Passing through King George County, he crossed the Rappahannock to Port Royal, on the banks of that river, and was shot in a burning barn near the village.

Section: Remington to Kelly's Ford Bridge
Counties: Culpeper, Fauquier
USGS Quads: Remington, Germanna Bridge
Difficulty: Class I–II with two Class II–III drops
Gradient: 12 feet per mile
Average Width: 35–150 feet
Velocity: Fast
Rescue Index: Accessible
Hazards: Occasional strainers, hydraulics at higher levels
Scouting: Sandy Beach Rapids, Piggly-Wiggly
Portages: None
Scenery: Good
Highlights: Scenery, wildlife, whitewater
Gauge: National Weather Service (Remington gauge), (703) 260-0305

Runnable Water Levels	Minimum	Maximum
Remington gauge	3.3 feet	6 feet
river gauge	0 feet	4 feet

Additional Information: None

Rappahannock River • Virginia

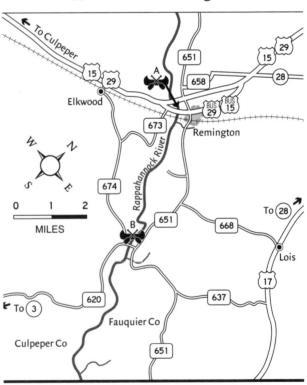

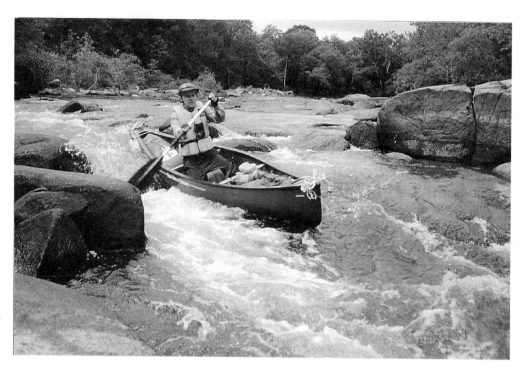

Richard C. Burke running
Sandy Beach Rapid.
Photo by Janice W. Burke.

The Rappahannock begins its existence in the coves and gaps of the eastern slope of the Blue Ridge in Fauquier, Rappahannock, and Madison Counties. The waters of the Rush, Covington, Thornton, Hazel, and Hughes Rivers join the upper Rappahannock near Remington while the Conway and South rivers join the Rapidan near Stanardsville. The latter mingles with the Rappahannock near the battlefield of Chancellorsville. The tributary streams are steep and rocky as they tumble off the Blue Ridge but flow sluggishly across the western piedmont. The Rapidan and Rappahannock, before their confluence, run between sandy or muddy banks with farmland straddling the streams for many miles. Downstream of Remington, however, the Rappahannock begins to tilt downward slightly and the stream accelerates enough to add some sporty action to the pleasant scenery.

After putting in at the Remington bridge (A) the paddler is teased by the river with a jaunty little ledge under the railroad bridge within sight of the put-in. After this brief chute through the remains of an old canal dam, the river remains quiescent for about two miles before rewarding the efforts of whitewater fans. This flat section is scenic, however, and runs along swiftly over a sand or gravel bottom. The wooded banks provide a sense of intimacy and shield the river from the fields surrounding the stream. Only the occasional sound of farm machinery or the mooing of the local bovine population will intrude on the paddler's privacy. The ambiance of this section invites the paddler to swing his feet over the gunwales,

rest his back against the thwart or aft deck, and drift with the gentle current, watching the trees overhead. This relaxation continues for about two miles before the sight of exposed rock and a pipeline notifies the voyager of a new mood of the river.

The remaining 1.5 miles to Kelly's Ford is an entertaining trip. A quarter mile below the pipeline, one comes to a short, easy rock garden followed by a pool. Then there is another gentle rock garden about 300 yards long. Look for a surfing spot on river right in this area. After a pool, a short rock garden, and another pool, one sees a line of rocks across the river as it bends left. This indicates that Sandy Beach Rapids ahead.

The rapid should be scouted the first time by novice and intermediate boaters. If the water is below roughly a foot on the Randy Carter put-in gauge, one can scout from the big, flat rocks just above the rapids. Better yet, a small group can have lunch there. If the water is higher or the group bigger, the lunch stop is a sandy beach on the bottom right of the rapids. The sandy beach on the bottom left is posted for no trespassing.

Basically, this Class II–III rapid can be run on the right or left at reasonable levels. The right has the cleanest chute, but you should still be careful of rocks on entry and on the bottom right of the runout. If the rapid is run left, either pick your way left all the way down or cut back hard right after entry. This way you avoid some rocks in the center of this channel, which widens substantially at the bottom.

A few minutes after Sandy Beach Rapid, the river turns right and becomes a good Class II rock garden known to local paddlers as the Maze. Go left or right, but the right has the best small chutes in the bottom through two big rocks. After the Maze, you have several mellow Class I–II rapids. The second of these has surfing possibilities if it is run to the right. The fourth drop is a rock garden. Run it center, but be careful to miss submerged rocks near the bottom.

With the take-out bridge (B) in sight, you are ready for the other main Class II–III rapid of note. This drop is called Piggly-Wiggly by old-timers. A good Class II way of running is to enter left of center going toward the right and cutting back left to finish. Alternately, if you are adventurous and competent, run the extreme left channel after scouting. This channel of pushy water drops three to four feet and is a moderate Class III because of the rock lurking in the center of the runout waiting to munch errant boats. Indeed, a former local outfitter (Ronnie Meadows) told me that he used to pull several pinned boats off this rock each year. Only two short, easy drops remain from here to the take-out. The first of these has a surfing spot on the left. Paddlers then go under the bridge and take out on river right.

The 1.5-mile whitewater section of this trip changes markedly with rising water levels. From 0 to 2 feet on the put-in gauge it is a Class II–III run suitable for shepherded novices and intermediates. Between 2 and 3.5 feet it becomes a continuous Class III run for experienced boaters. Approaching four feet it changes to a continuous Class IV run—the recommended limit for advanced boaters.

Kelly's Ford is very interesting historically. During the Civil War, troops of both sides forded the Rappahannock near here and many skirmishes took place close to this strategic river crossing. One battle was along an old wall that extended from river right above Sandy Beach Rapids to Route 674. Also, from the start of the rapids to the take-out, the trace of the old Rappahannock Canal from Fredericksburg to Waterloo comes close to the river at various places on river left.

Tye River

The Tye River packs a lot of variety into a comparatively short run. Beginning at Nash (A), just a mile or so below the mouth of Crabtree Creek, the Tye starts in a mountain pass, cuts through foothills, and then settles into an open valley. In the first couple of miles below the confluence of the North and South Forks at Nash the Tye is a steep boatbuster with abrupt drops and tight turns through boulder-strewn chutes. The scenery in this section is spectacular, with high rock formations and steep forested slopes on both sides. The road follows the river closely on the left but is not intrusive, and the paddler may bless its presence in the event of a rescue effort or a boat salvage operation. Rapids are almost continuous in

this stretch, with four memorable ledges that may have to be scouted depending upon water levels. The difficulty of these drops will be Class III in low water and Class IV at higher levels. You'll find a canoeing gauge on the North Fork at the Route 56 bridge at the confluence.

After passing under the first bridge at the confluence of Campbell Creek, the Tye relaxes a bit. Rapids continue to appear at regular intervals but they are not so threatening as those above Campbell Creek. The river valley widens somewhat and the gradient lessens as the Tye leaves the mountain pass it carved through Pinnacle Ridge at Nash and approaches its alluvial fan east of the mountains.

The rapids in this section consist of gravel bars and

Section: Nash to Massies Mill

County: Nelson

USGS Quad: Massies Mill

Difficulty: Class III–IV in the upper section, Class II–III in lower reaches

Gradient: 56 feet per mile average; 85 feet per mile in upper 1.5 miles

Average Width: 20–40 feet

Velocity: Fast

Rescue Index: Accessible

Hazards: Strainers, steep rapids, pinning possibilities on boulders, cold water

Scouting: All major rapids scoutable from road

Portages: None

Scenery: Beautiful

Highlights: Scenery, geology, whitewater

Gauge: National Weather Service (Buena Vista), (703) 260-0305

Runnable Water Levels	Minimum	Maximum
Route 56 gauge	0 feet	2.5 feet
Buena Vista gauge	5 feet	8 feet

Additional Information: The correlation between the gauges and the level on the Tye is indirect. In general, when everything else is ripping and roaring, go take a look at the Tye.

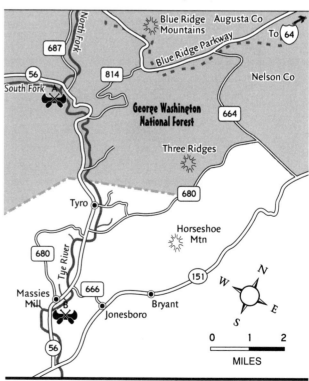

Tye River • Virginia

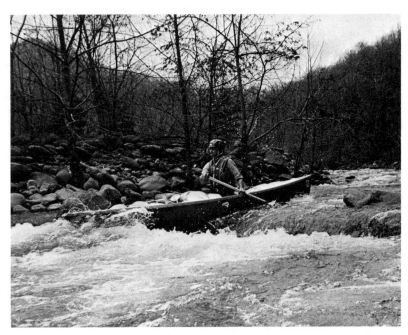

Ed Grove on the
Upper Tye River.
Photo by Bill Kirby.

occasional sizable ledges where the Tye runs up against rock bluffs on either bank. The difficulty of the rapids in this section is a step down from the upper region, in the Class II–III range. The scenery is still good but a few cabins and cleared areas begin to intrude on the view.

As the fourth bridge crossing approaches, the Tye leaves the steep terrain behind and begins meandering through a broad valley full of orchards and cattle. The river flows primarily through a channelized trough with bulldozed banks, only occasionally dropping over a Class II ledge or a shallow gravel bar, or through a narrow chute around a small island. The channelization in this section is not overwhelming because the river has been kept in its natural course. Hurricane Camille in 1969 caused great damage in the Tye River valley and the flood caused the stream to relocate its course in this lower section, according to locals. As Massies Mill (B) is approached the river broadens out over a gravel bed; at low-water levels the paddler may find him- or herself sliding and/or hiking for short stretches.

The water on the Tye is usually brilliantly clear and clean. The river is a popular trout stream and paddlers should make all possible effort to avoid conflict with these fellow friends of the river. As with many small streams in the state, it is probably best to be very careful in early spring when there may be many fishermen on the Tye. Once, some locals threatened to tow away the cars of some paddlers because "this is private property

and canoeing isn't allowed." This sort of comment is hard to swallow when the banks are lined with dozens of anglers who don't seem likely to have secured permission from all the landowners, but remember, the quiet word turneth away wrath. Getting into a shouting match on the banks of a stream is worse than useless. In this particular instance the cars were not towed, nor have any cars ever been towed, according to all the paddlers we consulted concerning this question.

The Tye drains a very small watershed which, even though it is almost completely forested, seems to lose water very rapidly. As a result the Tye can go from too high to too low in a day and the paddler must be alert and determined to catch this stream with a suitable flow. By the time the Buena Vista or other gauges show sufficient water to indicate good flow in this area, the Tye has most likely waxed and waned and may be unrunnable. But go take a look anyway; if there is sufficient water it will be worth it, and there are plenty of alternatives in the area if you miss the Tye (alternatives in the general area include the Piney River, the Pedlar, the Buffalo, and somewhat farther away, the Maury).

When in the neighborhood of the Tye, a short hike is a must for all lovers of falling water. Above the runnable section of the Tye, along Route 56 toward the Blue Ridge Parkway, lies a small U.S. Forest Service parking area. From here a trail leads up Pinnacle Ridge along Crabtree Creek to a spectacular cascade high on the mountainside.

Crabtree Falls consists of a steeply sloping curtain of water some 100 feet high where Crabtree Creek ends its meandering along the top of the ridge and falls abruptly into the valley of the upper Tye. The hike to the falls from the parking area is short but very steep, following lots of switchbacks beside the swift and clear creek. Those who struggle all of the way to Crabtree Falls are amply rewarded by the beauty and the breathtaking views available from the top of the rock dome over which the creek cascades.

Maury River

The Maury River is formed just above Goshen Pass where the Calfpasture and Little Calfpasture Rivers join. These two streams flow on a southwesterly parallel course along opposite sides of Great North Mountain until the Calfpasture turns southeast near Goshen. Just as the streams merge, the now-sizable Maury cuts across the spine of Little North Mountain and drops precipitously into the Valley of Virginia. This happy circumstance of a reasonably large amount of water flowing through a steep mountain pass provides whitewater paddlers with excellent scenery, easy access via interstate roads, splendid rapids, and sparkling water quality—a combination unsurpassed anywhere in the eastern United States. Luxuriant rhododendron stands, steep rock cliffs lining the river, and cascading tributary streams create a superb arena for the enjoyment of our sport. The Maury is therefore the quintessential Virginia whitewater stream and, if one were forced to choose the finest among the 10 best streams of Virginia, the Maury would be a strong candidate for such a title. The only negative aspect of this stream is that it's too short.

One aspect of the Maury that may be considered a mixed blessing is the presence of a paved road closely paralleling the river throughout the length of the Goshen Pass. The road, State Route 39, is usually dozens of feet above the stream; however, it does not detract very much from the wild character of the scenery. The presence of this artery will be appreciated by many who require assistance, who are forced to walk away from the river sans boat, or who have friends or family that wish to see what the devil their friend or relative has been doing on weekends for all these years. In addition, the fortunate location of the road provides the Maury with a delightfully short shuttle route, allowing multiple runs of the river in a single day.

The put-in (A) is shortly below the confluence of the Calfpasture and Little Calfpasture rivers, where the river runs up against the road and turns left into Goshen Pass. A dirt road here leads the short distance from the paved road to a convenient pool. Below the put-in the Maury flows swiftly over some entertaining, riverwide low ledges for a few hundred yards, a few short rapids and quick ledges, and another 100-yard rapid to the first of the named rapids, a mile below the put-in. Undercut Rock is a three-foot ledge, broken on the right and more abrupt on the left. Either side may be run but beware of the boulder on the bottom right that gives this rapids its name.

Shortly below Undercut Rock is Roadside, recognizable by a jumble of low boulders on the left forcing the river to the right against the roadside bank. Take a left course through this drop, easier at high levels when room is created for the passage of conservative boaters. This

Section: Goshen to Rockbridge Baths
County: Rockbridge
USGS Quad: Goshen
Difficulty: Class III (IV)
Gradient: 48 feet per mile average; 71 feet per mile in the Goshen Pass
Average Width: 40–60 feet
Velocity: Fast
Rescue Index: Accessible
Hazards: Strainers, keeper hydraulics at high levels, difficult rapids
Scouting: Devil's Kitchen, Corner Rapids, Brillo
Portages: None
Scenery: Exceptionally beautiful
Highlights: Scenery, wildlife, history, geology, whitewater
Gauge: National Weather Service (Buena Vista), (703) 260-0305

Runnable Water Levels	Minimum	Maximum
Rockbridge Baths	1.5 feet	5 (advanced), 6–7 (experts)
Buena Vista gauge	3.5 feet	7 (advanced), 9 (experts)

Additional Information: Added congestion makes swims at levels above 3 feet on the Rockbridge Baths gauge hazardous; levels up to 5 feet are not too difficult for advanced paddlers, and levels up to 6 or 7 feet are possible for crazed experts. James River Basin Canoe Livery, (540) 261-7334

rapid is a long wave field (100 yards) with a nice surfing wave three-quarters of the way down. You'll find excellent surfing waves at the bottom of this drop.

A long and pleasant Class II–III boulder garden appears below Roadside. This rapid is an example of the good nature of the Maury: it seems to be provided as a morale builder for the nervous paddler in preparation for the serious business that lies below. At the bottom of the boulder garden is a pool known as the Blue Hole. Running out of the Blue Hole the river disappears to the left, the road retreats high up on the right bank, and an unusually deep roar may be heard from the stream ahead. These clues, along with the sight of people in brightly colored helmets and nylon clothing scrambling all over the riverbanks, should indicate that something unusual lies ahead. This is indeed the case.

Devil's Kitchen is the object of all of these grave portents and it deserves them. This drop is a 100-yard-long heavy Class IV with almost every conceivable river hazard packed into a short distance. The river drops about 20 feet in this span, with steep drops, limited visibility, strong holes, undercut rocks, tiny eddies, fallen trees, and the possibility of strainers, making this spot by far the most serious rapid on the trip. The complexity of the series makes a detailed description impractical, but the general path is to start on the left side of the river and work right over seven to eight drops of two to three feet each to end up on river right at the end of the run. Avoid the temptation to sneak the heavy stuff by running through the more lightly watered channel to the right of an island because this route is festooned with strainers and studded with undercut rocks. Land above the entrance of Devil's Kitchen on the left, take a long, hard look at it on foot and portage left if it's too tough.

Below Devil's Kitchen the Maury provides another of the delightful Class II–III boulder gardens that make this trip such a pleasure. When these drops are navigated you'll find yourself at a picnic area, where, after Devil's Kitchen, some may wish to make use of the restrooms near the road. Leaving the picnic area, the highway, perhaps sensing more accurately than paddlers what lies ahead, again retreats from the river and cowers high above the canyon floor for over a mile. Just below the picnic area are two four-foot drops. Run the first on the right and the second left of center.

Soon Laurel Run falls off the right mountainside and enters the Maury, but it isn't noticeable unless you look for it. There are three small drops below Laurel Run that afford nice play spots. Corner Rapid, located after a sharp bend to the left, is formed from boulders cut from the cliffs on the right. The river is squeezed to the left and

through a boulder jumble. Paddlers should run the upper section on the left and then get to the right for the lower section. This section has lots of large holes to punch or avoid, depending on the skill or inclination of the paddler. You should scrupulously avoid being pushed too far right at the top, as you'll be squeezed into one of two violent channels. Also, the lower left is ugly, with pinning spots and scrapy channels.

A couple of hundred yards of Class II water follow and soon a smoothly sloping rock wall will be seen on the right. This indicates Sloping or Sliding Rock Rapids, a 100-yard-long ledge series. The route is straight through on the right. The channel is right next to the sloping rock wall, which runs uninterrupted into the water, and zooming down this bouncy channel with the rock within arm's reach on the right is reminiscent of looking out the window of a speeding subway. The eddies against the wall are very entertaining if they can be caught, and they provide opportunities for dynamic eddy turns, exciting surfing chances, and the possibility of customizing your boat by grinding off the bow on the unyielding stone. There are easier eddies on the left and some nice surfing holes here.

Downstream is a long Class III rapid that has some very nice surfing waves toward the end. About 100 yards later, the paddler will reach a calm spot known as the

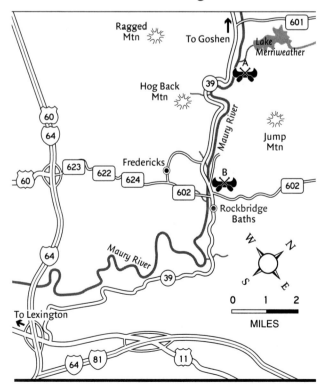

Maury River • Virginia

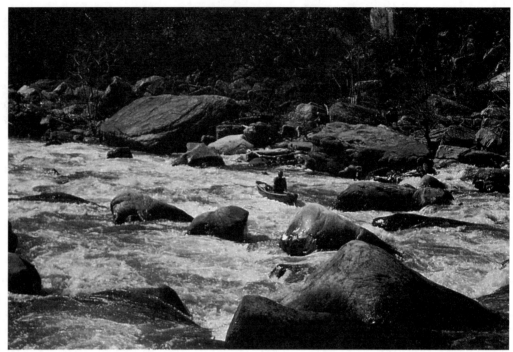

Scott Gravatt in Devil's Kitchen at Goshen Pass on the Maury River. Photo by Bob Maxey.

Indian Pool, recognized by a picnic table, a stone stair-way, and the road. Below Indian Pool is another Class II–III rock garden almost a half mile long that becomes rather bony at lower levels. This rapid has several play spots and a four-foot drop about two-thirds of the way down on river left. It is possible to take out soon after this rapid where the road reapproaches the river, but we recommend continuing into Rockbridge Baths unless you want to repeat the heavy-duty part of Goshen Pass.

Below Indian Pool the canyon opens out into the valley but the river has tenaciously retained enough gradient to keep the paddler entertained a while longer. Class II–III boulder gardens and ledges continue for a mile, with the river occasionally splitting around islands. These islands are deposited material, occurring where the steep gradient of Goshen Pass has receded, reducing the capacity of the stream to carry rock, rubble, and sand. This excess material settles out of the flow and forms the islands and braided channels of this section. These characteristic formations are found wherever a steep stream reaches a level of temporarily decreased gradient. The drops in this area tend to be technical and require careful channel hunting at lower levels. Near the end of this mile (below a house on river left) are a couple of zesty surfing ledges.

The last two notable drops on the run are easily recognized. They are both within a few hundred yards of the Route 39 highway bridge (B). The first is called Lava Falls, after the igneous rock intrusion that forms the rapids.

Lava is a Class II–III chute, run on the far right, with good surfing waves at the bottom. Shortly below is Brillo, an abrupt four-foot ledge. Scouting is in order here because the channel is difficult to see from above. The route of choice at low and medium levels is on the far left but even a perfect run will likely be accompanied by a grinding sound on the hull of the boat, providing an immediate answer to the question of the origin of the rapids' name.

The Route 39 bridge is now in sight, signaling the end of the run. Do not take out at the bridge, however; this is frowned upon by the landowners. Instead, continue downstream to the General Store on the left bank in Rockbridge Baths, a distance of a few hundred yards. There is a 150-yard-long Class II rapid before the store.

Now go back and do it again!

The Maury River is referred to on old maps and in old texts as the North River of the James. In 1742 the first bloodletting between Native Americans and the colonists in the upper James Valley occurred on the North River near its confluence with the James, near present-day Glasgow. A band of Native Americans from the north traveled, as was common at the time, along the Great Warpath to attack their enemies, the Catawbas, in North Carolina. This Great Warpath was also used by the colonists and later grew into the Valley Turnpike, now State Route 11. The marauding Native Americans apparently took some property from white colonists on their way to the south and the local militia gathered to punish them for this transgression. John McDuwell, commander of the local militia, intercepted them on North River and was killed along with seven of his men in the ensuing battle.

The North River was renamed in honor of Matthew Fontaine Maury, born in Virginia but raised in Tennessee. Maury obtained a commission in the U.S. Navy as a young man and sailed out of Newport News, Virginia. Over the following years he began a study of ocean winds and currents, which was to earn him the title "Father of Oceanography." The Civil War interrupted his scientific career, however, and he devoted his efforts to strengthening the minuscule Confederate Navy and destroying the ships on which he had formerly served. After the defeat of the South, Maury became a professor at the Virginia Military Institute at Lexington on the North River. There he fell in love with the Goshen Pass and he requested that upon his death his remains be carried through it. An honor guard of VMI cadets carried out this wish, and a monument to him stands on the road in the pass today.

While in the area, those with a historical bent will not want to miss a side trip to Lexington, Virginia, one of the most historically rich towns in a state that thrives on its past. The Virginia Military Institute, where Stonewall Jackson was a professor before the Civil War, Washington and Lee University, where Robert E. Lee spent his last years after the same war, as well as a wealth of historic buildings, monuments, and cemeteries bring the past alive. The James River and Kanawha Canal reached as far as Lexington until 1895 and provided reliable transportation between the tidewater region and the mountains.

Despite the engineered safety of the canal, river travel in the past had the same attendant hazards it has today. The famous tale of Frank Padget, a black slave employed on the canal, is a timeless story that modern whitewater paddlers are most equipped to appreciate (for a detailed account readers are referred to Blair Niles's *The James,*

From Iron Gate to the Sea [New York: Farrar, Straus & Giroux, 1940]). The basic story is as follows: A canal boat was attempting to pass across the mouth of the rain-swollen Maury on its way up the James to Buchanan, but it drifted into the James when its towline broke. It accelerated toward the Balcony Falls section, which is run by whitewater paddlers today for sport at lower water levels. The boat was headed for a dam; seven people jumped off the boat and swam for shore. Four reached shore but three were swept over the dam and drowned in the hydraulic. The packet boat, with some 50 people on board, then successfully ran the dam and continued on toward the rapids. Volunteers were called for to save the people who had jumped from the boat onto nearby rocks and those still on the boat itself, which was hung up on a rock in midstream. Five boat hands, including Frank Padget, took a bateau from the canal, dragged it over the towpath, and got on the river. They rowed the boat into the middle of the river, by all accounts using techniques of ferrying and eddy turns in heavy water as modern as this year's slalom boat, and retrieved most of the victims after several trips out and back. On the last trip, however, the bateau broached and wrapped firmly about a rock and all were thrown into the river. Frank Padget and the man he was attempting to rescue drowned in the flooded James. The contemporary account, from the Lexington Gazette, is astounding to read and shows evidence of whitewater technique that most present-day rescue squads would do well to emulate. A monument to Frank Padget still stands today along the railroad tracks that replaced the canal towpath near the scene of the accident.

The Maury lies virtually at the intersection of I-64 and I-81 and is easily reached from any area of the state. Route 39 crosses Route 11 at the ramp for I-81 off of I-64.

Other rivers in the neighborhood include the Cowpasture, Calfpasture, Bullpasture, and Jackson, all due west of Goshen Pass; the Upper James to the south; and the Tye, Piney, and Pedlar over the Blue Ridge to the east.

James River

The James River drains over a quarter of the land area of the Commonwealth of Virginia. At its fall line, the division between the piedmont and the tidewater geographic regions of the state, the James drops 100 feet through the "Falls of the James" section of the river. The Falls of the James are located entirely within the city of Richmond; here is an adventure-class whitewater river (which is commercially rafted) flowing directly through the center of a major city and state capital. Flows vary from typical late-summer levels of less than 2,000 cfs to massive flood surges in excess of 100,000 cfs. Therefore, the river is never too low to run and provides water-craving, summer boaters with a place to maintain their skills and sanity when most of the smaller streams in the state are as dry as a bone. Indeed, the paddler should beware of levels of too much water during the winter and spring. The James can rise extremely rapidly to a dangerous level. The ledges and broken dams that create the whitewater sport on this section of the James can become deadly when large amounts of water pour over them, creating dangerous hydraulics of great width.

As with the rest of our eastward-flowing rivers, the James meanders for many miles through farmland with no appreciable gradient before it reaches the edge of the bedrock underlying the North America continent. Here, the river tumbles off the continent onto the coastal plain, creating whitewater for our enjoyment. The city of Richmond was located here in colonial times because the fall line obstructed river travel. Many low dams were built across the river in the late 1700s to support an early canal and navigation system, in which goods were first transferred from boats to land and then to canal transport. Most of these dams have fallen into disuse and have fallen apart, creating chutes and broken ledges. The nature of the rapids on the James is largely determined by these structures, the original nature of the river bottom having been overwhelmed by the man-made alterations. The resulting run is as unique as it is convenient, and the

paddler must take care to realize the unusual hazards attendant to a primarily artificial whitewater course.

The James River makes up the heart of the state of Virginia. Along its banks were founded the earliest settlements in the western hemisphere. The tidewater planters created a society modeled on English laws and traditions, establishing the pattern for the continent-wide society that grew from these initial plantations. Later, Patriot and English armies marched through the James basin in the American Revolution, establishing Virginia as the birthplace of the American nation and presaging it as a major battle arena in a later war that nearly destroyed the nation.

When the Southern states seceded from the Union in late 1860 and early 1861, Richmond was chosen as the Confederate capital, both to bring the border states into the war on the Southern side and to emphasize the pre-eminence of Virginia among her Southern neighbors. As a result of this decision, the state became the center of the most destructive event in the history of the country. The banks of the James became the goal of the Union armies for four years of insane destruction, and Richmond lay in ruins at the end of this struggle. Factories on the fall line in Richmond churned out weapons, gunpowder, and supplies for the Confederate armies; Yankee prisoners were incarcerated at Libby Prison on the left bank of the James and on Belle Isle in midstream. In the end, of course, the Union prevailed, and the nation, begun in Virginia and symbolically rent asunder there, was restored to its previous state of unity. Students of ecology will notice while traveling through the countryside between Richmond and the Potomac that the land of Virginia is still recovering from the depredations suffered during the Civil War. Think of these things while paddling through the modern metropolis of Richmond on the James River.

There are two sections of the river within the city, each with different characteristics. The "Upper Section," from Pony Pasture Park to Reedy Creek, contains Class I–II rapids at normal river levels. The "Lower Section," from Reedy Creek to Mayo's Island, is generally a Class III+ run, although in high water the difficulty and danger of the four major rapids increase dramatically.

The put-in for the upper section is on Riverside Drive on the south bank of the James, at Pony Pasture Park (A). The river flows quietly for a mile or so to the first of the rapids. For a couple of miles the river flows through rocky islands and over numerous small ledges and rock gardens. After four miles you'll reach Reedy Creek (on the right), which is the take-out (B) for the upper section and the put-in for the lower section.

After leaving Reedy Creek, you soon reach the first of the major drops, known as First Break. First Break is actually two breaks in the old Belle Isle Dam, a masonry structure. The upstream break is dry in low water. The more often used lower break is a three- to four-foot drop into nice waves, a good surfing spot, but watch out for submerged rocks immediately below the surfing waves. Catch the eddy on the left to get back into the waves. Below here stay to the right, close to Belle Isle, to enter

Section: Pony Pasture Park to Mayo's Island
Counties: City of Richmond
USGS Quads: Richmond East, Richmond West
Difficulty: Upper Section, Class I–II; Lower Section, Class III+
Gradient: 7 feet per mile (Upper Section); 30 feet per mile (Lower Section)
Average Width: 200–400 feet
Velocity: Fast
Rescue Index: Accessible
Hazards: Iron bars, broken dams, hydraulics, strong rapids
Scouting: Hollywood, Second Break, Pipeline
Portages: None
Scenery: Urban but striking
Highlights: History, whitewater
Gauge: Richmond Recorded River Reading, (804) 649-9116 (updated several times daily)

Runnable Water Levels	Minimum	Maximum
Richmond-Westham gauge	4.2 feet (Upper)	7 feet (21,000 cfs)
	3.9 feet (Lower)	7 feet (21,000 cfs); permit is needed above 9 feet

Additional Information: National Weather Service recording (Richmond-Westham gauge), (703) 260-0305 or (757) 899-4200; Richmond Raft Company, (804) 222-RAFT

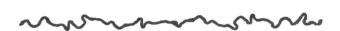

Hollywood Entrance, a pleasant Class II–III set of drops at normal levels. There are several nice surfing spots in holes and waves. Don't come out of your boat, however, because the big one, Hollywood, lies below.

Hollywood Rapids consists of a five- to six-foot ledge, broken and runnable on the right, followed by a mess of wet boulders in the outflow. The preferred route is to the left at the bottom but you will have to scamper to get there. The boulders can also be avoided on the right with some speed. Go either way, but make up your mind early. You'll find lots of entertaining waves and holes here. Scout Hollywood from the right bank.

The Robert E. Lee (Route 1/301) bridge is just downstream. Suspended underneath is a pedestrian and bicycle bridge allowing access to Belle Isle from Tredegar Street. The parking area for the Belle Isle section of the James River Park is a convenient boating access. Use the ramp adjacent to the Tredegar Iron Works, just upstream of Browns Island. Tredegar Iron Works produced over half of the cannon manufactured in the Confederate States of America during the Civil War. The gun foundry building is the one with the red brick smokestack visible from the river.

After passing under the Robert E. Lee Bridge, the VEPCO Levee Rapids is reached. This is an easy ledge,

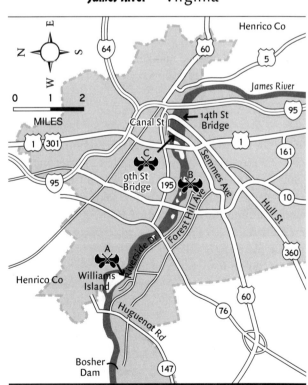

James River • Virginia

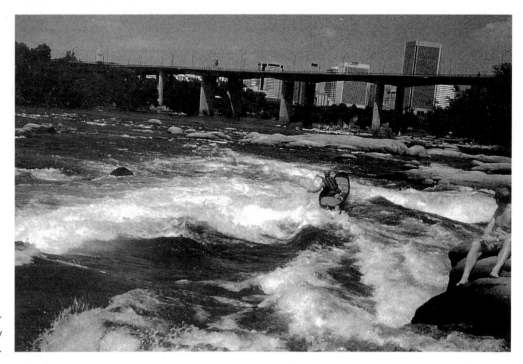

Hollywood Rapid near downtown Richmond. Photo by Ron Knipling.

but with more boulders in the outflow of the best channel. Soon the Manchester bridge is seen overhead and the Second Break Rapids looms. Second Break is a four- to five-foot drop through a break in an old VEPCO (Virginia Electric Power Company) dam. Although this is a straightforward drop, dead ahead at the bottom are broken-out chunks of concrete with exposed rebar (steel-reinforcing bars). Just as with Hollywood, go right or left but know before you go and don't mess with the rebar. After running Second Break, ferry to the far left to enter Pipeline Rapids.

Pipeline consists of four distinct drops. The third drop contains a great ender spot at reasonable levels, accessible from the eddy on the left at the bottom. From the eddy, just poke your bow into the hole and hang on tight. Again, don't come out of your boat because the fourth drop lies just below and would make an unpleasant swim. Pipeline Rapids is named for a sewer pipe suspended underneath a rail trestle, which may be used as a viewing platform for the rapids below. When the James exceeds seven feet, water starts pushing beneath the trestle piers. These produce a series of potentially lethal strainers, so it is advisable to avoid Pipeline at higher levels.

The most commonly used take-out for the lower section has been the Reynolds Metals lot immediately adjacent to Pipeline's third ledge (the end spot) on river left. However, this area is part of Richmond's riverfront re-

development efforts. Consequently, alternative take-outs have been created at either end of the 14th Street Bridge. An informal take-out at Mayo's Island also has been permitted by the owners. Boaters may also take out at Ancarrow's Marina on river right. This take-out requires a paddle under I-95 and across one half mile of tidal flatwater. Paddlers may also use the Richmond Raft Company parking area on river left (at 4400 East Main Street) with permission and avoid the paddle to Ancarrow's.

It should be noted that the above description is only a brief treatment of the most commonly paddled route through the Falls of the James. The many variations possible in the run through the lower section and the many access options available ensure that local paddlers are rarely bored by paddling on the James. Those unfamiliar with the river could, however, encounter some of the many potentially dangerous obstructions and hazards. Indeed, this river is so complex that a first trip down the Falls of the James should be in the company of experienced locals if at all possible, for both safety and enjoyment reasons.

The shuttle takes a little doing, but with patience you should find the desired put-in. From the north part of Richmond, head south on I-95 and take the Downtown Expressway (Highway 195). This is the last exit before you cross the James. Once on the Expressway, turn right on Canal Street. Once on Canal Street, you will pass the 14th Street Bridge (also known as Mayo Bridge or Martin

Luther King Bridge). You will take a left at the next bridge, which is Manchester Bridge. As you take the left, notice the Reynolds Metal parking area, which provides access to the lower James take-out. After you cross over the Manchester Bridge, continue on Semmes Avenue, take a right onto Forrest Hill Avenue, and shortly thereafter, take a right on 42nd Street. Proceed to Riverside Drive where it passes Reedy Creek—the put-in for the lower section and the take-out for the upper section. To reach the put-in for the upper section at Pony Pasture Park, continue on Riverside Drive upstream about 4.5 miles.

Appomattox River

The Appomattox is another of those gems of the eastern seaboard, a river that meanders over a mature landscape through pleasant and wooded scenery for many miles before dropping off the continental shelf. Where mills and other industry were once located, the river now flows through pretty scenery and drops over entertaining ledges and boulder gardens. Indeed, a great portion of this section has been preserved as a Virginia Scenic River.

The Appomattox is filled with Virginia history. Like the Rappahannock, the Appomattox played host to some of the earliest settlements in North America, in the days when the area west of the fall line was the frontier. Native Americans populated the area heavily, unlike the area north of the Rappahannock, and place names testify to their influence with early colonists. The Petersburg area was the site of the denouement of the Civil War, the city enduring a 10-month-long siege that produced severe civilian and military casualties. The Petersburg campaign is considered by many historians as the beginning of the concept of total warfare, which reached a fuller development in the wars of the twentieth century. The siege is interpreted by the National Park Service at the Petersburg National Battlefield south of the city. Following the break of the siege by Union forces, Robert E. Lee and his Confederate troops retreated west along the Appomattox, attempting to reach Danville and the much-needed supplies at the railroad there. The ragged remnants of the forces of the South were caught and surrounded at the town of Appomattox on the river of the same name and the four-year struggle was over for all practical purposes.

Putting in at Brasfield Dam (A), a Chesterfield County boat launching facility reached via Route 669, the paddler is allowed a mile of flatwater paddling for warming up before reaching the first obstacle: a six-foot dam with a required portage on the left. Once on the river and staying near the right, you will drop over three one-foot ledges in the first 100 yards. Just after this is a two- to three-foot drop (Class II). Then comes a long, mellow rock slalom. At the end of his slalom is Picnic Rapid (Class II+)—so named by all the float anglers who used to picnic and fish here. Enter this rapid left of center and work right toward the end to avoid some sneaky rocks in the runout. You'll find a good recovery pool at the bottom; nervous novices can look Picnic Rapid over from the right bank before running it. You'll then pass Woodpecker Island on the left after a river channel enters from the left. Woodpecker Island is a great spot to relax and camp for those so inclined. The river then breaks into three channels; the middle or right routes are generally best.

After the channels converge, paddle through a rock garden toward a large rock on the left bank. As you approach this rock you will see the Matoaca Cotton Mill Canal wing dam. The right half of the river bypasses the dam, and has two Class II channels running through it. Less experienced paddlers can take this route. If you continue on the left within the wing dam, you will go down the canal under a power line and enter Jughandle (Class II–III) as the current bends right and breaks out of the canal. You can scout Jughandle from the island on its right to make sure there are no trees in this bumpy three- to four-foot drop. Also, while you're on the island, notice the remains of the head gate of the Matoaca Mills Canal on the left and visualize the dam, which was built across to the island in 1830. Jughandle gets it name because of the left channel and island forming this rapid, which look like a jug handle on a map.

You enter a long, Class II rock garden just below Jughandle, so try to pick up the pieces of errant paddlers quickly. Halfway down this rock garden is a two-foot ledge. Just below this ledge, get over to river left for a very pleasant lunch stop if your stomach is growling. After the rock garden ends, you reach Matoaca Bridge, with two historic items of interest on river left here. First, if you walk a short distance north on Route 600 and turn left on Ferndale Road, you will see three buildings that were Matoaca Mills—a busy cotton mill complex

Section: Brasfield Dam to Campbells Bridge (Route 36)

Counties: Chesterfield, Dinwiddie

USGS Quads: Sutherland, Petersburg

Difficulty: Class II–III

Gradient: 13 feet per mile

Average Width: 40–90 feet

Velocity: Fast

Rescue Index: Accessible

Hazards: Dam one mile below put-in, deadfalls, spikes at old Spike Dam

Scouting: Jughandler, Pipeline, Target Rock

Portages: Dam below put-in

Scenery: Good

Highlights: Scenery, whitewater, history

Gauge: National Weather Service (Matoaca NWS), (757) 899-4200

Runnable Water Levels	Minimum	Maximum
Matoaca Bridge gauge	0 feet	4.5 feet
NWS Matoaca gauge	2.4 feet	6.5 feet

Additional Information: Appomattox River Company, (804) 392-6645.

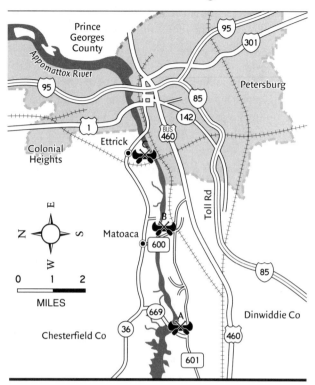

Appomattox River • Virginia

that operated for 100 years and employed 200 workers. Second, slightly downstream of Matoaca Bridge are the abutments from an old, turn-of-the-century, wooden toll bridge, which charged a nickel for pedestrians and 15 cents for horses and wagons.

A quarter mile below the bridge you'll enter a maze of delightfully beautiful islands with some large pine trees growing on them. Weave your way through the smaller maze of rocks in the right channel passing by these islands. Relax and enjoy this scenic mile while you look for great blue herons and other critters. There is good fishing here, too. The river reforms after these islands, and you may be able to see a silo on your left. This is a part of the Randolph Farm, which, in the late 1700s, was the childhood home of "John Randolph of Roanoke," a U.S. congressman and senator.

You then see a VEPCO transformer station high on the right, and you pass underneath some power lines. Rohoic Creek (formerly called Indian Town Creek) enters here on the right. This was the last Appomattox Native American village site. Indian Town Aqueduct (which was 42 feet high) used to support the Appomattox Navigation Canal as it crossed Rohoic Creek. Four toll locks upstream from the aqueduct lowered boats 33 feet from the upper canal.

After going under the power lines (you are now two miles below Matoaca bridge), look for a sign on an island warning of dam spikes. Go left of the island and run a Class II drop center as you do so. Don't worry about the spikes; you won't reach them for half a mile. Soon after this island you can take a far left channel (which has a two- to three-foot drop in it) around a second island, or go right of the second island. If you go right, stay near the right bank. Soon you will see a horizon line formed by the remains of Spike Dam (a crib dam that diverted water to a mill race on the right side of the river) and you will also see a small channel (an old mill canal) to the extreme right. Here you face another choice: You can take the intimate Class I–II old canal channel or look for a place to carefully bump down Spike Dam. Although this is technically a Class II–III drop, look out for spikes and nasty rocks if you decide to run it. Many boats have been damaged here. After the initial three-foot drop, there are a couple of rocky passages to negotiate before reaching the pool below.

Soon you'll cross under a railroad bridge. Notice the newer bridge built on top of the much lower, older bridge. After a good quarter mile you will pass a rock garden with stone canal walls on the right. Not far below, you will see the twin stone arches of a mill and a dam warning sign on the left. After exploring these arches, stay tight right. Just below is a five-foot dam (Battersea Canal) that, like Spiked Dam, diverts water to mill races on both sides of the river. You will see a pipeline on the right bank and a canal alongside it. After about 50 yards, the current breaks left through the canal wall into Pipeline Rapids—a mellow Class III with two good drops that are best run right of center to avoid the rocks in the left-side runout. There is an eddy on the right at the top of the rapids; here you can scout Pipeline, after pulling your boat up the large granite boulders on the right side of the canal break that leads into the rapids.

After getting your act together below Pipeline, you will soon come to a one- to two-foot ledge. About 50 yards below this on the left is Target Rock Rapids, a tougher Class III and very aptly named; paddlers without good boat control tend to crash into the center of this large rock at the bottom of the rapid. If the current isn't too pushy, you can scout from an island in the center of the river to the right of the rapid. Otherwise, you'll need to pull over to the left bank and get over to the rocks forming the left side of the rapid to scout. Paddlers generally run Target Rock Rapids on the left and catch a big eddy on the left below the main drop before being blown into Target Rock. This eddy is a great place to practice ferrying if you can avoid intimacy with Target Rock. On river left below Target Rock, notice the striking, 12-foot cascade as another canal break enters the river. Take the right side of the river to sneak Target Rock. However, beware of a

large hole that develops on the right at higher water.

Shortly below, you'll pass under Campbells Bridge (C, Route 36); the take-out is less than 100 yards below on river right. At high water, when a large, moving whirlpool forms beneath it, you may want to take out on river right well above the bridge. You don't want to swim the whirlpool at high water because a six-foot dam with a keeper hydraulic is lurking only 200 to 300 yards below the Route 36 take-out bridge.

Spend some time poking around the take-out. There are mill ruins on both banks of the river. On the right are the remains of Battersea Cotton Mill, which was several stories high, had a bell tower, and operated for over 75 years until 1918. On the hill overlooking the left side of the river is the campus of Virginia State University. This used to be known as Fleet's Hill—a famous dueling site in colonial times. However, do not leave vehicles unattended on the Petersburg (south side) of the river at the final take-out. There have been numerous instances of vandalism here.

Before starting, check the Matoaca Bridge gauge on the downstream side of the color-coded abutment. Green (zero to one foot) is for very carefully shepherded novices; yellow(one to three feet) is for intermediates with good boat control; red (three to 4.5 feet) is for advanced paddlers; and black (above 4.5 feet) is the time to take an alternative trip.

Johns Creek

This section of Johns Creek is a superb run for the advanced paddler in good physical shape. It should only be undertaken with careful attention to the river gauge, and paddlers doing it for the first time should go with someone who knows this tight, tough technical stream well. Please note that a change of only a few inches on this gauge can dramatically increase the difficulty of this river.

What can be seen of Johns Creek from the road is misleading. At the put-in, it looks like a drainage ditch, while the section immediately above the take-out looks like the Class II–III Nantahala River in western North Carolina. In between, hidden from view, is a ruggedly beautiful, two-mile gorge with an average gradient of 115 feet per mile, with some places exceeding 150 feet per mile. This gradient combines with a heavily obstructed riverbed to create a classic trip of very challenging water. The rapids in the gorge range from Class III to Class V and are mostly continuous, with only a few short, flat stretches offering a breather. Where possible, all of these rapids should be boat- or land-scouted.

After the put-in at the Route 311 bridge (A), there are about two miles of mostly flatwater leading into the gorge. The arrival of the heavy rapids section is heralded when the paddler reaches an overhanging rock wall on the right. Then, the river takes a sharp left bend and immediately picks up to a strong Class III level at two drops called Shubaloo I and Shubaloo II. After these "smaller" rapids, the proverbial bottom drops out.

The first major rapid in this hot-and-heavy section is a

Section: Route 311 Bridge to New Castle (Route 615)

County: Craig

USGS Quads: Potts Creek, New Castle

Difficulty: Class I–II for the first two miles; Class IV for two miles in the gorge (with one Class IV–V); Class II–III at the end

Gradient: 60 feet per mile; two miles in gorge are 115 feet per mile with one mile in gorge at 150 feet per mile

Average Width: 25–35 feet

Velocity: Fast

Rescue Index: Remote (with hostile landowners)

Hazards: Bambi Meets Godzilla (Class IV–V); numerous Class IV rapids; Fool's Falls; trees in river

Scouting: Boat- or land-scout all major rapids

Portages: Optional

Scenery: Beautiful in gorge

Highlights: Beautiful gorge

Gauge: Visual only; gauge on Route 615 bridge in New Castle

Runnable Water Levels

	Minimum	Maximum
	0 feet	1.5

Additional Information: None

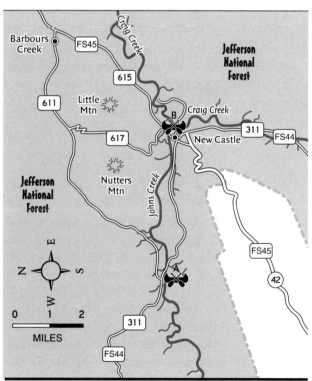

Johns Creek • Virginia

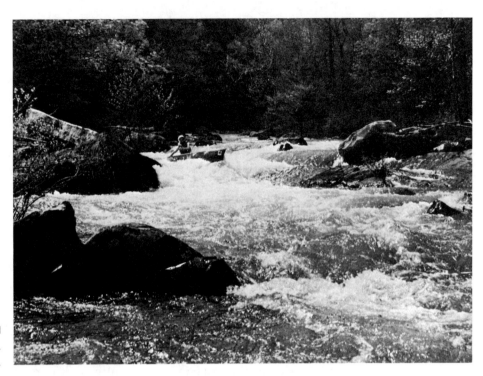

Liz Garland runs Found
Paddle Rapid on Johns Creek.
Photo by Ron Mullet.

steep Class III–IV S-turn from right to left over a succession of rocks, drops, and holes for about 75 yards. Locals have christened this rapid Sirius, the Dog Star, an abstract but somehow very appropriate name.

The paddler is soon confronted with a picky entrance to Class III Royal Flush. The entry requires a slalom around rocks and pourovers, setting the stage for a fast blast from left to right where the main flow piles into a boulder on the left. Some very fast ferries and dynamic eddy-hopping can take place at the bottom of this drop.

Immediately after, an island splits the river again, with a shallow channel on the left and a steep, blind chute on the right. (The left channel is very shallow if the Route 615 gauge is below one foot.) You enter by dropping down on the right and catching a small eddy on the right bank just downstream of a large rock. Downstream is a rock in midchannel. Run just left of this rock and quickly cut back right below it to miss a big hole at the bottom left. Running right of the rock is not recommended because strainers are often found there. Indeed, the whole right channel of the river should be scouted for trees after high water. This tough, Class IV rapids has informally been called "Coke Island" as it is certainly "the real thing."

Shortly thereafter is another strong, steep, Class III–IV sequence terminating with a large padded rock dividing the current into two chutes. The right chute is more easily run by dropping off at an angle and surfing down a wave/hole into the bottom eddy. The left chute is more difficult and should be scouted carefully before attempting it. Locals have dubbed this rapid "Little Heinzerling" due to its similarity to Heinzerling rapids on the Upper Yough in Maryland.

Just below is the granddaddy of the rapids on Johns Creek. One colorful name (among several) applied to this Class IV–V rapid by local paddlers is Bambi Meets Godzilla. One may assume that "Bambi" is the innocent paddler. This rapid is a real heart-pumper with a total drop of about 15 feet in 30 yards. Here the flow channels to the right and narrows, with a tongue that drops over a five-foot slide into a boiling hole. Then comes another drop next to a boulder and a final drop into another hole before reaching the pool below. Run this last drop right or left to avoid a pinning rock. Blind Man's Bluff is around the next bend. This Class IV rapid is simply a jumble of boulders. The paddler's predicament is to guess which channel is clear and safe. Watch out for logjams blocking the path. Run the left side of the center chute and then cut back right.

Next is a Class IV rapid called The Separator. Here the river funnels to the left and plunges steeply over a jumble of rocks. Halfway down is a four-foot drop. Immediately below is a screaming right-hand turn to avoid a pillowed boulder. The current then continues over another drop into a hole that requires a sharp left turn. The final chute deposits paddlers into a small pool where they can regain their breath and composure.

Just below a short pool, Typewriter Hole spans the

width of the stream; sneak it against the far left bank or on the right, or be prepared to punch it in the center. This hydraulic can get very sticky at higher levels and scouting is advised for first-timers.

Typewriter is followed by a series of ledges and pourovers known as Found Paddle. Take care here, as the last large drop has a pinning rock in what looks like a clean chute; run tight left to avoid a nasty vertical pin. Fast water carries the paddler from Found Paddle to a smooth horizon line that announces Fool's Falls.

Fool's Falls is the last and biggest individual drop; it has been described as unrunnable by some previous guide books. However, with proper care and appropriate water levels, a path can be found over this Class IV six-foot drop into a rock garden. In popping over the drop and overshooting its hydraulic immediately below, proper boat angle is critical to avoid a vertical pin. Run right with your boat pointed to the right, and be really cranking when you go over the drop.

The river changes character immediately after this drop and soon becomes Class II to the first take-out a half mile below Fool's Falls at the rescue squad station near New Castle. A second take-out option at the Route 615 bridge (B) in Newcastle lies a half mile farther down.

The only difficulty with this delightful trip are problems with local landowners. From Bambi Meets Godzilla to the take-out the left bank is posted against trespassing while the right bank is similarly posted between Typewriter and a good quarter mile below Fool's Falls. Indeed, local landowners can be very hostile; there have been instances of paddlers being threatened by a landowner brandishing a shotgun. When planning a run down Johns Creek, check with local boaters to ascertain the latest information about this situation.

One final word of warning. At levels above 1.5 feet, Johns Creek is one megarapid (with very few eddies) from Blind Man's Bluff to Fool's Falls. Consequently, anyone contemplating this run at or above this level should be an expert paddler who makes this trip with fellow experts who know the river well.

Whitetop Laurel Creek

Born at the confluence of Big and Little Laurel Creeks, Whitetop Laurel cascades down Whitetop Mountain (near Damascus) in what can best be described as whitewater ecstasy. Characterized by some paddlers as the premier whitewater stream in southwest Virginia, its only drawbacks are a relatively short season and its distance from most paddlers (3.5 hours south of Roanoke). With an average gradient of about 72 feet per mile, Whitetop Laurel flows through intimate gorges of magnificent scenery, excellent water quality, and continuous rapids. Basically a Class III–IV run of 12 miles, Whitetop displays a broad spectrum of treats for the advanced boater: big ledges, steep tricky rock and boulder gardens, some uncharacteristically big holes, and eddies and other play spots galore.

Another special treat for the boater as well as spectator is the Virginia Creeper. Although it winds around quite a bit, the Creeper is not a vine known to gardeners but is the remains of an old, narrow-gauge logging railroad that runs the entire length of Whitetop Laurel. The U.S. Forest Service maintains the area as a hiking and cross-country ski trail, providing recreation for the nonboating crowd. The Creeper is also quite significant to boaters—not only as an access route, but also because of the numerous railroad trestles crossing the stream, some at unusual angles to the river flow. These trestles can provide some heart-stopping moments at high levels.

Most trips on Whitetop Laurel begin at Creek Junction (A), just downstream of its confluence with Green Cove Creek and near the Appalachian Trail. Creek Junction is 1.5 miles from Route 58 on Route 728, a dirt road made from the old logging railroad. As you follow Route 728 for a mile to the Green Cove confluence, notice the beginning of Whitetop Laurel's first gorge. Not recommended for boating, this gorge contains falls over 15 feet; tight, boulder-choked rapids; and strainers. The preferred Creek Junction put-in is a half mile further down at the end of Route 728, where you'll also find sites suitable for primitive camping.

Soon after you put in here, the river goes under the first railroad trestle. About 150 yards downstream, the river bends slightly left. Before venturing further, the boater should eddy out on river left, walk downstream, and scout The Slot, an eight-foot (Class IV+) drop. In low water it can be run center through the slot. Higher water allows a more difficult run over a turbulent S turn (Class IV–V) on river left. For those not wishing to attempt this rapid, an easy carry and put-in below The Slot are available on river left.

For the next mile, the river is fairly narrow and creates some interesting holes. Not far below trestle number eight, the river picks up with a series of bigger rapids culminating in a four- to five-foot drop into an intimidating but benign hole. Just run this Class III+ drop down the center.

In a few more miles, the paddler will notice the gorge opening up, and as the river bends hard to the right, signs of civilization appear. This is Taylors Valley, and you are about to encounter the rapid of the same name (Class IV). You can't really see all of this rapid until you are in it, so be ready to scramble for an eddy, preferably on river right. At most levels, the best route is also along the right bank. Higher water opens up a left-side run over a sloping diagonal ledge. On one trip, someone had installed a log bridge across this rapid; it would be wise to look before committing a group to run it. There are two road bridges in this valley. Immediately below the second one, on river right, is a pretty community wayside, perfect for a lunch stop. This marks the halfway point of the trip.

Leaving Taylors Valley, Whitetop Laurel enters its second gorge. The rapids are much like those before, only a little steeper. Another high ledge (Class IV) awaits paddlers a few miles downstream. Easily spotted, it can be run on river right in low water or left-of-center at higher water. At low water this latter route has nasty rocks at the bottom.

Somewhat below here, the river briefly braids around several islands, with some channels blocked by fallen tress. Look before you leap here! These islands are a sig-

Section: Creek Junction (off Route 728) to east of Damascus (US 58)

Counties: Washington

USGS Quads: Whitetop Mountain, Grayson, Konnarock, Laurel Bloomery, Damascus

Difficulty: Class III–IV with three Class IV and one Class V–VI rapids

Gradient: 72 feet per mile

Average Width: 20–40 feet

Velocity: Fast

Rescue Index: Remote

Hazards: The Slot (Class IV+), Big Rock Falls (Class V-VI), occasional fallen trees (particularly one place in second gorge where river braids)

Scouting: The Slot (Class IV+), rapids below trestle number eight (Class III+), Taylors Valley (Class IV), a high ledge (Class IV) and braided area somewhat below second gorge, Big Rock Falls (V–VI)

Portages: Possibly the Slot (on left), definitely Big Rock Falls (on right)

Scenery: Exceptionally beautiful to spectacular

Highlights: Two beautiful, intimate gorges; Virginia Creeper trail; Mount Rogers National Recreation Area; Appalachian Trail

Gauge: Visual only at railroad bridge gauge at take-out

Runnable Water Levels	Minimum	Maximum
	0 feet on gauge or if the river is barely runnable at the take-out; South Fork of Holston gauge should be over 1,200 cfs	1 or 2 feet on gauge or if river is easily runnable at take-out

Additional Information: Call Marc Raskin of the Coastal Canoeists, (540) 947-5576; South Fork of Holston gauge, (800)238-2264, press 3 on touch-tone phone.

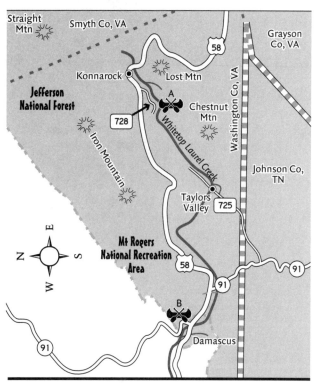

Whitetop Laurel Creek • Virginia

nificant landmark for the paddler: less than a mile beyond them, the river is again crossed by a railroad trestle. As you go underneath, quickly move to river right and catch an eddy above Big Rock Falls. Big Rock (Class V–VI) is a two-step drop of 10 to 12 feet. It has been run tight left by demented experts, but is better left alone. A mistake here could be costly. A fairly easy carry can be made on river right, where you'll find a piece of narrow gauge rail track to use as a ladder.

Just downstream, about 10 miles into the trip, Whitetop Laurel finally comes back to the US 58 highway. The water in the remaining two-mile stretch to the take-out is very deceptive, especially when viewed from the highway. It is turbulent with some very rambunctious holes that are best avoided at higher levels. The take-out (B) is just below the third railroad trestle after the river comes to the road.

Below the recommended take-out, the river eases up considerably. It joins with the Tennessee Laurel at the US 58 intersection with Route 91, and becomes Laurel Creek. Laurel Creek then travels through the town of Damascus on to its confluence with the South Fork of the Holston.

There is a gauge on the railroad bridge at the Whitetop Laurel take-out. However, its distance from most boaters still requires a long drive to ascertain whether there is sufficient water to run this stream. If there's been heavy rain or snowmelt in the spring, it's a good bet Whitetop Laurel will have enough water. It comes up easily, but, unfortunately, goes down quickly. Also, because this is one of the most popular trout streams in southwestern Virginia, late March and early April runs are to be avoided. Find out when fishing season opens to avoid an unfortunate experience. Call Coastal Canoeist Marc Raskin at (540) 947-5576 if you are planning a trip.

If the lucky boater comes to the area and finds water in Whitetop Laurel, there are several nearby streams to paddle as well. Go up Route 91 from its junction with

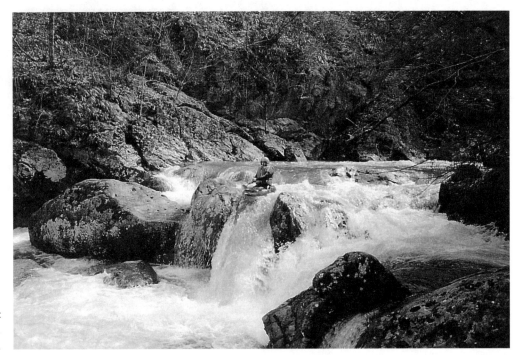

Bill Hat running The Slot
on Whitetop Laurel.
Photo by Mayo Gravatt.

US 58 and you immediately find Tennessee Laurel on your right. More difficult to catch with water than Whitetop Laurel, it is also steeper with a gradient of over 80 feet per mile. Scout from the road and put in as high up this Class III stream as you feel comfortable. However, in Virginia near the state line, be alert for Triple Drop (Class IV+).

For an easier trip, drive into Damascus and find your way to Backbone Rock State Park. The stream running along your right is Beaverdam Creek. Dropping 55 feet per mile, this is a fun, Class III run. Just put in as far up this stream as your nerve and the water will allow. However, it has a few surprises to keep and boater alert. (For example, by Backbone Rock State Park, the river runs underneath the highway—which you can scout on the shuttle.) Also available are numerous Class I–II runs on the Holston and its forks. With some time, water, and topographic maps, the exploratory boater could spend several days exploring the creeks running out of the mountains around this area.

WEST VIRGINIA

Gauley River

Upper Gauley

The Upper Gauley is one of the finest runs in the eastern Appalachians. It's big, tough, dangerous, and intoxicating. The river flows through a magnificent, steep-walled gorge with few easy access points. At 2,800 cfs the rapids are complex and intense. There are eight major rapids in the Class IV+ to V category on the stretch from Summersville Dam to the Bucklick take-out with innumerable "minor" Class III–IV drops. But although the whitewater is challenging, the fast water is separated by long pools. These provide a welcome break in the action, allow for rescue, and provide time to appreciate the cliffs and forests of this remote, unspoiled canyon, now managed as a national river by the National Park Service.

A few intrepid explorers rafted and canoed the Gauley during the 1960s, before the Summersville Dam was built. In 1968, with the dam in place, the river was attempted by a group of world-class paddlers in kayaks and C-1s. Running on a 1,500-cfs release, they ran the entire 26-mile stretch in a single day. In the early 1970s only a few dozen people went down each weekend. The river became a qualifying cruise for the title of expert boater. Paddlers gradually became more skilled and better equipped, and now thousands run the Gauley each year. The river is home to many commercial raft outfitters and is considered one of the best commercial trips in the world. All this leads to big crowds during fall release weekends.

The Upper Gauley, for the purposes of this guidebook, consists of the stretch from Summersville Dam (A) to Appalachian Wildwater's take-out at Bucklick (D). Despite its growing popularity, the Gauley is still an intense and dangerous river. The Upper Gauley has many undercuts and sieves that must be avoided, making it impractical for most first-timers to pick their way down. Don't attempt this run without the skill, confidence, and endurance that makes the Cheat Canyon or New River Gorge seem easy. If you still have doubts, try the Lower Gauley first. Then make your first run with experienced paddlers who know the upper section well and are willing to serve as guides. Even with their help, a number of rapids deserve scouting.

Here's a description of the primary rapids of the Upper Gauley at the normal fall release levels of 2,400–2,800 cfs:

After several big, Class III warm-up rapids you'll encounter Initiation (Class IV), the first major drop. After a long lead-in the river drops over a high, sloping ledge into a medium-sized stopper. It looks like you could run it anywhere and the smooth wave at the brink of the drop looks tempting to skilled surfers. But a hidden boulder sieve on the right has been responsible for two fatalities and dozens of narrow escapes in the past 20 years. Run to the left of center, then keep working left to avoid the stopper if desired. Don't even think about surfing the top wave; it will throw you into the sieve if you lose control. The right side of the bottom hole is surprisingly sticky at low levels (1,200 cfs). There are several fine Class III drops below here with great wave trains. Rafters should watch out for Bud's Boner (Class IV), which is formed when the river squeezes to the right and plunges over two drops. There are potential pinning rocks in both drops for rafts; the second drop should be run on the left to avoid a strong pour-over on the opposite side of the chute. Rafters should go left after the first drop and run the second drop with a strong right-hand angle to avoid a sticky hole on bottom left.

Two miles into the trip, a high sandstone wall looms ahead, signaling your arrival above Insignificant (Class V). This rapid was named because the 1968 party reported "no significant rapids above Pillow Rock." Later parties, running at higher flows, encountered unexpected difficulties. Insignificant is one of the most difficult on the river at fall release levels. At the top, a huge pour-over in the center and another slightly downstream on the left often separates paddlers from their boats. Then the flow sweeps up against a huge sloping rock on the right and into a wave train. A nasty ledge lies on the left side of the river just upstream of this rock. First-timers and marginal

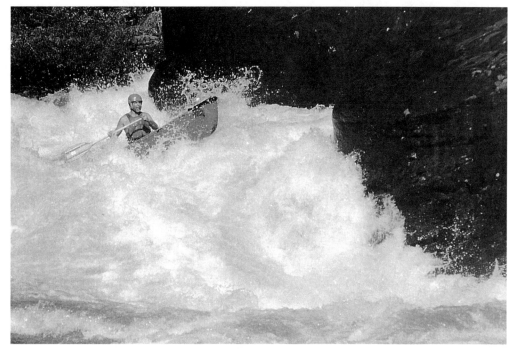

John Deardorff
getting upclose
and personal with
Pillow Rock on
the Upper Gauley.
Photo by Ed Grove.

players can easily scout this rapid on the far right.

There are several possible routes. Hard boaters usually start at the center of the rapid, drop down just to the left of the top two pour-overs, and cut quickly to the right to avoid the nasty ledge on the left downstream. Rafters typically cross the river just upstream of the center pour-over, then run down on the right. There's an excellent sneak route on the far right that avoids the big holes in the upper part of the rapid. A vigorous wave train at the bottom is fun to play if traffic permits.

After two lesser rapids, Iron Curtain (Class III+) awaits. The rapid is named for the iron oxide stains on a sandstone cliff on river right. The water is channeled toward the left side and you'll find big holes on the right and center. The left chute has a fast wave train and a superstrong left-hand eddy. Rafts should avoid the undercut Sperm Whale Rock, lurking downstream. You can now see the overlook at Carnifex Ferry State Park on the top of the ridge on river right. Pillow Rock Rapid lies just downstream.

Pillow Rock Rapid (Class V) is an impressive 25-foot drop, creating over 50 yards of big waves, large holes, and impressive turbulence. The entrance at the top is rocky, offering many possibilities. Halfway down you'll encounter a series of nasty holes and very confused, aerated water. The hole on the far right side is extremely deep. At the bottom the water piles up against a huge rock wall, creating the impressive pillow that gives the drop its

name. Then it roars around and over Volkswagen Rock. There's a lot happening in here, and it's a good idea to scout on the right side. On fall release weekends large crowds gather to watch the show.

There are two reasonable routes down Pillow Rock and a third that's nothing but trouble. The best hard-boat route is down the center. Enter just right of a boulder at the top center, then hug the left sides of two successive rocks downstream. Now work right, grazing the left side of the big hole near bottom right. Cut in behind this second hole to catch the right-hand eddy above Volkswagen Rock, then take a second to decide how much of the downstream craziness you want before peeling out. If you miss this eddy, brace into the pillow at the bottom and ride the current around the rock. The left side of Volkswagen Rock has a very powerful ender spot on the left.

Most rafts prefer the right channel, cutting left to follow a distinct wave train that terminates in the big hole on the far right. Large rafts punch the left side of the hole to slow down so they don't get pushed up on the pillow. From there you can move across the river and slide past Volkswagen Rock on the left.

Unless you like big-time craziness, avoid the left side "hero route" on Pillow Rock. It lines you up for the top hole, then carries you directly into the pillow. Most boaters flip here, and usually it's all right to hang in your boat upside down and wait for things to calm down. But the river could deposit you in the Room of Doom, a ter-

Upper Gauley • West Virginia

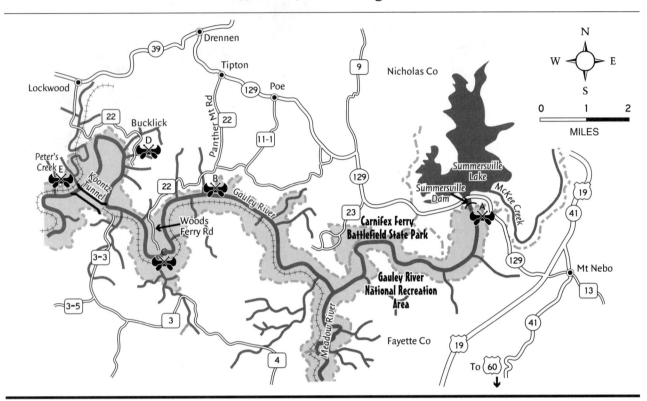

Section: Summersville Dam to Bucklick

Counties: Nicholas, Fayette

USGS Quads: Summersville Dam, Anstead

Difficulty: Class IV–V, with one Class V–VI

Gradient: 28 feet per mile

Average Width: 75–100 feet

Velocity: Fast

Rescue Index: Remote

Hazards: Undercut rocks, long Class V–VI rapids, high water

Scouting: Insignificant, Pillow Rock, the second drop and Tumblehome in Lost Paddle, Iron Ring, Sweet's Falls, Woods Ferry

Portages: Perhaps Iron Ring (especially below 1,500 cfs)

Scenery: Beautiful

Highlights: Unique expert whitewater river, spectacular gorge and rock formations

Gauge: National Weather Service in Charleston, (304) 529-5727, Monday through Friday, 8 A.M. to 4:30 P.M. for Belva; Summersville Dam (dam release and Meadow River), (304) 872-5809

Runnable Water Levels	Minimum	Maximum
Belva gauge	2.4 feet (800 cfs)	4.5 feet (5,000 cfs)

Additional Information: National Park Service, (304) 465-0508

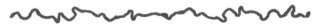

minal, box-shaped eddy to the left of the pillow. Many hapless boaters have spent anxious moments in here wondering why their buddies told them to run it on the left. A few had to be pulled out from above with ropes! If you are in over your head, the steep trail to the overlook at Carnifex Ferry departs at the top of the rapid on river right.

There are several milder drops before the Meadow River comes in on the left. Like most of "easier" Gauley rapids, you must stay alert for undercut rocks and large holes. Rafters should beware of the last Class II–III rapid above the Meadow, known as Flipper's Folly. Marked by an island at the top of the drop, the right side funnels through Toothpaste Slot, which is too narrow for all but the smallest rafts to negotiate. The left channel has some pinning rocks on the left side at the bottom, so start left of center and work right for a clean run.

Lost Paddle (Class V) is the longest rapid on the river. Also called Mile-Long Shoals, it's full of waves, ledges, undercuts, and holes. It's difficult to scout and a murderous carry along the railroad tracks on the left. It consists of four distinct drops, with the second and the fourth being the most difficult. Always check the flow of the Meadow River when running the Upper Gauley; any-

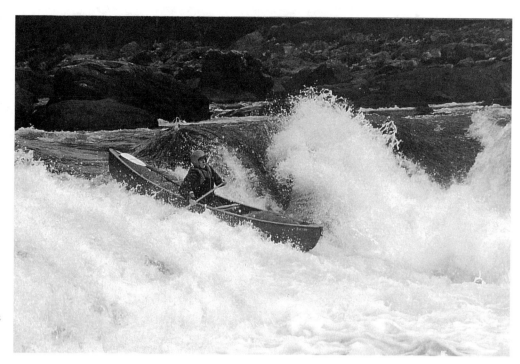

Liz Garland running Sweets
Falls on the Upper Gauley.
Photo by Mayo Gravatt.

thing more than a minimal inflow (200–300 cfs), when added to the fall release, makes Lost Paddle pushy and rescues become difficult.

The first drop is pretty straightforward; a 200-yard boulder garden with a strong hole at the bottom. Enter to the left of a pyramid-shaped rock at the top and work left, split two holes, and catch the eddy at the bottom. A second eddy is about 50 yards below on river right, just above the second drop.

The second drop is the steepest, shallowest, and most turbulent part of Lost Paddle. Easily boat-scouted from the eddies above, the top of the drop consists of a large, curling wave extending from the left shore to the center of the river. The wave hides a steep ledge; the best route is just to the right of this crest, no more than two boat lengths from the left shore. This takes you past the hole into the waves below. There is also a tight, rocky sneak route on the far right that should be scouted from shore first. The rock in the center of the wave train at the bottom (Decision Rock or Six Pack Rock) can be run on either side; this rock and the ones on the left shore are undercut, so swimmers should stay in the center and float with the current.

The third drop is an easy chute with a big hole at the bottom right. Run down the left, easily avoiding a hole on the top left. Quickly pick up swimmers and gear in the calm, but swift water below. Watch out for commercial rafts in the right eddy.

The fourth drop is also called Tumblehome and must

be run with care. The chutes over the ledge at the top left are badly undercut and were the site of a fatality in the 1970s. A large rock sits in the center of the river above this rapid. Rafts like to run to the right of this rock, punching or skirting a hole, then cutting to the left to catch the next good chute over a rocky ledge. Hard-boaters with good skills can set up in an eddy on the upstream left, then aim for a very narrow chute at right center. They could also catch a weak eddy behind the big rock, go one chute over, and pick up the raft line. Below here the routes converge; head for the center chute at the bottom of the rapid. There's a great ender spot on the left side of the chute. The next chute over to the right (the mail slot) is very narrow and potentially dangerous.

Some easy, but deceptively dangerous rapids lie below. Conestoga Rapid is easy Class III unless you take the blind chute at river center. A dangerous hole at the bottom, backed up by a rock, is called Darrow's Doucher and is very strong. Take the left chute, then work quickly to the right to avoid some pinning rocks. Table Rock Rapid (also called Shipwreck Rock) is another Class III, but the rock itself is undercut and extends across two-thirds of the river. Most of the river goes under it, creating a deadly trap; this is the site of two deaths and several narrow escapes. The normal route starts on the left of a rocky island, runs through some large waves, then works through several hundred yards of small waves to the far right side of Table Rock. Be sure to swing to the left to avoid Razor Rock, which is hidden behind the top wave.

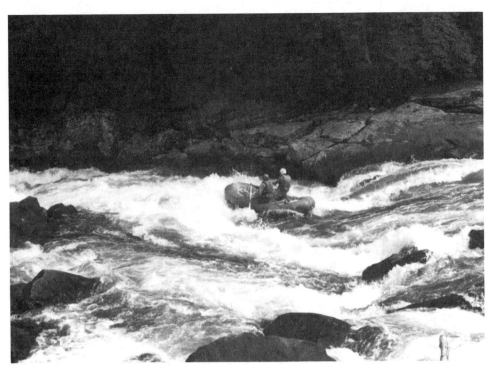

Two-person raft on the big tongue entering Iron Ring on the Upper Gauley. Photo by Ed Grove.

Below here there's plenty of time to paddle (or swim) to the right. When looking for a safer approach, the top of the rapid can also be run on the right.

Not far below Table Rock, the river bends right and the current is compressed along the right shore by a point of rocks. This is Iron Ring (Class V–VI), named for an iron ring set in the rocks on the left (stolen in 1988). It was used during an attempt to create a log-floating passage here in the early 1900s. Dynamite blasts created an irregular midchannel obstruction. The river sharply constricts on the right and drops down a six-foot-high slide into a hole a boat length above the obstructing boulder (Woodstock Rock). The current welling up out of the hole mostly slips down the right side. Some splashes over the now-smooth, man-made block, and about a fourth flushes under and around the left side of Woodstock Rock in a channel between it and its mother stone. The channel is crooked, turbulent, and powerful enough force to fold an errant paddler and boat together. Carry on the left or scout carefully and run from left to right. The proper line is very clean but leaves little margin for error. You start from the left, skirting the right side of two hydraulics to line up for the main rapid. Then you work carefully from left to right (bow angled right) on a large tongue to slip between the Woodstock Rock obstruction on the left and Backender Hole on the right. Don't relax too soon at the bottom because a lot of current slams into rocks on the bottom right. Throw ropes can be set on the left below the holes. At lower water levels, Iron Ring becomes meaner; most paddlers walk it below 1,500 cfs.

The next mile is easy except for a word of caution about Fingernail Rock Rapid (Class III), three-quarters of a mile below Iron Ring. The rock on the far left is badly undercut. Run right. About eight miles into the trip you reach Sweet's Falls (Class V). Here the Welsh sandstone, shale, and thin strata of Sewell coal rise straight up from the right side of the river. The river jogs right, then left, and drops over a cliff of this sandstone as heavy, steep, 10-foot falls. It was named for John Sweet, who ran it on the initial Gauley trip in 1968.

The left side of the falls is a technical boulder garden—a Class IV sneak. To run the falls proper, take out on the right well above the entrance for a difficult scout, or run carefully behind someone who knows this drop well. The entrance is three to five feet to the right of an easy hole followed by a small wave train continuing to the lip of the drop just downstream. A large eddy is on the left. The main route to run the falls is very narrow. If you follow the wave train to the lip of the falls, you'll be too far right; here the drop is steepest with a terrible hole below. Running from the calm of the eddy will put you too far left with Snaggletooth Rock and another bad hole as a consequence. The safest line is a tongue or tube just below the seam or small depression where the wave train current and eddy current join. Run the seam. Some paddlers angle right with a strong left brace, others angle left.

Talk to someone who has run this drop to determine your route. After the big plunge, recover quickly to avoid being swept into the rocks below. Rafters should move right to avoid being blown into Postage Due Rock or the nasty Box Canyon on the left. Catch swimmers quickly because the main current blasts diagonally left.

The river calms down for several miles after Sweet's Falls. There are several excellent play spots about a mile below Sweet's Falls. A large pool with a giant, right-side eddy marks the beginning of Class VI River Runners' Mason Branch Road and the steep trail up Panther Creek. The section from Mason Branch to Bucklick is sometimes called the Middle Gauley, a Class II–III run with a number of delightful play spots. At Guide's Revenge the river rushes left toward a large, diagonal hole. It's easy to miss, but if you have some dry passengers aboard it's a good place to get them wet.

Woods Ferry Rapid, sometimes called Little Insignificant, is the hardest drop on the Middle Gauley. This very deceptive Class IV drop starts as a rather inoffensive boulder garden, then picks up speed. A large hole extends out from river left, forcing hard-boaters to swing out to the center to avoid it. But just downstream a big flat rock called Julie's Juicer forces most of the water to the left, and paddlers must make the move or suffer the consequences of dropping into Julie's Juicer hole just left of the rock. Large rafts often punch the hole to be sure they make it through the slot. Hard-boaters can also get past the Juicer by running the entire rapid down the far right. A short distance below here is the Woods Ferry take-out on the right.

Ender Waves rapid is just below the Woods Ferry pool. It's a snappy Class III wave train with some dynamic surfing opportunities. Then the river alternates between easy rapids and long pools for several miles. Suddenly, the river narrows up against giant boulders and rushes into a large hole at the bottom. This is Back Ender (Class IV). The hole is strongest at flows in the 1,200 cfs range and starts to wash out around 3,000 cfs. Most boaters start by running this drop down the center, cutting to the right to miss the hole. Appalachian Wildwater's Bucklick take-out is just downstream on the right. This is a popular boundary between the upper and lower run.

A word about water levels. Although most people run the river during fall releases, there are many opportunities to run the river at other times. Hard-boaters report good runs with 500 cfs or less! The big rapids are steep and technical, but lack the push of the higher levels. At the other extreme, the run is paddled regularly at 4,000–6,000 cfs. At these levels, the big drops become huge and pushy, making them suitable for experts only.

Lower Gauley

The Lower Gauley from Bucklick (D) to Swiss (E) is the best advanced level, big-water run in the East. It may be more beautiful than the upper stretch, and the rapids are more open and considerably easier. There are five rapids of Class IV or greater difficulty and many easier drops with excellent play spots. At release levels the biggest waves and the biggest holes on the river are found on this section. It's good fun from 1,000 to 8,000 cfs. At low water it's a good run for intermediates; mostly Class III–III+. At high water levels experts will encounter long wave trains, massive holes, and scores of giant surfing waves.

Here's a description of the rapids at release levels of 2,400–2,800 cfs:

Koontz Flume (Class IV+) has a tricky entrance and big waves. The huge rock on river right is undercut and a few careless paddlers have been pushed underneath it. There's a large hole on the top left center; most paddlers skirt it to the right, then work quickly left to catch the main tongue. This maneuver can be tricky because a wave at the right edge of the hole kicks the other way. Alternatively, hard-boaters can catch a large but deceptive right-hand eddy and ferry out into the flume. This leads to the main drop, a smooth ride into a big wave train. Whatever you do, don't run the vertical drop on the far right side of the flume; it takes you under Koontz Rock! For the more cautious, the rapid can be scouted and run on the left. There's also a sporty, hole-studded run down the center. Five Boat Hole, at the base, is a bit sticky, but is still a fine play spot. Watch out for oncoming rafts!

Canyon Doors (Class III) is ornamented with beautiful sandstone cliffs on the right. Run far right, then work left toward the bottom for a good surfing hole. Immediately downstream is Junkyard (Class III)—usually run on the left. There is a safe route on the far right that ends with a good ender spot.

After four minor rapids, the Peters Creek trestle (an alternate put-in), and 3.5 miles of paddling, you come to the Mash brothers, Upper and Lower. Upper Mash (Class III+) is a complex and torturous bump-and-grind over and through a steep, shallow boulder garden. It is perhaps best entered in the center to the left or right of a large rock. In low water, avoid a pinning rock below the two- to three-foot ledge on the left of this rock by staying to the left. After picking your way down the technical center channel, eddy right or left at the bottom. These eddies are your last chance to scout Lower Mash—a big wave train (Class IV) with a big breaking wave that's hard to

Lower Gauley • West Virginia

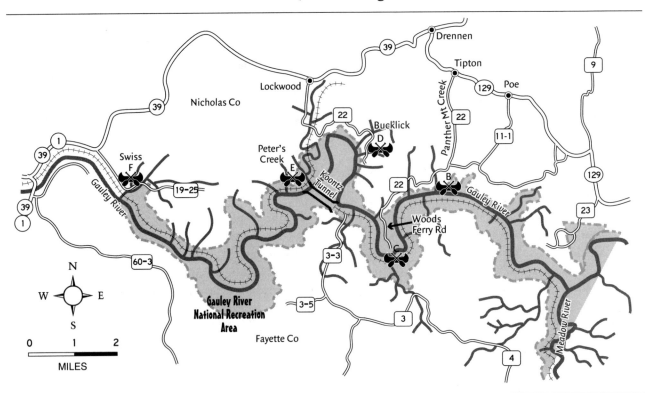

Section: Bucklick to Swiss

Counties: Nicholas, Fayette

USGS Quads: Ansted

Difficulty: Class III–V

Gradient: 26 feet per mile

Average Width: 100 feet

Velocity: Fast

Rescue Index: Remote to remote but accessible

Hazards: Long rapids, high water, undercut rocks, strainers

Scouting: Koontz Flume, Lower Mash, Gateway to Heaven, Riverwide Stopper, Pure Screaming Hell

Portages: None

Scenery: Beautiful

Highlights: Classic trip through pristine gorge, cliffs at Canyon Doors

Gauge: National Weather Service at Charleston, (304) 529-5127, Monday through Friday, 8 A.M. to 4:30 P.M. for Belva gauge; Summersville Dam (dam release and Meadow River), (304) 872-5809; National Park Service, (304) 465-0508

Runnable Water Levels	Minimum	Maximum
Belva gauge	2 feet (700 cfs)	9 feet (10,000 cfs)

Additional Information: National Park Service, (304) 465-0508

avoid. The most conservative route starts left of center and ends right, in the eddy below the ledge. Beware of an undercut boulder sieve at the bottom left, well below the ledge. At high water levels, run right of center and watch out for big reaction waves crashing in from the left. Rescue flipped boaters quickly because the river continues to flow fast and rocky for several hundred yards downstream.

After being "Mashed," the paddler reaches Diagonal Ledges (Class III), which has some good surfing holes. A chute between two rocks forms an ender slot just to the right of the first drop. Even open boaters can get enders here, but swimmers will not escape without assistance. Below here, Maui Wave (a.k.a. Hawaii Five-O Wave) forms at the bottom left at high water. It's a great surfing wave that easily surfs (and flips) rafts at high water.

Gateway to Heaven is a long, Class IV rapid where the river necks down and gets squeezed between two large rocks that form the gate. Begin the run by threading your way through the boulder garden at center, then cut left to avoid a nasty ledge/hole that blocks the right side of the river. After passing this boat-eating monster, work right and catch the wave train headed for the Gate. Take the right side of the chute and angle your bow right for the best run. If you stray to the left, the water slams you against the left-hand "gatepost." The entire rapid can be snuck on the left, finishing to the left of the gates; this is the best high-water route and avoids the huge hole that forms in the gates. At high flows do not run through the Gateway, but stay on the far left.

After Gateway to Heaven are three Class III rapids. The first is Rocky Top; run it on the right and look out for a hidden hole right of center near the bottom that gets larger as the river gets higher. To miss it, work left in the lower part of the rapids. You'll find a good ender spot, "Chicken Ender," below Rocky Top on the left. Picture Rock is next—a real sneaky rapid upstream of a large, midriver rock. The current goes over a sloping ledge from right to left and can push you further left than you want to go. Just as you go over the bottom of the drop, water coming in suddenly from the left shoves you to the right—sideways into a hole that will flip you upstream unless you have a strong low brace ready on your left. Upper Stairsteps rapid follows, a wave-train roller coaster on river left. Look out for a large hole in the center halfway down, which gets bigger at higher levels.

Next is Riverwide Stopper (also known as Lower Stairsteps or The Hole). This is a larger Class III–IV wave train. Run it center with a large, riverwide crashing wave midway down. Punch this squarely and with vigor to avoid a fisheye view of the river. At low water you can sneak the hole to the right or left of center.

The next good Class II–III wave train is called Rollercoaster. There are three more Class III rapids. The first is Cliffside: easy on the right and fun on the left. It can be recognized by the cliffs on the left. If you run it on the left, angle right and brace left into a diagonal curler after you enter. Below is Rattlesnake—a long rapid with a rattler on the end. Enter right of the island, and work right for the most conservative route. The last of the trio is Roostertail, which should be run left to avoid a pinning rock on the bottom right.

After a short pool (7.5 miles into the trip), you'll arrive at the top of Pure Screaming Hell (Class IV–V), the last of the major Gauley rapids. This appropriately named rapid starts on a curve to the right and ends on a left turn that is far, far below. The trick to running this rapid successfully is to stay in the center of the main flow. Starting right of center, pass some large holes on your right, then start looking for a larger hole extending out from river left. Skirt the edge of this hole, then cut behind it to avoid hitting an even bigger (almost riverwide) hole just downstream. Although none of these holes are keepers, they play rough! A more serious danger is a bad rock sieve on the outside of the turn, just above the final hole. If you find yourself drifting or swimming in this direction, work back toward the center fast!

Kevin's Folly, the last named drop, appears after a few miles of easy rapids and short pools. A bouncy run at

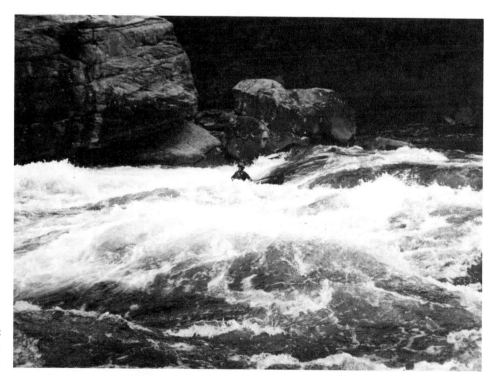

Scott Gravatt running Koontz
Flume on the Lower Gauley.
Photo by Court Ogilvie.

release levels, it has some big waves and holes at high water. A mile and a half below, on river right, is Omega Siding, just above the town of Swiss. There are a number of take-out options here.

Access Points for the Upper and Lower Gauley

The first paddlers to run this river assumed that the surrounding area was mostly trackless wilderness. This was never true, and today many of the jeep trails and wagon roads have been rebuilt to provide access for outfitters. Many of these companies permit their use by private paddlers, but remember to follow the directions of outfitter personnel and stay clear of the large trucks and buses that the roads were built to accommodate. Be prepared for some traffic jams on busy fall weekends.

The put-in for the Upper Gauley is easy to find: it's at the base of Summersville Dam (A). Go left on Route 129 from Route 19, about ten miles south of Summersville. The turn-off to the "tailwaters" of the dam is well marked; during Gauley season, park rangers staff a checkpoint a few hundred yards below it. The huge torrents of water coming from the tubes at the base of the dam have been a humbling spectacle for paddlers since the 1970s. By the time you read this they may be stilled, sacrificed to a hydroelectric project operated by the town of Summersville. Most people choose to run their shuttle on river right, where most of the take-out options are.

A few miles west Route 129 makes a sharp turn at Carnifex Ferry Battlefield State Park. Confederate troops under General Floyd camped here; when probed by a large contingent of Yankee soldiers, they decided they were outnumbered and retreated. Under cover of darkness they traveled down from the heights, across the Gauley, and up the Meadow River Valley. A steep trail leads from an overlook down to the top of Pillow Rock Rapids, and the remains of the old ferry road wind from the heights to a point opposite the mouth of the Meadow. Believe it or not, this was once an important travel route!

Eight miles into the trip, you'll reach the most popular take-out for the Upper Gauley (B). The Mason Branch Road and the Panther Creek Trail are both owned by Class VI River Runners. The road is private, and the trail, while beautiful, is extremely steep. Both are reached via the Panther Mountain Road (WV 22), which turns off Route 129 behind a church a few miles west of Carnifex Ferry Park. American Whitewater and the West Virginia Rivers Coalition work together with the Class VI River Runners to provide a shuttle service during the fall season. At other times you'll have to carry your boat up the

trail or continue downriver. The next access point is Woods Ferry (C), 12 miles into the trip on river right. It can be reached by traveling further down Panther Mountain Road and taking the left fork. The last half mile is extremely steep and rough.

The Bucklick access (D), owned by Appalachian Wildwater, is 15 miles below the dam. It can be reached by turning off WV 39 at the old Otter Creek School (WV 22), where Peter's Creek turns away from the highway. After the blacktop ends, turn left, then choose the right fork. This winding dirt road is heavily traveled by private vehicles and outfitter trucks and buses; expect delays. After several miles you'll arrive at the top of a well-maintained dirt road dropping into the canyon. Vehicle access is limited during Gauley season, but Imre Szilagyi, the owner, has generously permitted walk-ins at this point for many years. The rules are simple: park where you won't cause problems for the trucks and buses, then carry your boat a half mile down the access road.

The best way to get to the Bucklick access from Swiss is to use Rusty's Shuttle Service (call 304-574-3475). Rusty meets paddlers at the first parking area and runs them and their boats all the way to the river. The cost in 1996 was $7. You can call to reserve a space or show up and take your chances.

Two miles below Bucklick the Peter's Creek trestle (E) crosses the Gauley. Before other access points were built, paddlers running the Upper Gauley left their boats beside the river here and hiked two miles up the railroad tracks to a muddy clearing in the woods. This walk crosses two other trestles and passes a 20-foot waterfall on Peter's Creek. The trestles have walkways, and this hike is pleasant. To reach the clearing, turn off at Otter Creek School, turn right after crossing Peter's Creek, then take the right fork. The road is badly rutted and requires a high-clearance vehicle.

On the far side of the Peter's Creek trestle the railroad plunges into the 0.9-mile-long Koontz Bend Tunnel, emerging five miles upstream just below Ender Waves. After some boats were stolen from the mouth of Peter's Creek in the mid-1970s, many paddlers decided to shorten the Upper Gauley run and improve security at the same time. They left their boats at the far end of the tunnel and walked the tracks to Peter's Creek. The tunnel was an unpleasant and scary walk even if they remembered to bring flashlights! They stubbed their toes on the ties, splashed through the muddy ditches, and lived with the ever-present fear that a train would come roaring through the mountain. Then they were forced to lie face-down in the filthy ditches while the boxcars clattered past. Needless to say, nobody wanted to do that again! The railroad is now abandoned but the walk is still unpleasant.

The take-out for the Lower Gauley run is the small hamlet of Swiss (F). Turn left on a side road about eight miles down WV 39 from the Otter Creek School on river right. Several short trails run from the river to the road. During Gauley season a few landowners rent parking spaces in their fields and yards. Because vehicles left just upstream at Omega Siding have been burglarized, it's a good idea to patronize these folks. Be sure to walk from the parking lot to the river so you'll know where to get out. If you do park along the road, all four wheels must be off the pavement or you'll be ticketed. Be sure to park at least five feet from the railroad tracks; the rail cars overhang the rails considerably and can do some serious damage. You can also take out in Jodie, a mile downstream on river left.

River Levels

Flow information on the Gauley River can be obtained from the National Weather Service in Charleston (call 304-529-5127) or from the U.S. Army Corps of Engineers at Summersville Dam (call 304-872-5809). The Belva gauge combines the flows in the Gauley and Meadow Rivers, Peter's Creek, and all other tributaries coming in above Swiss. The Gauley season begins the week after Labor Day and runs Friday through Monday for six consecutive weeks. For more information call the National Park Service in Glen Jean (304-465-0508). American Whitewater's Gauley River Festival is typically on the third release weekend; for more information call them at (301) 589-9453.

Although most paddlers run the Gauley during the fall releases, the river runs over 2,250 cfs 35 percent of the time in May, 10 percent of the time in June, July, and August, and over 50 percent of the time November through March. It runs over 800 cfs, a great level for the Upper Gauley, even more often. To predict the flows, you'll need to know the lake flow and the pool level. If the lake is over 1,575 feet during November–April and over 1,652 feet in May–August, the inflow to the lake is passed through the next day. The Craigsville gauge provides the inflow information. All three numbers are on the Summersville Dam number. But beware: big flows of 6,000 cfs or more with considerable inflow from side streams are not uncommon! If the Meadow River is running over 1,000 cfs, regardless of the dam release, the Lower Gauley is boatable.

Gauley Conservation Efforts

The whitewater of the Gauley River remains available today only because of the efforts of a few private boaters and commercial outfitters with strong support from the West Virginia congressional delegation.

To the U.S. Army Corps of Engineers, which operates the Summersville Dam, the project and the river held great potential for the construction of a hydroelectric power plant. During the early 1980s, the Corps of Engineers made a big political push to build a "long tunnel" hydro project for taking water from Summersville Lake to a powerhouse to be constructed just above Pillow Rock. The project would have dried up several miles of the best whitewater on the Gauley. At the same time, the Corps of Engineers claimed that whitewater releases from the dam were not within the project's authorized purposes, which include flood control and pollution abatement. However, to gain the support of river users for its proposal, the Corps of Engineers promised that a hydroelectric power plant would enhance rather than detract from whitewater opportunities on the Gauley.

A group called Citizens for Gauley River, made up of private and commercial whitewater boaters, was quickly formed to fight the Corps of Engineers' proposal and to work for scheduled whitewater releases from Summersville Dam. David Brown of Knoxville, Tennessee forged this group into an effective and powerful political force, just as he had in an earlier, successful battle to save the Ocoee River in Tennessee. Under Brown's skillful leadership, the Citizens for Gauley River succeeded beyond all expectations.

In early 1984, U.S. Representative Nick J. Rahall of Beckley, West Virginia, threatened to amend a funding bill for the Corps of Engineers with a provision prohibiting any further consideration of the proposed hydroelectric power project and vowed that Congress would never authorize its construction. Almost immediately, the Corps of Engineers withdrew the proposal and ceased further planning for Gauley hydroelectric developments. Rahall proceeded with legislation to authorize whitewater recreation as a project purpose of Summersville Dam. Enactment of this provision later that year set a precedent. The Summersville Dam became the first of many Corps of Engineers water projects to have whitewater recreation as one of its official purposes.

To further enhance whitewater recreation on the Gauley, Rahall also added a provision to the 1986 Omnibus Water Projects Authorization Bill that would guarantee whitewater releases from Summersville Dam at 2,500 cfs for a minimum of 20 days during the six-week period following Labor Day each year. This legislation was enacted by Congress and signed into law in November 1986. In the years that followed, the Gauley became a national river administered by the National Park Service.

New River

The New has a little something for everyone in its three most popular sections. The uppermost section from Sandstone to McCreery (15 miles) is the least paddled and consists of Class II rapids and some seemingly unending pools. It's a good run for open canoes and can be combined with the succeeding Prince-to-Thurmond run at moderate levels for canoe camping. This latter section sports more continuous Class II and borderline Class III water than the section above and is a longtime favorite of novice and intermediate paddlers in both decked and open boats. Below Thurmond the bottom falls out as the river runs through the celebrated New River Gorge. This is one of the premier Class IV-V whitewater runs of the eastern United States. Contrary to its name, the New is the oldest river in North America and is one of the few large rivers in the world that flows north.

Sandstone to McCreery

The section from Sandstone (A) to McCreery (B) is a very long run consisting of several nice impressive rapids, but, as with much of the New, these are interrupted by long expanses of flatwater. It is a big powerful river, very beautiful, always up in the summer, with plenty of excellent fishing. Numerous campsites are available for overnight trips. The rapids are mainly long chutes dropping gently over ledges. Although the waves are large, not much maneuvering is required.

Open boaters and novices will encounter only two places that may cause trouble. The first of these occurs at the top of Horseshoe Bend, which can be viewed from Grandview State Park. The entire river necks down, creating big waves that can swamp open canoes immediately. This one is located about a half mile downstream from the obsolete concrete bridge piers at Glade (the second rapid from there). The river heads to the left and turns sharply back to the right. In this curve you'll find some very heavy water including a Class III+ stopper. After the rapids have pushed their way to the right, they

straighten out and more heavy turbulence is found midstream. Amid these waves is a mean hole that's large enough to eat a whole canoe. You will need a lot of drive to get through this one. Open-boaters or novices may avoid all of the heavy water by maintaining control and staying to the far right.

The second potential trouble spot is a delightfully long Class III rapids at Quinnimont just before reaching the railroad station. It is not difficult, but open canoes might swamp due to its length. Such canoeists should consider dumping excess water halfway down. Near the bottom, a huge drain pipe enters from the right. Just before this there is a powerful hydraulic in the middle of the river, followed by 20 yards of flatwater, and then another very deceptive wave that camouflages a hole deep enough to set a C-2 in. Fun, but surprising!

Access at Sandstone is not ideal, but folks are neighborly and are normally happy to grant you access to the

Section: Sandstone to McCreery
Counties: Summers, Fayette, Raleigh
USGS Quads: Meadow Creek, Beckley
Difficulty: Class I–III
Gradient: 8 feet per mile
Average Width: 125 feet
Velocity: Slow to moderate
Rescue Index: Accessible to remote
Hazards: None
Scouting: None
Portages: None
Scenery: Generally beautiful
Highlights: Excellent fishing, camping
Gauge: For Hinton gauge information, call Bluestone Dam, (304) 466-0156; National Weather Service, Charleston, (304) 529-5727

Runnable Water Levels	Minimum	Maximum
Hinton gauge	1.75 feet	2.50 feet

Additional Information: National Park Service, (304) 465-0508

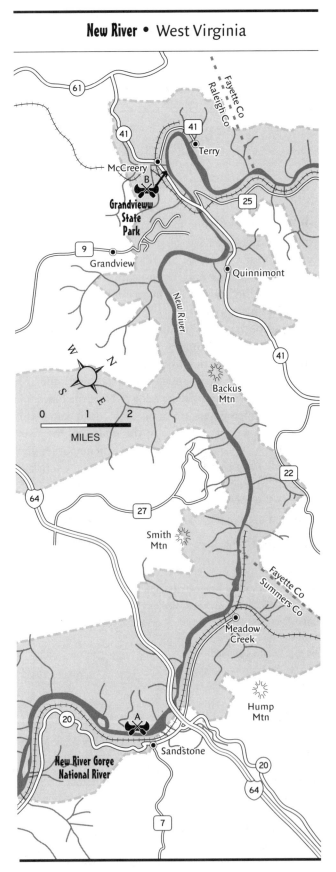

New River • West Virginia

river. To drive to the take-out, take WV 20 out of Sandstone to Meadow Bridge, turn left on CR 31 to Danese, and turn left again on WV 41 to McCreery. The take-out is easiest at a very large, sandy beach located on the left, two rapids beyond the WV 41 bridge. It may be reached in a car by turning right off WV 41 onto a dirt road where WV 41 turns left to go up the mountain.

Prince to Thurmond

The stretch from Prince (B, just below McCreery) to Thurmond (C) is characterized by more rapids and more long, flatwater pools. Generally the individual rapids are heavier than those in the upper river. The river is wide and powerful at 2.5 feet on the Hinton gauge, and it would be unwise for novices or open-boaters lacking substantial experience or flotation to proceed at this or higher levels. Each rapid is a riverwide, long stretch of big waves with few obstructions. Occasionally a ledge is encountered at one side or the other, but is always eroded in the heaviest current. Consequently, although large stopper waves and an occasional hydraulic are found, very little maneuvering is required.

Intermediate paddlers with heavy-water experience should encounter no difficulties or unexpected surprises, but this is a tough place for beginners. More than halfway along and after a particularly long flat stretch, four sand silos appear on the right bank of a left-hand turn (the sand in the silos is used for making glass). Just below this, very large Class III+ waves are found along the right bank. Another long, flat stretch, two minor rapids, and a zesty chute over a ledge bring the paddler to the take-out.

You can put in at the McCreery beach mentioned above or at a developed put-in across the bridge over McCreery Creek. The easiest take-out is on the sandy beach 200 yards above a bridge located a mile above Thurmond (the first bridge you'll encounter). This take-out, located on the left side of the river, is reached by a dirt road. The water is pretty flat from this bridge to Thurmond itself, although you'll find a nice Class II rapid right under the Thurmond bridge. Although there is a dirt road connecting Prince to Thurmond, we don't recommend using it when setting shuttle. Take WV 41 from Prince toward Beckley, turn right on WV 61 to Mount Hope, turn right onto WV 16 for about a mile, and then make one more right turn at CR 25 leading to Glen Jean and Thurmond.

For water information call the Bluestone Dam at (304) 466-1234 or (304) 466-0156. The Hinton gauge reading takes into account the output of the Greenbrier; for a computerized reading of this gauge, call (304) 465-1722.

Section: McCreery/Prince to Thurmond

Counties: Fayette, Raleigh

USGS Quad: Beckley

Difficulty: Class II–III

Gradient: 10 feet per mile

Average Width: 150 feet

Velocity: Slow to moderate

Rescue Index: Accessible

Hazards: None

Scouting: Large waves below four sand silos on river right, waves can be avoided on the left

Portages: None

Scenery: Generally beautiful

Highlights: Big river; rapids are mainly waves, the biggest over halfway into trip below four sand silos

Gauge: For Hinton gauge information, call Bluestone Dam, (304) 466-0156; National Weather Service, Charleston, (304) 529-5127

Runnable Water Levels	Minimum	Maximum
Hinton gauge	1.75 feet	2.50 feet

Months Runnable: All year

Additional Information: National Park Service, (304) 465-0508

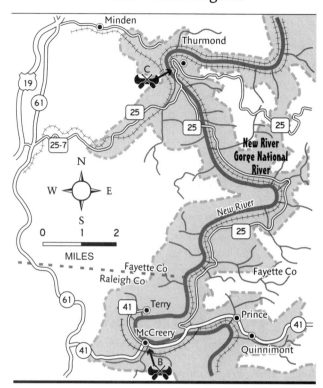

New River • West Virginia

The river seldom drops below 1.75 feet and is often at this level in the summer. Approach the entire river with great caution if over 2.5 feet.

Thurmond to Fayette Station (The Gorge)

The New River Gorge from Thurmond (C) to Fayette Station (E) contains the biggest whitewater in the southern Appalachians. The river flows through an immense gorge. Steep slopes and rugged cliffs can be seen throughout the run. The first half of this stretch alternates long, flat pools and easy Class II–III rapids that could be run by conventional canoes at low water levels. Below Cunard the drops get bigger and the turbulence increases. Most rapids are straight shots through big waves, with little maneuvering required. There are six drops in the Class III+ to IV+ range. This is a hugely popular commercial raft run and becomes very crowded on summer weekends. A reliable roll is recommended for all hard-boaters.

There's a Class II rapid under the bridge at Thurmond with some medium-sized waves, then several miles of flatwater broken by a small rapid at Buzzard's Bend. About four miles into the trip one particular rapid deserves respect—the famous Surprise Rapid (Class III+). At the top it looks like another straight shot over a gravel bar, but the water rapidly converges toward a huge set of waves. There is a big hole between the first and second waves that swallows kayaks and sets rafts on end at moderate levels. Hit the left side and angle slightly to the right if you want to punch it, but be prepared to swim out! The hole is easily skirted to either side, with the left side being easier. At high water levels all but the largest rafts opt for the left-hand route.

Three miles below Surprise the National Park Service improved the old four-wheel-drive road to the Cunard put-in (D). People interested in the best whitewater begin their trip here. A half mile away you'll be able to see a railroad trestle downstream. Upper Railroad Rapids starts about 200 yards above the bridge. This rapid has two distinct parts: the top section has a huge hole on river right called the Cunard Stripper. It's a keeper at levels over three feet at Fayette Station, but it can be easily missed on the left. At lower levels there is a tongue that's hard to see from upstream. If you plan to surf this hole, post a lookout upstream to warn off commercial raft traffic and get ready for one hell of a ride. People who swim out of the hole should head for deep water. The second part of the drop features a wave train on the left and a shallow boulder garden on the right.

At the other end of a short pool a horizon line marks the start of Lower Railroad. This steep boulder barrage can be run in several places, but the route is blind and first-timers should scout it. Paddlers typically start one-third of the way over from the left and run right over a big water hump, then work over to the right to miss the hole at the bottom. At low levels (below zero at Fayette Station) there are some deadly undercut rocks in this drop that cannot be seen from upstream. Two boaters have been killed here, so everyone should get out and scout!

Four easy wave rapids, separated by pools, await downstream. These are big fun at high water levels and always offer excellent surfing. The second one is frequently occupied by kayakers playing chicken with oncoming rafts. The third has a nasty hole on the right side that only the most daring boaters will want to try.

After nine miles of paddling you should be warmed up for the big stuff, the Keaney Brothers. Upper Keaney (Class III+) can be recognized by the huge, smooth boulder (Whale Rock) coming in from river left. Run through the waves and angle into the eddy behind Whale Rock to set up for Middle Keaney (Class IV). At higher levels the eddy is hard to get into, so you may want to head directly into the next drop. Middle Keaney has three large, breaking waves in the center channel. The easiest route is just to the left or right of these monsters. At two feet or lower, rafts can aim for a black rock in the bottom right center, while open boats can shoot past a dry, camel-back rock at left center. There are holes on the left and right sides, so don't try to sneak this one! At levels higher than four feet the waves are eight feet high and this rapid merges with the biggest drop of the three, Lower Keaney, which lies downstream.

Even experienced New River paddlers like to get out and scout Lower Keaney (Class IV+) on river left. It cannot be lined or snuck, and it's a nasty carry over giant boulders, so you might as well figure out how to run it. The river has necked down on the left side to one-third its normal width, concentrating the action enormously. The waves at the bottom surge ominously, bombarding a huge rock (Wash-up Rock) on river left and exploding into a giant wave train. The size of the wave varies with the level; they're big at one foot; wash out slightly at two feet, and come back bigger than ever at three feet. The trick is to start at the center of this huge chute and work quickly over to the right. You can then ease back into the waves if you're looking for a thrill. At certain levels you'll find a roostertail in the center of the chute; you must get to the right of it to avoid being pushed into the rock. There's a small drop about 50 yards below here with a nice surfing wave and an eddy line infested with huge whirlpools. If you have swimmers, pick them up fast.

Dudley's Dip (Class III) follows. Above 0.5 feet on the gauge, begin this rapid left of center. As you enter, look for a pour-over rock and run just to the right of it. Below 0.5 feet, enter on the far right and work diagonally to the left; the route is easier to read from this angle. Go between the two pour-over rocks on left and right of center. The large, upside-down-canoe–shaped rock on the right side and the slanting rock on the left side are undercut.

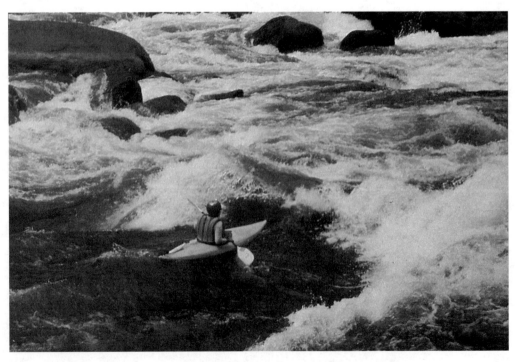

Keith Merkel on Lower Keeney Rapid. Photo by Bob Maxey.

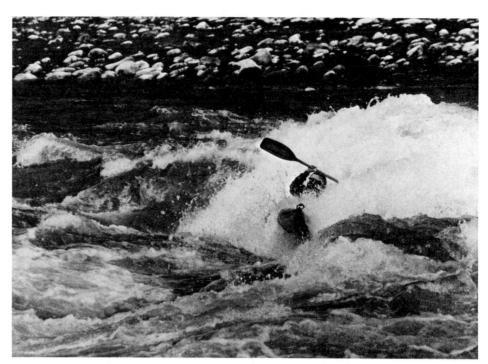

Diana Kendrick in Surprise
on the New River.
Photo by Paul Marshall.

Next comes Sunset, or Double **Z** (Class V), the most technical rapid on the river. Over 10 miles into the trip, it's marked by a chain of rocks extending halfway across the river from the right. First-timers can pull over to the right above this chain of rocks and scout before entering the rapid. Enter the rapid and eddy out behind the rock chain in order to reach the far right channel and avoid a nasty, complex **V**-ledge and hydraulic in the center. The right channel will take you diagonally to the left, but it tumbles steeply through a field of holes and boulders, ending with a mean pour-over and powerful hole below at bottom center. At levels of up to two feet, try to run this rapid close to the right bank. Over three feet, it's best to run left of center down a big "**V**" that forms. At levels above four feet, watch for a nasty hole in the middle of the rapid. At all levels, avoid the huge boulder toward bottom left that is undercut and has a powerful current under it.

The next rapid is Old 99 or Hook (Class III). This can be run right, middle, or left. Right gives a sliding-board feeling, middle is a backward **S** turn, and the left is the straightest. Just below is Bear's Rock or the second part of Old 99 (to some paddlers). Left of center is a smooth chute just to the right of a semidry rock. After running the chute, angle left to pass a large, violent hole on your right.

Work far left or far right after running this rapid because Greyhound Bus Stopper is just below. This aptly named monster could probably stop a bus at high levels and has a dangerous recirculation even at moderate flows. It can be avoided to the far left or right at any level. At levels of 1.5 feet or lower, look for dynamic enders just right of the rock forming Greyhound. Eddy behind Greyhound Rock and work back up to the spot where the river pours off the right edge. Enjoy!

Next comes Upper Kaymoor or Upper Tipple (Class II), which is easily read. At levels below zero the ledge on the far right side creates a steep, strong hole. Lower Kaymoor or Lower Tipple (Class III) can be run right (following a wave train) or left of the large rectangular rock in the middle (a more technical run). If running left, watch out for the squirrelly curler just to the left of the big rock.

Miller's Folly or Undercut Rock (Class IV+) follows, after 12 miles of paddling. Scout from the left. Avoid the temptation to begin at the far right, but instead begin in the center and paddle toward the left side of the big rock on the right (which is, of course, undercut). Stay in the left of the chute and then cut sharply left before you reach the rock, following the flow of this channel. Just below this you'll encounter some enormous, fun waves. At moderate levels, expect to find large eddies on the left and right that you can use to scout the lower part of the rapid. The best route is just left of center. Watch for an **L**-shaped hole at the top, run just to the right of it, then angle left to avoid going over Invisible Rock and hitting its accompanying steep, nasty hole. To sneak this lower

Section: Thurmond to Fayette Station

Counties: Fayette

USGS Quads: Thurmond, Fayetteville

Difficulty: Class III–V

Gradient: 15 feet per mile; the first seven miles at 11 feet per mile and the last seven miles at 19 feet per mile

Average Width: 150–200 feet

Velocity: Moderate to fast

Rescue Index: Remote

Hazards: Upper Railroad, big hole on river right; Lower Railroad, pinning rocks on left; Double **Z**, undercut rock at bottom left; Greyhound Bus Stopper, huge hole; Undercut Rock/Miller's Folly, undercut rock on top right and Bloody Nose on lower left

Scouting: Lower Railroad, Middle and Lower Keeney, Double **Z**, Undercut Rock; Fayette Station Rapid

Portages: None at lower levels

Scenery: Generally beautiful

Highlights: Biggest whitewater river in West Virginia, immense gorge

Gauge: Call Bluestone Dam, (304) 466-0516; National Weather Service, Charleston, (304) 529-5127

Runnable Water Levels	Minimum	Maximum
Fayette Station gauge	-1.5 feet	12 feet

Though it has been run down to -3 feet, more dangerous, pinning rocks appear; for expert open-boaters, the cutoff is 3-4 feet, although it has been run at 10-foot levels

Additional Information: National Park Service, (304) 465-0508

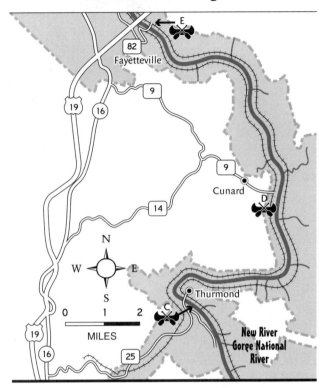

New River • West Virginia

part, run right. The far left is appropriately called Bloody Nose and should not be run.

Shortly after this rapid you will see two bridges—one crossing the gorge high above. Soon, you will reach Fayette Station Bridge; just below is Fayette Station Rapid (Class IV), which should not be missed. Run right of center. It is a multiholed roller coaster with some deceptively vigorous drops hidden by big waves. Be ready to hit the waves squarely. You can scout from the left. Take out on river left at the National Park Service Fayette Station access point after running this rapid. Other than one or two minor rapids (the second one requiring care to avoid the pour-over on the left side) the next four miles to Hawk's Nest Dam are mostly flatwater and seldom run. There is an outfitter's take-out a mile below Fayette Station at Teay's Landing on river right.

The shuttles for the New River Gorge are very straightforward. Fayette Station can be reached from Route 19 via WV 82. This area gets very crowded on summer weekends and parking is at a premium. Thurmond is also reached from Route 19 via Route 12. To find the Cunard access point, take the Main Street/Fayetteville exit off Route 19, drive through town, take the first left past the beer store, and follow signs. The road is steep but very well maintained. Park in the private boater section. Rusty's Shuttle Service (304-574-3475) will take you to Cunard and drop your car off in Thurmond for $7.

New River Dries

The New River Dries, a five-mile stretch from Cotton Hill to Gauley Bridge, is a little-known but very enjoyable section of whitewater through the most beautiful part of the New River Gorge. The Hawk's Nest tunnel diverts 9000 cfs of water to the power plant, so the Dries only run when there is water spilling over Hawk's Nest Dam. This happens whenever the New is flowing above 9,000 cfs or when the hydro plant at Gauley Bridge is not running at full capacity. At levels of 1,000–3,000 cfs this is Class II+ open-boatable. From 3,000–10,000 cfs it is suitable for intermediate decked boats and advanced open-boaters. From 10,000–20,000 cfs large holes and standing waves start to form and only paddlers comfortable with big water (like the New River Gorge at four to eight feet) should attempt the run. Above 20,000 cfs the sheer canyon walls constrict the flow into huge exploding waves and holes. At this level, the Dries should be attempted by experts only.

The rapids here are long but readable, with one exception. Entrance Rapid is rocky on the right and sports Broken Paddle Hole at bottom left, but it is easily run down the middle. Then comes Foreplay, a long stretch of smooth surfing waves at levels above 8,000 cfs. The river then bends to the left for Preparation, a half-mile series of Class II–III drops. After a short pool the river turns sharply left for Mile Long, which has the biggest water at high levels. Watch out for Multi-Bender-Bowl-Hole under the overhanging ledge at the bottom right at all levels and for Hatch's Hole at bottom left above 18,000 cfs. A long pool is followed by Landslide Rapid; scout this from river right at low water or river left at higher levels. Enter through the right slot and pick your way through the squirrelly, technical water below. Staying right all the way is safe but other options are possible. The Dries finishes with Afterplay, a series of nice, playable waves and holes.

Due to the unpredictability of water levels on the Dries, it is advisable to check with Hawk's Nest Dam for the most current information before putting in.

New River Gorge High Water Information

When the water gets really high (between five feet and twelve feet on the gauge), the New River Gorge changes dramatically. Huge holes, waves and other factors affect many of the rapids, dictating much more scouting and care in running the river. The river is substantially pushier and tougher. The following two examples show how different the gorge becomes.

A new rapid called the Halls of Karma (Class III) only exists between seven and nine feet on the Fayette Station gauge. This is the short narrow section of the river between Double **Z** and Old 99 (Hook). The sudden extreme narrowing of the river creates some dynamic waves and currents with large waves that are pulsating and moving. Most of the time, luck and quick reactions get paddlers through.

Also, at higher levels Upper, Middle, and Lower Keeney merge to become The Keeney (Class V+). At 10 feet, Whale Rock at Upper Keeney becomes Whale Hole—awesome. Between 8 and 11 feet, is a huge pulsating, crashing wave called The Mouth (downstream of Whale Hole in the center of the river where Middle Keeney used to be). It rises up, opens wide, and crashes down—even eating rafts on occasion. Below this (above seven feet), the rocks at the top right of Lower Keeney become Meatgrinder, a long, nasty hole; the rocks at the bottom left of Lower Keeney create another strong hole called Lollygag

(worst between three and seven feet).

The expert paddler should first scout The Keeney. Enter it far right so that Whale Hole does not swallow you. Then run to the right of The Mouth to avoid being eaten. Now start working left, but watch out for two very large, breaking waves angled downstream toward the left. They can easily flip you if you have too much left angle. After this, the river seems to calm down, but not much. Set up for what used to be Lower Keeney. Meatgrinder, the long nasty hole extending from the right, begins fairly small in the center of the river. To

New River Gorge Water Level Conversion (correlation) Table

Fayette Station (feet)	cfs
-3	544
-2	1,072
-1	1,704
0	2,440
1	3,352
2	4,436*
3	5,820*
4	7,550*
5	9,550*
6	11,400*
7	14,100
8	17,200**
9	20,200
10	23,800
11	26,800
12	30,000

Source: Dave Bassage

*Note: At these levels, the Fayette Station reading is approximately one-half of the cfs level, rounded to the nearest thousand. For example, 4,436 to 5,000 cfs equals 2 feet on the Fayette Station gauge; 5,820 to 6,000 cfs equals 3 feet; 14,000 to 14,100 equals 7 feet.

**Note: Calling the Thurmond gauge at (304) 465-0493 gives a system of beeps, which can be converted to Fayette Station equivalents. First, translate the beeps into a reading: you will hear a series of four groups of beeps. A long first beep means zero; a short first beep means one, heavy water. Write down the numbers of each series of beeps, and put a decimal between the second and third numbers, for example, 03.62, or 3.62 feet at the Thurmond gauge. To convert to Fayette Station equivalents, multiply the Thurmond reading by four-thirds (1.33), then subtract 4 2/3 (4.66) from the result. Your answer will show the equivalent reading at Fayette Station.

Example: A Thurmond reading of 3.62 times 1.33 equals 4.81 minus 4.66 gives 0.15 feet as the Fayette Station equivalent. This formula works for levels up to 7 or 8 feet at Fayette Station.

avoid it and its downstream companion, Lollygag, run just left or clip the left side of Meatgrinder (where the hole is still relatively small) and angle right. Drive hard to the right so you can miss Lollygag, which extends from the left side of the river. Then collapse from exhaustion or enjoy a king-sized adrenaline high in the calm area below.

At levels above eight feet the largest wave on the river is found on the left side of Fayette Station Rapid; it shouldn't be missed. Enter in the left V at the top. Halfway through, a huge, smooth wall of water blots out the sun. If you are good enough to have made it this far, you won't be flipped and the ride is rivaled only by Hermit rapid on the Colorado River.

Middle Fork of the Tygart River

Look at the rapids under the bridge at Audra State Park (A), look at the lush, sylvan surroundings, subtract the road, bridge, and bathhouse at the park, and then you'll know what to expect for the first 2.6 miles of this run. It's a beautiful, busy, boatbuster. If the water is low, the rapids under the bridge can be run on the right side, heading straight for the retaining wall of the swimming area, then slipping to the left down into the pool. When the water level is high, it is more entertaining to fandango down through the center.

Below the pool the Middle Fork of the Tygart takes off through a delightful mix of ledge and boulder rapids. You

can "read and run" most of them from your boat. At low water, the rapids are scrapy; at higher levels they pack some punch. It's a good place for newcomers to get a feel for technical paddling and prepare for runs like the Big Sandy, Blackwater, and Upper Yough. The water, though polluted with acid, is sparkling clear.

About an hour into the trip you'll paddle through a long rapid ending in a series of well-formed, playable, sliding ledge holes. After you're through messing with them, follow the river as it bends right around a hemlock-covered island. You'll encounter a long slide rapid into a powerful stopper. A rock just downstream makes a flip in the stopper more exciting, and it directs floating debris into an aggressive, left-side, whirlpool eddy. It's easy

Section: Audra State Park to Tygart Junction
County: Barbour
USGS Quad: Audra
Difficulty: Class IV
Gradient: 2.5 miles at 72 feet per mile
Average Width: 35 feet
Velocity: Fast
Rescue Index: Remote
Hazards: Continuous rapids; rocky, steep, technical paddling
Scouting: Last half mile of Middle Fork (three big rapids)
Portages: Possibly one or more of the three big rapids in the last half mile
Scenery: Beautiful
Highlights: Lush, wooded surroundings
Gauge: Visual. The government gauge just upstream of the bridge at Audra State Park has been partially washed away, so you must extrapolate

Runnable Water Levels	Minimum	Maximum
	3.3 feet	5.0 feet

Additional Information: National Weather Service, (412) 262-5290 (Pittsburgh) or (703) 260-0305 (Washington, DC area); the Belington gauge should be a minimum of 5 feet; Audra State Park, (304) 457-1162; Waterline, (800) 297-4243, #541319.

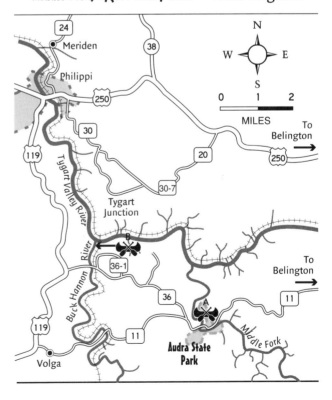

Middle Fork, Tygart Valley River • West Virginia

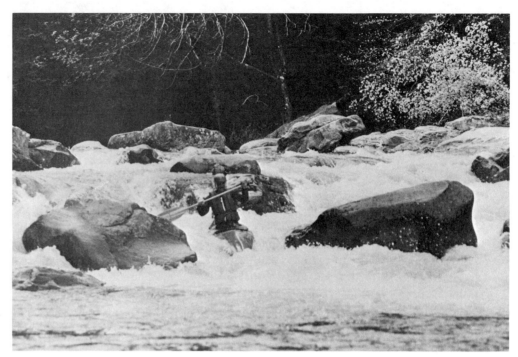

Jon Wright on the
Middle Fork of the Tygart.
Photo by Charles Walbridge.

enough to avoid the excitement by working right to miss the stopper.

Downstream you'll encounter three rapids that are significantly harder than anything upstream. The first one is a long, boulder rapid culminating in an impossibly sharp left turn around a broken ledge. The ledge can be run, but the channel is narrow and it should be scouted. The next big rapid is easily recognized by a huge boulder on river right. The right side offers a tight but clean run through narrow chutes between huge boulders. The route at the bottom is not obvious from above, but you can scout on the right with little trouble. The final rapid, just above the junction with the Tygart, consists of a steep, sliding ledge backed up by a vertical rock wall. Many people have lost some skin trying to make this move! How you get by depends on water levels, but the obstructed boulder garden on the right is not much better.

The river empties into the Tygart Gorge at about its midpoint, and the only way out is to paddle the remaining four miles to the mouth of the Buckhannon (B). This results in two interesting trips for the price of one. First is the steep, rocky, technical paddling of the lower Middle Fork and then the much heavier, pushy Tygart with its tripled volume.

Audra State Park can be reached from Belington; take a right turn at the light in the center of town and cross the new bridge over the Tygart. The take-out is the same as for the Tygart Gorge section. The riverside campgrounds at Audra State Park were created during the Depression by hundreds of workers using hand tools. The sites fit perfectly into the riverside environment and offer what is unquestionably the finest riverside camping in West Virginia.

The USGS Audra gauge is about 50 yards upstream from the bridge at Audra State Park on river right. Paddlers often check the water level while running a shuttle from Belington; they head for the Tygart gorge if the Middle Fork flow is insufficient. Because of the beautiful surroundings this section is often run low; I've had a good day on the river with Audra reading 3.2 feet. Conditions at the bridge rapid are pretty indicative of what will be encountered downstream.

Tygart River

The Gorge

The Gorge is the most rugged section of the Tygart, filled with many complex and bodacious rapids. The river runs through an isolated gorge civilized only by a set of worn-out railroad tracks on the right. These tracks have been used many times for walking out. The water is clear though acid-polluted, and flows through second-growth deciduous forest.

At the Belington put-in, the river is flat, then gradually picks up speed and flows through easy rapids down to an alternative put-in at Papa Weeze's. Immediately below here the river drops over four big ledges. At the first rapid, Keyhole (Class IV), the river tumbles between boxcar-sized boulders separated by four-feet-wide sluiceways. The center slot has been run, but is narrow and nasty. Most paddlers prefer the far right opening, a sharp left turn in a narrow channel. The channel widens and actually becomes easier at moderate flows (5.5 feet at Belington). The next two ledges are clean, but you should scout carefully to find the right chute.

The final ledge, Hartung Falls (Class V), was named for "Crazy Dave" Hartung, the first to run it. The water roars over a 10-foot-high sliding ledge on the left and caroms off the wall behind it to form a huge, nasty-looking diagonal hole. Boaters with enough moxie to run it can brace into the foam and ride it down to the big, exploding wave at the bottom. At moderate levels the ledge can be snuck in the center of the river. The water tends to carry you from right to left, so pick a line that takes this into account. At high water levels this section is very pushy and it may be a good idea to carry the entire section on the tracks at river right.

Below here the river alternates between exciting boulder drops and less obstructed, easier rapids. A few are memorable. Let's Make A Deal (Class IV) is a pushy rapid that culminates in a row of boulders that create three distinct chutes. Take the center door, please; the left goes between undercut rocks and the right, while open, is a real scramble to reach. Further down you'll see a pyramid-shaped rock that forms part of The Room (Class IV-). As you run down the left side, the left eddy at the bottom looks tempting, but it tends to throw you out as fast as you come in. Instead, eddy right. Large boulders now surround you on all four sides. Paddle across a boil and leave via the back door.

The river calms down again for a mile or two, then picks up below the mouth of the Middle Fork. The river's volume grows by 50 percent, increasing its power noticeably. After several interesting play rapids the river pools, then turns left and drops into a boulder barrage. This is S-Turn (Class V-), which drops 25 feet in its twisting, boiling, 75-yard course. Most paddlers start in the center or far left and pick their way down to a point above a ledge

Section: Belington to Mouth of Buckhannon or Phillippi
County: Barbour
USGS Quads: Belington, Audra, Monongahela National Forest
Difficulty: Class III–V
Gradient: 37 feet per mile; 1.25 miles at 80 feet per mile
Average Width: 100 feet
Velocity: Fast
Rescue Index: Remote
Hazards: Vision limited by huge boulders, undercut rocks, Hartung rapids, Shoulder Snapper has pinning possibilities
Scouting: Keyhole, Hartung, S-Turn, Shoulder Snapper, Hook
Portages: Usually Hartung
Scenery: Pretty to beautiful in spots
Highlights: Big boulders, second-growth mixed forest
Gauge: National Weather Service (Belington gauge), (703) 260-0305

Runnable Water Levels	Minimum	Maximum
Belington gauge	3.5 feet	7 feet

Months Runnable: Spring (but can be run in the summer after extended rains)
Additional Information: National Weather Service, Pittsburgh, (412) 262-5290; Audra State Park, (304) 457-1162; Waterline, (800) 297-4243, #541471

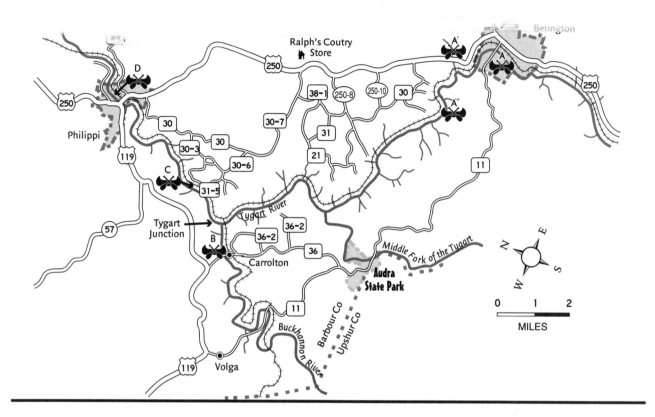

that juts out from river right. Skirt this hole, then sprint for the far right of the bottom chute. This allows you to miss two very powerful pour-overs sitting just out of sight at the bottom of the drop. At high water (six feet and higher) the entire drop can be snuck down the far right channel. If someone is having a bad day at low to moderate levels you can run them down this section and carry the last drop.

On the other side of the pool is the impressive Shoulder Snapper Falls (Class IV+), an eight-foot ledge drop broken out on the right. The name stems from an incident involving John Sweet, one of the strongest paddlers in the late 60s. Sweet broached against a boulder near the top and dislocated his shoulder, but managed to crawl out on a midstream boulder. Sweet, who hated to swim, was then forced to jump off and float the rest of the drop so his buddies could pick him up. At low water there is a submerged rock in the preferred channel; one boater hit it so hard that he slipped out of his foot brace and impaled his shin. Despite these horror stories, the right center line is a pretty straight shot. The drop is blind, so scout it on river right. At high water, pay attention to the powerful rapid just downstream. A hole at top right pushes hapless boaters left, lining them up for a big stopper hidden between two waves. You can avoid embar-

rassment by immediately cutting back to the right.

A few miles below here is Hook Rapid (Class IV+), the last major drop. The top of this rapid is full of holes, several of which are capable of stopping a boat and recirculating a swimmer. Then the river curves sharply to the left between two more holes. At low levels a nasty suckhole lies on the inside of the turn. A large rock on river left gives you a good view of the drop; pick a line through the center of the rapid and follow the water as it makes the turn. The next drop is Instant Ender (Class III), a dynamic play spot at levels between 4.0 and 4.3 feet at Belington. From here it's an easy float through moderate rapids to the mouth of the Buckhannon.

For access to this river section, put in at the bridge in Belington (A) or at a pullover spot north of town where the river leaves the road (A'). To avoid three miles of easy whitewater, turn left at the south end of the Belington fairgrounds from US 250, then take the second left down a dirt road to Papa Weese's Paradise, a fishing camp (A''). This is rather time consuming, and isn't really any faster than paddling the river.

The Mouth of Buckhannon take-out (B) is at the end of a mile-long stretch of railroad tracks that run along the Buckhannon to the covered bridge in Carrolton. It's a tedious hike, exhausting for open-boaters. The tracks are

Arrive, an then your own and are open for running. To get in Carrolton, turn right at the traffic light in downtown Belington and follow Country Road 11 to Audra State Park. Drive across the Middle Fork, turn right, and 2.5 miles later take the next right onto Country Road 36. Follow this to the covered bridge. It's about five miles from the Middle Fork to Carrolton, a reasonable length for a walking or bicycle shuttle.

There is an alternate take-out (C) for the Tygart River Gorge (one mile below the confluence with the Buckhannon on river right). Head toward Phillipi from Bellington, turn off Route 250 opposite Ralph's Country Store onto Old Route 250 (Country Road 30-7). Take the first right and proceed 3.3 miles to a sharp left turn. Just after the turn, the Union Church will be off to your left. Proceed 0.8 miles to a point where the main road curves sharply to the right at a cinder-block building with a network of outside stairs called the "Garden Apartments" by locals. Take the road to the left here and 0.1 mile later, take a right and keep going right down to the railroad tracks on the river bank. Proceed carefully; it's easy to get lost here.

Below the Buckhannon the Tygart runs a bit over five miles to Philippi (D). The first three miles have several Class II rapids; the last two miles are pretty flat. You can cover this distance quickly at high levels (5.5–7.0 feet), and the shuttle from Belington to Philippi along US 250 is fast and direct. There's a small park on river right where you can leave vehicles and load up afterwards.

Arden Section

The Tygart in the below Philippi. The Arden Section (E) are ... this section is strewn with huge boulders and drops over big rock ledges and reefs as the Tygart descends 170 feet before reaching the reservoir behind Grafton Dam. All but the last three miles of the run below Arden may be scouted from a secondary road on the right; this runs from Philippi downstream to the ancient concrete bridge at Teter Creek (F). However, don't take out at Teter Creek unless absolutely necessary because some of the best water is in the remaining three miles to the reservoir (G). At high levels (over 4.5 feet), this eight-mile section becomes expert decked-boater country only.

About a mile below Arden is a ledge channeled on the left. The current continues down the left side for 50 feet, dropping over a boulder and ending in two stoppers. This rapid is called Gallaway by local paddlers and can be scouted from the left. The larger upstream wave must be skirted to the right if one is to maintain the alignment and speed necessary to run a ledge and the second stopper. The second rapid downstream from Laurel Creek (which enters from the right under a steel bridge) is called Deception. Here the river narrows and piles over a rapid succession of three ledges with unavoidable, five-foot, standing waves. Three hundred yards below Deception,

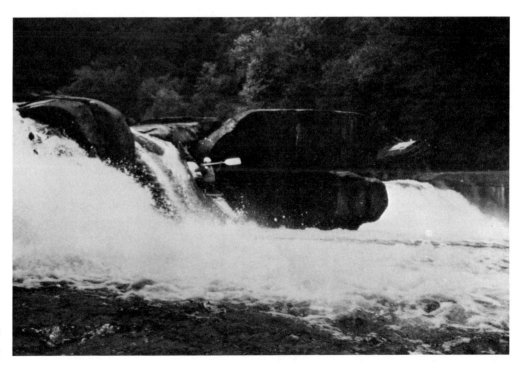

Ollie Fordham running Valley Falls. Photo by Mayo Gravatt.

Tygart River • West Virginia

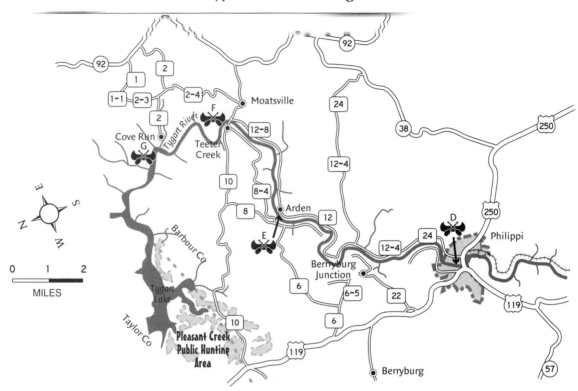

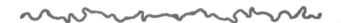

Section: Arden to Cove Run

County: Barbour

USGS Quads: Philippi, Nestorville

Difficulty: Class III–V

Gradient: 27 feet per mile

Average Width: 125–150 feet

Velocity: Fast

Rescue Index: Accessible for the most part

Hazards: Undercut Rock, Moat's Falls, Classic, Wells Falls; very difficult at high water

Scouting: Gallaway, Undercut Rock, Premonition, Moat's Falls, Classic, Wells Falls and rapids below

Portages: Depending on water levels and experience, Undercut Rock, Moat's Falls, Classic, and maybe Wells Falls

Scenery: Pretty in spots, good to fair otherwise

Highlights: Big ledges and large rapids, runnable Moat's Falls, big water at Wells Falls

Gauge: National Weather Service, Pittsburgh (Philippi gauge), (412) 262-5290

Runnable Water Levels	Minimum	Maximum
Philippi gauge	3.5 feet	7.0 feet

Additional Information: National Weather Service, Washington, (703) 260-0305; Waterline, (800) 297-4243, #541474

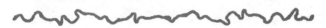

the river funnels over a ledge to the left and undercuts a shelf of rock on the left that has a one-foot clearance. This rapid is fittingly called Undercut (Class IV–V depending on water levels) and should be scouted from the right. Be careful when running this rapids to guard against being blown to the left underneath the undercut rock shelf. Expert paddlers can get enjoyable enders here below four feet on the Philippi gauge. A few hundred yards below Undercut is a riverwide three- to four-foot ledge that should be scouted from the right before running it. The right side of this ledge (called Premonition by local paddlers) is a particularly dynamic drop with a curler that forces a quick left turn.

A hundred yards or so farther downstream, the river spills over a good 15-foot riverwide falls called Moats Falls. Very experienced paddlers are now carefully running this falls over the middle—a 15-foot drop into soft suds with a good-sized pool below. Those contemplating running the falls should first scout the launch and landing points carefully. At low water you can go left over the rocks at center. For the squeamish or less advanced boater, an honorable option is to carry along the road on the right and put in just below the falls.

About 500 yards below Moats Falls is a rapid called Classic (Class IV–V at higher water levels) by genteel paddlers and unprintable names by salty boaters. Get over on river left to scout this drop (it can be really nasty at higher levels) and carry it if you have any doubts. The river is narrow and split by a partially submerged, house-sized boulder in a powerful drop. After this rapid, the Tygart is fairly flat until the ancient Teter Creek bridge.

Below Teter Creek bridge is a nice wave train appropriately called Rodeo Rapids. After numerous other good rapids, the river pools behind a natural rock dam, turns left, then immediately right, all the time being necked down considerably. There are big, diagonal stoppers pushing to the right in this turn, and as you regain alignment around the last corner, you are faced with a huge tongue of water called Wells Falls (Class IV at moderate water levels; Class V at high levels), dropping 10 feet over a slide into a formidable stopper. If you slide off the left-side tongue to the right, you will slam into a four-foot wall of water. This is the most powerful of the runnable rapids in the entire Monongahela Basin and should be scouted each time. The next rapid is also mean; it is a sheer drop into another nasty hole. Both Wells Falls and the rapids below are runnable, but they are also easily carried on the right. However, one does have to contend with poison ivy on the portage. The remaining rapids below Teter Creek are nice Class III drops that offer no special problems in low water.

Regarding the shuttle: use the dirt road on the right from Arden because it has been repaired. Drive about two miles upstream to the first rapid for an easy put-in. Inex-

perienced paddlers should take out at Arden bridge. One can also take out at Teter Creek for an easy shuttle with a road alongside throughout. To reach the Cove Run take-out, turn right at Teter Creek and go out to the main highway, WV 92, and turn left onto it. Take Cove Run Road "2" to the left, then take a right, another right, and then a left at the succeeding forks. The last part takes you down a very steep, unimproved road to the river. Be sure you recognize this point from the river. You will not find rapids on the lower part until the first of October. Peak drawdown is generally reached about the last of February. At such time there is another 1.8 miles of rapids dropping thirty feet per mile. You then have to paddle another two miles of flatwater before taking out on the left side at Wildcat Hollow Boat Club.

Valley Falls Section

This one-and-a-half mile section of the Tygart requires close scrutiny of the dam discharge from Grafton by highly experienced boaters. The major difficulty in addition to the 60-feet-per-mile gradient is the fact that this section of the river has been narrowed by 80 percent as it enters the steep gorge. This is a very heavy descent for such a large volume of water.

The put-in for the Valley Falls section of the Tygart is in Valley Falls State Park (H). It's easily found by following signs from Fairmont or Grafton from WV 310 or Country Road 31/14, respectively. Boaters have negoti-

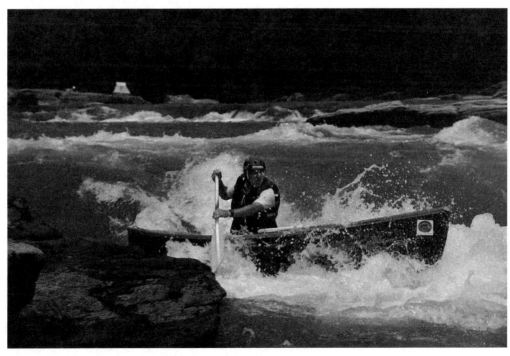

Ollie Fordham at Undercut Rock. Photo by Andre Derdyn.

Tygart River • West Virginia

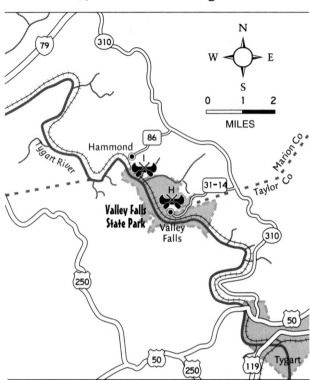

Gauge Conversions

Tygart River at Belington

3.5 feet	443 cfs
4.0 feet	708 cfs
4.5 feet	975 cfs
5.0 feet	1,250 cfs
5.5 feet	1,560 cfs
6.0 feet	1,910 cfs
6.5 feet	2,260 cfs
7.0 feet	2,610 cfs
8.0 feet	3,400 cfs
9.0 feet	4,270 cfs
10.0 feet	5,270 cfs

Middle Fork at Audra

3.0 feet	255 cfs
3.5 feet	455 cfs
4.0 feet	690 cfs
4.5 feet	980 cfs
5.0 feet	1,280 cfs
5.5 feet	1,620 cfs
6.0 feet	2,030 cfs
7.0 feet	2,990 cfs

Section: Valley Falls to Hammond
County: Marion
USGS Quad: Fairmont East
Difficulty: Class II–VI
Gradient: 60 feet per mile
Average Width: 150 feet
Velocity: Fast
Rescue Index: Generally accessible
Hazards: First two ledges, Hamburger Helper
Scouting: First two ledges, Hamburger Helper
Portages: None
Scenery: Beautiful
Highlights: Steep gorge and huge drops
Gauge: Grafton Dam, (304) 265-1760

Runnable Water Levels	Minimum	Maximum
	350 cfs	1,000+ cfs

Additional Information: Valley Falls State Park, (304) 367-2719

ated an agreement with park management that specifies the following procedure: First, stop at the park headquarters, a short distance beyond the entrance, and sign in, giving the name, address, and phone number of all members of your party. Next, drive down to the river and make a 200-yard portage from the parking lot, cross a bridge over the railroad tracks, and arrive at the pool above the first drop. Lastly, unlike previous years, boaters are allowed to scout and make multiple runs of the various falls if they wish. But deliberate swimming in the park, with or without PFDs, is not allowed.

Several major drops in this section start just below the put-in. The first ledge is a riverwide, 10-foot drop that at low water levels has three distinct chutes. The sloping right chute and the far left chute can both be run, but scouting is essential. The next Valley Falls ledge of 12 feet is sharp and appears unrunnable. However, at low water it can be run on the left of the right side. The third ledge is called Punk Rock, a Class III rapid with two runnable channels. Both channels require right-angle turns to the left after running tight along the right bank.

The fourth ledge is clearly Class V at even moderate water levels. Aptly called Hamburger Helper, the river here narrows to a single channel and drops eight feet over a boulder with a thin flow at the center and a boiling flume at each side. The fifth rapid (Twist 'n Shout) is a series of three drops in rapid succession in a 20-foot channel. The last two have huge souse holes up against the undercut right shore. The remaining three ledges (colorfully called This, That, and It by local paddlers) are straightforward; the last one can be reached from the take-out.

The Valley Falls section never gets too low to run due to the discharge from Grafton Dam. If several gates are open, however, the rapids would be a nightmare. Always call the Grafton Dam (304-265-1760) before starting. Several outfitters who run summer trips use 750 cfs as a cutoff point. Kayakers will often run at higher levels, exercising caution when running the bigger drops. The Hammond take-out is found at the end of a yellow brick road (CR 86) which leaves WV 310. However, the run is so short that many local boaters find it easier to simply portage their boat back to the park along the railroad tracks.

Laurel Fork of the Cheat River

All things considered, this may be the best intermediate run in the Cheat River basin. It is a long trip through uninhabited and virtually inaccessible country in the high valley between the Middle and Rich Mountains. The remnants of an early logging railroad play tag with the meandering river for the first of a series of two- to four-foot ledges. The ledges continue regularly for the next two miles to the granddaddy of them all, a 12-foot waterfall (runnable by demented experts only!), which you should portage on the left along the tramway bed. A November 1985 flood eroded a big chunk of the left bank below this waterfall, making this portage more difficult. After lunch at the foot of the falls, be ready for seven miles of continuous Class III rapids to the mouth.

There are a total of eight bridge crossings on the run.

Section: US 33 bridge to Jenningston
Counties: Randolph, Tucker
USGS Quads: Harman, Monongahela National Forest
Difficulty: Class III–IV
Gradient: 9 miles at 71 feet per mile
Average Width: 50 feet
Velocity: Fast
Rescue Index: Remote
Hazards: Keeper hydraulics in high water; 12-foot falls halfway through trip
Scouting: Several of the larger rapids
Portages: 12-foot waterfall
Scenery: Pretty to beautiful
Highlights: Scenic high valley, 12-foot falls
Gauge: Visual; on the right side of the Route 33 bridge abutment

Runnable Water Levels	Minimum	Maximum
	0.3 feet	1.5 feet

Additional Information: National Weather Service, (412) 262-5290 (Pittsburgh), (703) 260-0305 (Washington, DC area); Parsons gauge should be at least 5 feet

None of the bridges remain but the abutments are readily spotted as landmarks. Between the seventh and eighth bridges there is a 50-yard tunnel from one limb of a half-mile loop to the other. The water visible at the mouth is typical of the entire river from the falls down. This is an exhilarating run among some of the least spoiled scenery of West Virginia. After being flushed out into the Dry Fork, it is just a quarter mile to the Jenningston bridge.

Spotting the falls from upstream should be no problem. It takes about one and a half hours of paddling time to reach the falls. You'll see six bridge crossings to the falls; the sixth one is about a mile above the falls. The falls are just around a right turn. Fluorescent strips have been tied in the tree branches on the left above the falls. The only other difficulty is the fatigue brought on by 13 miles of wilderness travel, including nine miles of continuous maneuvering. Near the end is a cluster of several memorable hydraulics, not far from the Jenningston bridge. At high water levels the hydraulics below many of its ledges become keepers. The Laurel Fork has killed people in its holes, so be careful.

The put-in is at the US 33 bridge (A). The take-out is at the mouth downstream along the left side from the Jenningston bridge (B). The best route from the put-in to the take-out goes west along US 33 four miles to Alpena, then north on "12" by the Glady Fork and Sully. You'll find a gauge painted on the rightside abutment of the US 33 bridge. The water will not be high enough unless the Parsons gauge reads over five feet.

Laurel Fork of the Cheat River • West Virginia

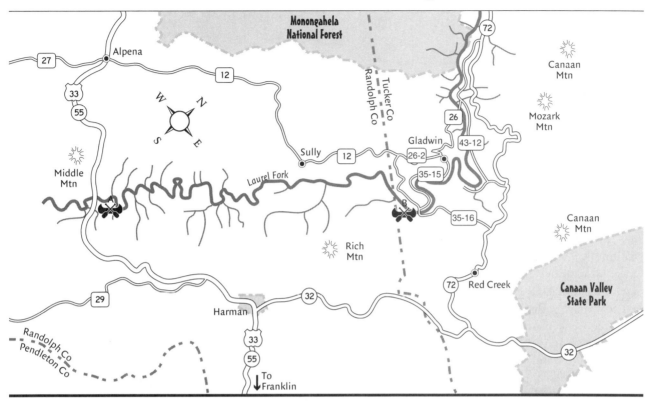

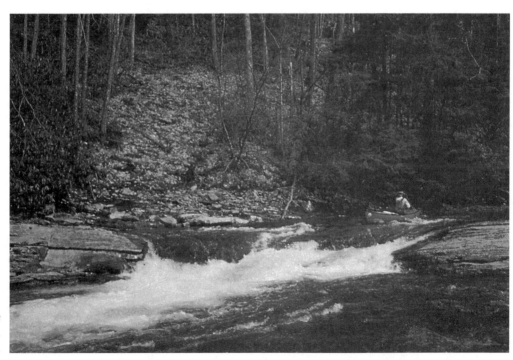

Frank Fico running the
Laurel Fork of the Cheat.
Photo by Bob Maxey.

Blackwater River

Caution: River under construction! The 1985 flood substantially changed the Blackwater River and made it significantly more difficult. Previously, it was a Class IV trip. Now it is a Class IV–V river with numerous rapids like the Upper Yough and somelike the more difficult Lower Meadow in West Virginia. Although the individual drops are not as large, the continuous nature of this river makes it tougher than the Lower Big Sandy (see below). Since the flood many of the drops have become more complex with numerous pinning possibilities. Substantial rock slides and fallen trees make this a river for experts only who continually scout and take all safety precautions. Many of the rapids are unstable and continue to change.

The Blackwater from North Fork Junction to Hendricks (seven miles) is West Virginia's longest rapid. It flows through a narrow, steep defile draining the Canaan Valley, a flat, upland swamp on the west side of the Allegheny Front.

Multiple branches of the upper Blackwater funnel the 15-square-mile drainage basin into two main forks that pass the former logging capitals of Davis and Thomas, respectively. Near these nineteenth-century towns, they suddenly leap off the mountain as two falls, 50 feet each, and begin their unrelenting rush to the Dry Fork, eight miles and 1,000 feet below. Its two main headwater streams, the upper Blackwater and its north fork, are extreme, steep-creek runs. They join a few miles below their initial drops and slow their descent to a more "realistic" paddling gradient. Here the rhododendron rise 30 feet high along the river, and spruce-topped cliffs tower 1,000 feet above. Both falls, one preserved by a state park and the other on the North Branch are worth seeing.

From the recommended put-in at the junction (A) followed by only minimal veering from left to right, the river is one continuous blind bend—downward. The paddler never sees more than 50 yards ahead before the river disappears over the edge of the world. It has a fantastic 112-feet-per-mile gradient for five miles to Lime Rock, an abandoned community two miles upstream from Hendricks. Fortunately, this descent is not broken into alternate stretches of rapids and pools but is generally evenly distributed. It is a gigantic sluiceway between mountains rising 2,000 feet on either side with almost no riverside beach.

Paddling the Blackwater is a constant challenge of reading and negotiating chutes over staircase ledges randomly strewn with 5- to 10-foot boulders. The paddler is constantly maneuvering in the ever-pushing current. Moving side eddies are the only rest or rescue spots along the course. The waters of the river are a nonsilted brown covered with suds—a form of pollution noted since the time of Thomas Lewis, a 1746 explorer who appropriately called this stream the "River Styx." The tannin color is attributed to organic acids from the upland swamps that leach iron oxide from the red shale that lines much of the riverbed.

The action starts immediately, then picks up about 200 yards below the put-in. The first drop, Krakatoa, is a double ledge, each one leading into a large hole. Fortunately this Class V drop is easily carried on the left. At the next major drop the river narrows to about 25 feet and drops over a six-foot ledge into a horrible hole. "The Ledge" can be carried on the left. A number of steep, blind, boulder drops below must be run with precision. One of these, Rock and Roll, is a long, steep Class V rapid created by the 1985 flood. It keeps changing, so scout from a rocky island on the right. A mile and a half into the run the water accelerates for 75 yards over a flat, sloping, red shale ledge. The current reaches incredible speeds before slamming into a hole at the bottom. Most of this rapid is too shallow to paddle, so you have to be on the correct line right from the beginning. Scout and portage on the right. Tub Run, a tributary, enters just downstream on river right.

The river is a bit easier below here, alternating between fast Class III+'s and blind, boulder-strewn Class IVs. Some of these rapids change significantly from year to year. You'll see evidence of recent landslides throughout the run, and downed trees are a continual hazard. At the three-mile point you'll encounter a shallow, 12-foot-high sloping falls. Some people run this mess; others choose to carry on the left. Below these falls is a steep drop that funnels into a big hole. You'll want to look this one over on the right before running it. After about five miles the gradient lets up to about 48 feet per mile. From here it's an easy, two-mile float to the take-out.

Although people traditionally leave the river at the Route 72 bridge in Hendricks, this is private land and there have been complaints about paddlers parking and changing in this area. The American Whitewater Affiliation (AWA) recently purchased a piece of land on the Dry Fork, just downstream of the mouth of the Blackwater. Turn right at the first street by the Post Office as you enter town and drive three blocks to the Dry Fork. You'll see a swinging bridge over the river; the take-out (B) is just upstream of the bridge.

The shuttle is straightforward, but the put-in is a bear! From the take-out, drive out Route 72 to US 219 north. Turn right and follow the road through Thomas, then bear right on a road marked "Douglas 27." You'll start to run along the North Fork of the Blackwater to where the old railroad bed meets the road. Bear left and drive a half mile to a locked gate. Drop your gear, then drive back

upstream and find a place to park. To reach the river from here you'll have to carry your boat a half mile down the railbed, past the junction of the North Fork, then slide it 300 feet straight down a 300-foot-high, 45-degree incline to the river. There have been several landslides here since the flood and the entire area is steep and unstable. The last 10 to 20 feet are almost vertical, and you'll probably need ropes to lower your boats. The railbed runs alongside on river right all the way to Hendricks. Although high above the river and not visible to paddlers, it provides a fast way out in case of trouble.

An alternate access puts you in below the first big drops. Continue on the Forest Service road past Douglas until you are high above the river on the side of the gorge. You may see a sign marked "put-in" or tape on a tree. Although you'll have to slide your boat further (almost 400 feet to the tracks) the slope is not as steep and the footing is better. This route was marked in 1986, but may not be easy to follow these days.

An old gauge painted on the bridge at Hendricks was sandblasted off during the 1985 flood. A second gauge painted on the rail bridge upstream was buried a few years later by another period of high water. This area is very unstable and changes from year to year. But because the rapids in the canyon are so narrow, we can safely say that if the take-out looks scrapy but passable, the river

Section: North Fork Junction to Hendricks

County: Tucker

USGS Quads: Mozark Mountain, Monongahela National Forest

Difficulty: Class IV–V, VI

Gradient: Five miles at 112 feet per mile; two miles at 48 feet per mile

Average Width: 30–50 feet

Velocity: Fast

Rescue Index: Remote

Hazards: Continuous technical rapids, trees in chutes, many pinning possibilities

Scouting: Both boat- and land-scouting are continuous

Portages: Several

Scenery: Beautiful

Highlights: West Virginia's longest continuous rapids

Gauge: Visual; levels below refer to Davis gauge on Blackwater

Runnable Water Levels	Minimum	Maximum
	2.6 feet	3.5 feet

Additional Information: National Weather Service, (412) 262-5290 (Pittsburgh), (703) 260-0305 (Washington, DC area); Waterline Service, (800) 297-4243 (#541132)

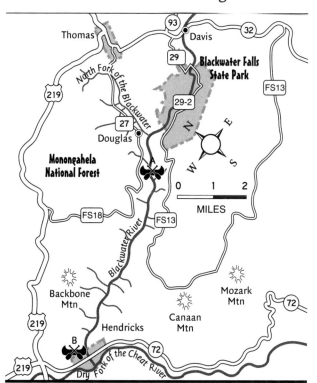

Blackwater River • West Virginia

can be run. If there's plenty of water here, the gorge may well be too high to run. The Davis gauge above the put-in is on the Pittsburgh Weather Service phone. It indicates roughly 50 percent of the flow at the put-in and is a good indicator of the levels on the Blackwater. At 2.6 feet (220 cfs), the river is low and abusive. I've found that 3.1 feet (350 cfs) is a good, medium level, and 3.5 feet (455 cfs) is getting high. The Parsons gauge typically needs to be between 4.5 and 5.5 feet for the Blackwater to run.

Gauge Conversion Table

Blackwater River at Davis

2.50 feet	197 cfs
2.75 feet	257 cfs
3.00 feet	320 cfs
3.50 feet	455 cfs
3.75 feet	527 cfs
4.00 feet	605 cfs
4.50 feet	780 cfs
4.75 feet	867 cfs
5.00 feet	960 cfs

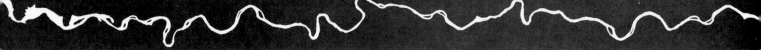

Big Sandy Creek

Upper Section, Bruceton Mills to Rockville

As this little stream tips down beside Chestnut Ridge to the Cheat Gorge, it provides six miles of progressive slalom training starting at Class I and working up to Class IV. This run is suitable for strong intermediate paddlers at lower water levels, but flotation is recommended for open canoes. Automobile camping is provided at nearby Cooper's Rock State Park or at Cheat Canyon Campground in Albright.

Hazel Run Rapids is the first problem and appears as an impassable barricade of boulders. Try the second passage from the right. Below the mouth of the Little Sandy (on the left), you'll encounter a long slide rapid where the water zips quickly over very shallow rock tables and then terminates in several wide hydraulics. About 500 yards from the confluence with the Little Sandy is six- to eight-foot Falkenstein Falls. It can be recognized easily by the large rock shelf jutting out from the left and forming a dam. The first shelf can be carefully run by cutting hard left below this ledge, then back across to near center for the main ledge. At higher levels you can run straight over the left or far right.

Several long rapids occur just below the falls, and this is where the best action is found. Steep drops over ledges around blind bends require quick decisions and paddle responses. This continues until the take-out. The last rapid is usually a good, Class IV run except in very low water. Intermediates should take out at the rustic cabin on the right just below the mouth of Sovereign Run and Corner Rapids. The approach to the bridge is tricky. At normal water levels, it's easiest to start in the center and then cut sharply to the right. At high levels the far left is no problem.

Put in below the dam at Bruceton Mills (A). To reach the take-out at Rockville Bridge (B), take Route 26 south and turn right on Hudson Road. Drive straight through the four-way intersection at Mount Nebo, pass Glen Miller's house, and follow the road around a sharp curve and across the wooden bridge over Sovereign Run. Take the first left, and follow a rough dirt road down to Rockville. As of this writing the road going out on river right is four-wheel drive only! Mr. Miller will run your shuttle for a reasonable fee; call him at (304) 379-3404.

Lower Section, Rockville to Cheat River

The most stunning aspect of the Lower Big Sandy is that it has five of the most distinctive and most memorable Class IV–VI whitewater rapids on the entire East Coast. These are Big Sandy Falls (Wonder Falls), Zoom Flume, Little Splat, Big Splat, and First Island. These rapids are truly unique. Add a pristine mountain setting and you have a truly stupendous trip for expert paddlers. The Lower Big Sandy is an exciting, beautiful, piquant mistress who shows occasional flares of bad temper to even the most experienced paddlers. However, this five-and-a-half mile trip contains the most scenic and most interesting whitewater in northern West Virginia. Although the banks are choked with rhododendron, the necessary scouting and portaging is not difficult. If a walkout is necessary, you'll find an old railroad bed on the right to within a mile of the Cheat River. The old railroad bridge is washed out but the path continues on river left to Jenkinsburg.

There are countless difficulties on this trip and numerous Class III–IV rapids not described here. Some drops are hazardous and require scouting or carrying. At 1.5 miles there is a rather difficult sequence terminating in 18-foot-high Wonder Falls. The Class III–IV rapids approaching the falls has a fairly steep, three-part drop on the left into a pool just above the falls. Scout and use safety measures; carry the falls on the right. At normal levels, Big Sandy Falls can be run on the left side of the main current. If running the falls, it is critical that the vertical angle of your boat be 45 degrees as you drop over the falls. Too vertical an angle means you could dive too deep and crunch your bow on submerged rocks below the falls. Too horizontal an angle could mean a very flat landing at the bottom, which could injure your back.

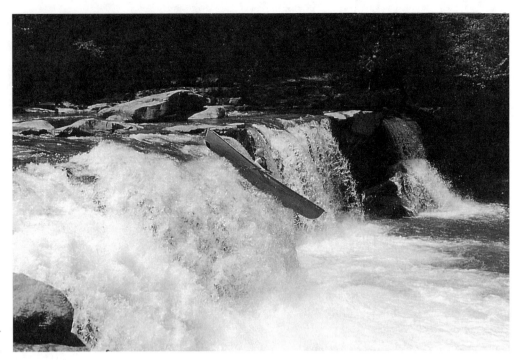

Liz Garland running Wonder Falls. Photo by Mayo Gravatt.

The next series of rapids is busy for a quarter mile, followed by a broad ledge split by a large rock in midstream. This is known as Undercut Rock rapids (Class IV). Scout this rapids. The passage on the right ends in a big curler that throws even good boaters under an undercut rock. Run just to the left of a huge midstream boulder, dropping over a six-foot ledge.

The next biggie is Zoom Flume, a steep, sloped, 8- to 10-foot Class IV drop that is easier than it looks and even more exciting. Scouting on the right is recommended to see the twisting flume. You can enter from river left to avoid being disoriented by the holes and ledges that interfere with a straight shot down the flume. Then work over to catch the flume properly. The cheese-grater rock shelf below has taken off a lot of elbow skin.

Get back out of your boat, if you are still in it, and scout the next rapids, Little Splat. This is one of the most complex and tricky Class V+ rapids anywhere in West Virginia. The upper part can be boat-scouted. At high water you can cut over to the right side. The center route has a reversal that has thrown boats into a nasty pinning rock. At lower levels (below six feet) the easier route on the right dries up and you're forced to run a very tight, twisting channel on the far left.

Big Splat is next. Very aptly named, it is a complex double rapid dropping a total of over 25 feet. Although run by the most skilled boaters, this is clearly a Class VI rapid. If you find yourself wanting to run Big Splat, you should seriously question not only your skills but also your motives. The risks are significant and the margin for error is alarmingly small.

The 8- to 10-foot drop guarding the approach to Big Splat falls below is perhaps the most dangerous feature. When scouting from the right bank, the dangers in the

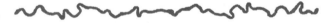

Section: Bruceton Mills to Rockville

Counties: Preston

USGS Quads: Bruceton Mills, Valley Point

Difficulty: Class I–IV

Average Width: 60 feet

Velocity: Moderate to fast

Gradient: Four miles at 9 feet per mile; two miles at 45 feet per mile

Rescue Index: Remote

Hazards: 6- to 8-foot falls and long rapids below Little Sandy, trees in river

Scouting: Falls and long rapids below Little Sandy

Portages: None

Scenery: Pretty to beautiful

Highlights: Progressive slalom in wooded setting

Gauge: National Weather Service, (412) 262-5290 (Pittsburgh)

Runnable Water Levels	Minimum	Maximum
Rockville gauge	5.8 feet	7 feet
Bruceton Mills gauge	0 feet	2.5 feet

Additional Information: National Weather Service, (703) 260-0305 (Washington, DC area)

Class V+ approach rapid are well concealed. Beginning as a sloping ledge, the current drops directly toward an undercut, partially submerged slab rock. The right side of the chute ends under the downstream corner of another large, undercut boulder. Almost all of the current then drops into a dangerous, horseshoe-shaped hydraulic.

However, one glance at the base of Big Splat falls should convince anyone that swimming here is simply unthinkable. After a short and very fast pool, the entire river drops 16 to 18 feet onto Splat Rock. Some of the water goes through sieves on the right, some underneath Splat Rock, and some pillows off Splat Rock—forming a frightening hole at the base of the falls. This area is fit for neither man nor boat. Fortunately, no one has been trapped in the approach rapids yet and most injuries have been limited to ankles bent by pitoning on Splat Rock. Portage both Big Splat drops on the right, lowering boats and bodies over a ledge.

Below Big Splat are a number of challenging Class IV+ rapids. The first two are steep and obstructed, but can be boat-scouted on the far right. The third drop, Roostertail, starts with a right-hand chute that feeds you into a complex, rocky rapid. Go to the left of the roostertail, then shoot down the right through a powerful chute and

Section: Rockville to Cheat River

County: Preston

USGS Quads: Bruceton Mills, Valley Point

Difficulty: Class IV–V with one Class VI

Gradient: Two miles at 30 feet per mile; four miles at 80 feet per mile

Average Width: 60 feet

Velocity: Fast

Rescue Index: Remote

Hazards: Wonder Falls, Undercut Rock, Zoom Flume, Little Splat, Big Splat, First Island

Scouting: All six of the above rapids, at least

Portages: Possibly one or more of the six major rapids

Scenery: Beautiful

Highlights: Five unusually distinctive rapids in a spectacular gorge

Gauge: National Weather Service, (412) 262-5290 (Pittsburgh)

Runnable Water Levels	Minimum	Maximum
Bruceton Mills gauge	0 feet	2 feet
Rockville Gauge	5.2–5.8 feet	6.5–7.0 feet

Additional Information: National Weather Service, (703) 260-0305 (Washington, DC area); 5.2 feet can be very technical: open-boaters and some decked-boaters prefer a minimum of 5.8 feet)

quickly catch an eddy below before getting pushed into a rock jumble. Then you'll have to ferry across the river to finish on the left. After a couple of easier drops you'll encounter a series of medium-sized ledges. You'll have to start on the left, then cut over to run the final drop on the right.

The river eases up a bit until you come to First Island, a Class V drop. This drop is on the right side and should be scouted. It's actually made up of two drops: a steep chute and a ledge where the runout is obstructed by downstream boulders. Angle your boat to the right when going off the top chute to avoid a pinning rock, then scramble downstream and boof the ledge on the far right. This is easier said than done because the current upstream of these drops is often uncooperative. Many people find it useful to catch an eddy (or two) on the way down.

Below First Island is a second island with a slalom boulder garden (Class IV+) that should be run right. Three and a half miles and 272 feet (down) later, the paddler, who may be hiking by now, will reach the Cheat River near Jenkinsburg.

The shuttle is done entirely on rough dirt roads. From the put-in at Rockville (B), drive up on the river left road, then turn right at the intersection. Drive past Glen Miller's house to the Mt. Nebo intersection. Turn right, pass a large A-frame house on the right, and follow the

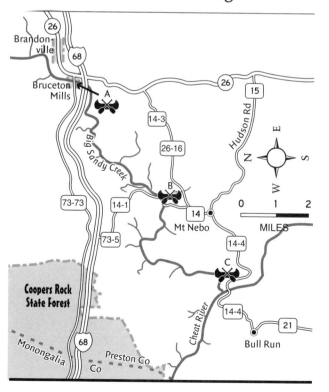

Big Sandy Creek • West Virginia

road into the Cheat Canyon. The take-out is at Jenkinsburg Bridge (C) where the Big Sandy meets the Cheat.

The gauge generally used is a government gauge on the bridge at Rockville, which is now available on the phone via satellite. The National Weather Service telephone number is (412) 262-5290. The river is rocky and technical from 5.2–5.8 feet. Ideal conditions are 6.0–6.2 feet; over 6.5 feet the river starts to get pushy and powerful. Anything over seven feet is high water.

There is also a paddler's gauge under the Bruceton Mills bridge. The correlation between the two is complex but reliable. Rockville = 3/4 (Bruceton + 1) + 5. The recommended levels for Rockville at Bruceton are zero to two feet. The Lower Big Sandy is often runnable in the spring.

Cheat River

The Cheat River is the largest undammed watershed east of the Mississippi. It passes through steep mountain country where the water runs off quickly. Locals say it got its name by rising without warning, taking away clothing and gear left along its banks. Because the headwaters are so far from the main stem, rain there can cause the river to rise in sunny weather. It's a large river that holds its water well, and it is often runnable well into the summer.

The countryside that the Cheat flows through is unspoiled for the most part. The last major tributary comes in above Parsons. The stretch between Parsons and Rowlesburg is flatwater, passing through unspoiled rural countryside. From Rowlesburg to Cheat Lake outside Morgantown the Cheat remains attractive despite considerable mining and timbering activity. The water quality is pretty good until the first acid stream enters at the take-out for the Narrows. At the mouth of Cheat Canyon two more acid streams, Muddy Creek and Green's Run, enter the river. The acid is not noticeable to most paddlers except at very low summer flows.

In November 1995, the Cheat River drainage was ravaged by a great flood. First, the area received four to six inches of rain on November 4. Late that evening a strong, low-pressure cell stalled at the headwaters, dumping another six to eight inches of rain in a short time. This caused a massive flood that forever altered the river. The entire watershed, including Shavers, Laurel, Glady, Dry, and Blackwater Forks, was scoured by the water. The unprecedented high water in the Cheat, Potomac, and Greenbrier watersheds had tragic results: 40 people dead, 2,600 homeless, and 29 West Virginia counties declared disaster areas. These waters changed the riverbed and rolled giant boulders in Cheat Canyon.

Despite this assault, the river is remarkably scenic. Anyone who runs the Cheat will surely love it! If you want to help with the clean-up efforts, Friends of the Cheat is a local group working to restore, preserve, and promote the outstanding natural qualities of this river.

Their current focus is on cleaning up acid-mine drainage. Send $20 to Friends of the Cheat, P.O. Box 182, Bruceton Mills, WV 26525.

The Narrows

The Cheat leaves the town of Rowlesburg quietly but soon becomes narrower and begins to pick up speed. The put-in (A) for the Narrows is opposite a worked-out limestone mine approximately three miles below Rowlesburg. Here you'll encounter the first big waves below Rowlesburg, called Cave Rapids. For the rest of this five-mile trip, the rapids become increasingly more difficult. There are good rescue spots after each rapid, but in high water it's not so easy. After passing several Class II rapids, the paddler enters a long series of harder rapids, properly called the Narrows.

In the first significant rapids, the entire river is necked down by an automobile-sized boulder (Calamity Rock) in midstream. Those unfamiliar with this Class III–IV rapid should scout it. Although this boulder is largely out of the water at roughly 1.5 feet on the Albright bridge gauge, it is completely submerged when the reading is around 2.5 feet. This should give the paddler a healthy respect for what just a few inches' increase in water level means on the Cheat. Usually this boulder should be passed on the right. At very high levels, however, it's best to run along the left bank, whether in boat or on foot. Keep in mind that there are two problems—entering the passage correctly (not always easy due to the combination of waves immediately above it) and managing the powerful drop at the end of the chute. This passage will swamp an open canoe without flotation at any level and flip a raft in high water.

There are three major rapids below this boulder that also pass through narrow confines, creating huge turbulence and powerful cross currents. In high water you simply blast through the standing, five-foot waves and try to maintain stability; at lower levels you must be more precise when maneuvering around the exposed boulders. Paddlers inexperienced with big water might be fooled into thinking that they can "sneak" down the sides of these narrow rapids in relatively calmer water, but they'll usually get sucked over into the big stuff by the high velocity of the main channel (sort of like Bernoulli's principle).

The first of these major rapids (Wind Rapids) is the most difficult in high water and consists of a wide hydraulic before reaching the chute. This hydraulic is best taken on the far left. There is also a severe hydraulic about halfway down the chute on the left, always an interesting scene. The second rapids (Rocking Horse) is the longest narrow passage, 100 yards of turbulence. The last rapid is less severe but still interesting. There is not much left before taking out at Lick Run (B) after an enjoyable five-mile trip. Note that the land at the take-out is private property, but landowners have been cooperative in the past.

The Cheat Canyon

The Cheat Canyon from Albright to Jenkinsburg was explored by John Berry, Bob Harrigan, and Dan Sullivan of Washington, DC, in the 1950s. Their first run took two days. In the 1960s it was considered one of the most challenging runs in the East. Although it seems less difficult when compared to the hardest rivers being run today, the rapids are still formidable. The hard rapids of the Narrows are like the easier ones in the Canyon. The rafting

Section: Narrows (below Rowlesburg to Lick Run)
County: Preston
USGS Quads: Rowlesburg, Kingwood
Difficulty: Class II–IV
Gradient: 20 feet per mile
Average Width: 100–150 feet
Velocity: Fast
Rescue Index: Accessible
Hazards: Big waves in high water (3–4 feet on the gauge)
Scouting: Calamity Rock
Portages: None
Scenery: Fair to pretty in spots
Highlights: Limestone caves near put-in
Gauge: Visual only; Albright bridge, Route 26

Runnable Water Levels	Minimum	Maximum
Albright bridge	0.5 feet	4.5 feet

Additional Information: National Weather Service, Pittsburgh, (412) 262-5290; Parson's reading (see above)

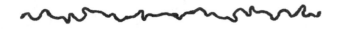

business in the area has been declining since the late 1970s, eclipsed by the growing popularity of the New River. The river is now a delightful, uncrowded big water playground.

Only fools take the Cheat Canyon lightly. The challenges that faced the pioneers of the 1950s must still be dealt with. Low-water runs are tight and technical, with visibility obstructed by huge boulders. The many pools between drops have no current, making the run seem longer. Moderate levels open up the rapids, but the water is considerably more powerful. Really high water brings huge pillowed boulders, boiling eddies, and monster holes. Although the river superficially resembles the Lower Yough, the Cheat has many rapids as difficult as the tough ones on the Yough and five that are significantly harder. A smash-up or injury puts a paddler on foot in very rough country. Walking out of the canyon straight up would take at least two hours, and you would still be miles from the nearest house. There is a good trail on the right, but it is high above the river and intervening cliff bands may make access difficult.

The most challenging aspect of this trip is the number of complex rapids in the inaccessible setting. A detailed description of each rapid is impractical as there are still over thirty (count 'em) rapids rated Class III or higher. Accordingly, scouting is not feasible in many cases. Also,

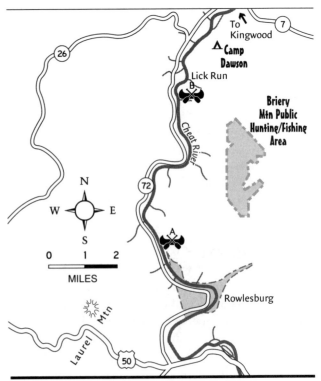

Cheat River • West Virginia

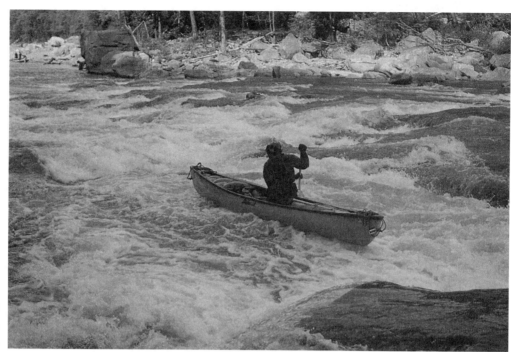

Scot Gravatt entering the left side of High Falls. Photo by Ed Grove.

several of the Class IV rapids are separated only by short pools or no pools in higher water. The remoteness of the canyon and the cold water in winter and spring make the Cheat a Class IV–V run in high water (over four feet).

The first rapid is Decision (Class III+). It is 1.5 miles below Albright, where the Canyon begins. This rapids starts as a wide rubble bar and gradually narrows as it drops over smaller rocks and ledges, forming several holes. Through this upper part, a left-of-center line is easiest, with an interesting chute on the right. Then move right toward a house-sized boulder through a short pool (or wave train at higher levels) before the river drops over a set of large eroded ledges. This rapid is similar to numerous others in the Canyon and is certainly easier than many. If Decision is too much, please carry out now. Your body and boat will thank you.

After about another mile of pools and three significant smaller drops comes Beech Run (Class III–IV). Enter this long rapid on river right before moving left to dodge rocks or holes depending on water level. About two-thirds of the way through and just below the steepest section, a group of closely spaced rocks obstructs the main channel at levels below about 3.0 feet. Run these on the left.

The next big rapid, and one to sway the minds of those who haven't seen any significant changes from the 1985 flood so far, is Big Nasty (Class IV at medium levels and Class IV–V at higher levels). About a half mile and two easier rapids below Beech Run, the river forms a large pool just before a right-hand bend. The left bank is a steep, high mountain here. At water levels above 3.0 feet, first-timers and those with foggy memories should scout from the left bank.

Above Big Nasty, flooding deposited many small and medium-sized boulders, building up the entire riverbed and raising the level of the pool there. The small rapid below Big Nasty has also been obstructed by rubble. In between these pools, the entire river has been channeled toward the right bank and over a ledge. The result is a steep, fast rapid aiming all of the Cheat's water and anything on or in it into one big hole. At 2.0 feet the question "what hole?" seems appropriate, but at 3.0 feet, the hole is hard for decked boats to punch and is fully capable of holding or recirculating floating objects. Around 3.5 feet, it becomes truly nasty, flipping and holding 10-man rafts and recirculating swimmers more than once. At 5.0 feet, Big Nasty is a real circus. First, rafts and boaters must take a tightrope line on the approach. Then, for those who slip off the tightrope, the hole pulls repeated stunts like violently flipping and juggling up to three large rafts at once. Finally, the megahole pulls a true disappearing act with swimmers—making them disappear, then reappear up to 50 feet downstream. Above 5.0 feet, the hole is fortunately too violent to recirculate swimmers; it just gets bigger! Regardless of the water level, successful lines all aim to the extreme left. Still, it is necessary to negotiate several lateral waves or diagonal holes constantly pushing toward the hole. At very high water a left-side sneak appears. A portage is an honorable option.

Even though Maui wave above Big Nasty is gone, a super surfing wave/hole still remains 200 yards downstream on river left. You'll find it after you cross the cobble rapids forming the pool below Big Nasty. This usually benign hole is called Typewriter because you can easily move back and forth on it. Covering the left half of the river, it is gentle on the right edge, sticky on the left.

After one more rapid, the paddler reaches Even Nastier (Class III–IV). This long rapid is entered just right of center and propels all comers through a respectable wave train leading to the left. From here it is either boiling eddies or ultraquick boat-scouting for the remaining 100 yards to avoid two offset boulders and holes. This rapid can also be entered on river left.

The middle third of the trip (a good three miles) is known as the Doldrums. Here you have Prudential Rock, great playing waves, and lovely scenery. This "flat" section with half a dozen significant lesser rapids ends as you enter the last third of the trip. This last section is the most demanding because it has several complex heavy rapids.

After Cue Ball, a Class III boulder drop with a great surfing wave on the left, the river begins to act more seri-

ous. Anticipation, with a fast, narrow chute up against a cliff on river left, is just downstream. After passing through the chute, work over to the center where the river opens up again. As you move through an easy boulder rapid toward a great surfing hole, notice the high cliffs in the distance on river left. Below here is Teardrop, a deceptive rapid that may lure you into a tricky chute on the far right or trash you in a nasty hole in the center. The easiest run is on the far left, to the inside of the turn.

By now the approaching cliffs and a growing roar signify your arrival above High Falls. Note the high, thin ribbon of water coming in on river left, then get ready for action. This drop is Class IV+ even at moderate levels. Scout from the right shore. There's a sneak route down river right, too shallow at low water, but a good choice when the river is high. There's a tricky route down the far left that flips many boats. The preferred center line is scrapy at low water and rambunctious at higher flows. Start a boat length to the right of a washed-out eddy above the drop. This turns into a small wave at high water. Look for a smooth wave at the lip of the drop and paddle through the left shoulder of the wave, angling your boat left. A few forward strokes will carry you between a huge pour-over on the right and a large stopper on the left. Ride the waves over the last ledge into the pool below.

Section: Cheat Canyon, Albright to Jenkinsburg
County: Preston
USGS Quads: Kingwood, Valley Point
Difficulty: Class III–V
Gradient: 25 feet per mile
Average Width: 100–150 feet
Velocity: Fast
Rescue Index: Remote
Hazards: In low water, some undercut and pinning rocks; in high water, heavy water and big holes; the toughest rapids are Big Nasty, High Falls, and Upper Coliseum
Scouting: At least Big Nasty (left), High Falls (right), Upper Coliseum (right), and Lower Coliseum (Pete Morgan's Rapid) at left
Portages: Possibly these same rapids at very high water levels
Scenery: Pretty to beautiful
Highlights: Beautiful gorge marred by acid-stained tributaries near put-in, and the scouring of the November 1985 flood
Gauge: Visual only; Albright bridge, Route 26

Runnable Water Levels	Minimum	Maximum
Albright bridge gauge	1.0 feet	6.0 feet
Parsons gauge	2.3 feet	

Additional Information: National Weather Service, (412) 262-5290 (Pittsburgh), or (703) 260-0305 (Washington, DC area)

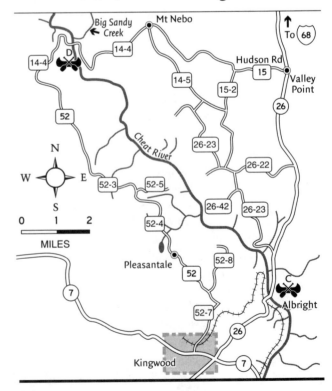

Cheat River • West Virginia

Maze Rapid is just downstream. At low levels the preferred route winds between giant boulders and is tight in places. Higher water opens up the passages, but huge, pillowed boulders and nasty holes complicate the route. Work from left to right to miss the deviously arranged boulders, then cut right at the bottom to finish. Solve the puzzle and win a chance at a trip down the hardest rapid in the Cheat Canyon: Coliseum Rapid.

Upper Coliseum Rapid (Class V) was formed when the 1985 flood completely filled in the right side of the river. The left chute, formerly a high-water line, now carries the full flow of the river. This wild drop has changed several times in the last decade; don't trust my description or your memory! Eddy out upstream on the right, just above a gorgeous tributary waterfall, and work your way downstream on foot and scout this drop carefully. The best view is from the top from a large rock on river right; the best portage route is on the left.

Here's the way things looked in 1998: Recyclotron, a giant hole that seems to get worse each year, dominates the top of the rapid. There is a clear, left-side route complicated by a breaking wave. After you thread your way between these obstacles you'll confront a powerful chute moving from left to right between two offset holes. The right-hand hole is very dangerous and the left side pourover could cause problems at some water levels. Some paddlers like to run to the left of a breaking wave at midstream, then cut to the right. Others like to catch a left-hand eddy, then ferry back out into the chute. The run-out of the drop is fast and powerful and it will be hard to recover swimmers. Boaters should consider setting a safety rope.

Now the river enters Lower Coliseum, cutting left and roaring through a short, complex boulder garden. A huge, pyramid-shaped rock (Coliseum Rock) looms downstream. There are huge holes on the left, but the right side is much easier. The river still does not let up, moving at full speed into Pete Morgan Rapid. This drop honors the owner of the gas station at the Albright bridge; he gave river gauge readings to inquiring paddlers for many years in the 60s and 70s. The gas station washed away in the 1985 flood, which also rearranged the rapid. The best route is down the left chute, starting on the right side and cutting left to avoid an aggressive stopper at the bottom. It's easily scouted from a cobble bar on the left. Pause for a moment in an eddy and note the unique fluted sandstone columns on the left side of the run-out before moving downstream.

After Pete Morgan Rapid you'll encounter several long Class III+ drops before the river calms down as it approaches the Jenkinsburg bridge. About a mile from the take-out a clear stream cascades in from river right. The slate outcrops at the mouth of this little stream are a great place to look for fossils and catch some sun. Paddle under the bridge and take out on river right.

There is a painted gauge on Route 26 where it crosses the Cheat in Albright. The river can be run at well below a foot; two to four feet would be considered moderate levels, and anything above that is high water. The gauge readings have fluctuated considerably since the 1985 flood, but we now think that it reads about three inches higher than the pre-1985 level.

After Pete Morgan's gas station washed away in 1985, the Albright bridge gauge could not be reported to the National Weather Service in Pittsburgh. There is a gauge under construction in Jenkinsburg, but it is not available yet. The Parsons gauge, 50 miles upstream, is available by phone. Three and a half feet (900 cfs) at Parsons equals about two feet at Albright; 4.5 feet (1,900 cfs) equals three feet at Albright. The actual flow at Jenkinsburg will be roughly 33 percent greater than at Parsons.

The Albright Power Station Gauge is reported on the flow phone operated by the National Weather Service in Pittsburgh (412-262-5290). This gauge previously gave erratic readings, but it was reset and upgraded in 1997. Steve Ingalls, an Ohio boater, worked with several active Cheat River paddlers to create a conversion formula between the Power Station and Bridge gauges. The formula is: Bridge Level = (1.6 x Power Station Level) + .1. The reliability of this formula for levels under 2.0 feet at the Albright bridge gauge has not been determined.

Put in at the Albright bridge (C) or, to avoid a mile or two of flat, uninteresting water, at one of the two campgrounds downstream. The take-out at Jenkinsburg (D) is hard to find and involves some travel on rough dirt roads.

Gauge Conversion Table

Cheat River at Parsons	
3.0 feet	530 cfs
3.5 feet	900 cfs
4.0 feet	1,350 cfs
4.5 feet	1,930 cfs
5.0 feet	2,620 cfs
5.5 feet	3,440 cfs
6.0 feet	4,370 cfs
7.0 feet	6,550 cfs
8.0 feet	9,440 cfs
9.0 feet	12,700 cfs
10.0 feet	16,700 cfs

From the put-in, take Route 26 north to Valley Point. Turn left on Hudson Road, then take a gradual left turn when you reach the four-way intersection at Mount Nebo. The road turns to dirt, passes to the right of a large A-frame house (the Clarks), then descends steeply into the canyon. It is passable by ordinary vehicles but becomes slippery in wet weather. The river can also be reached from Route 7 in Masontown via Bull Run Road; turning left at the first intersection, right at the second. This road is also steep and rough. The Cheat shuttle takes about an hour and a half to run. Glen Miller (304-379-3404) will pick you up in Jenkinsburg and run you back to Albright for a reasonable fee. It saves time and vehicle wear.

Meadow River

The Meadow River contains several sections of excellent whitewater alternating with long stretches of flatwater. The upper segment is quite isolated and difficult to reach, but contains a long stretch of Class IV rapids. The popular middle section part is easier, with many Class III–III+ rapids leading to a take-out at the Route 19 bridge. Below here is a very dangerous Class V–VI stretch that runs into the Gauley River above Lost Paddle Rapid.

Upper Meadow

The Upper Meadow contains seven miles of continuous Class IV–IV+ rapids in a remote, forested valley that is not easy to reach. Eight miles of flatwater separates Russelville and the start of the rapids at Burdette Creek, but an obscure system of dirt roads allows paddlers to bypass the flatwater and get right into the good stuff. This run starts to get pretty serious at high water, so

Section: East Rainelle to Russelville
Counties: Greenbrier, Nicholas, Fayette
USGS Quads: Rainelle, Corliss, Winona
Difficulty: Class III–IV+
Gradient: 32 feet per mile
Average Width: 75 feet
Velocity: Fast
Rescue Index: Remote
Hazards: Natural Weir
Scouting: Natural Weir
Portages: Possibly at very high water levels
Scenery: Beautiful
Highlights: Continuous rapids
Gauge: Mt. Lookout gauge

Runnable Water Levels	Minimum	Maximum
Mt. Lookout gauge	5.2 feet	6.6 feet

Additional Information: Summersville Dam, (304) 872-5809; Huntington District of U.S. Army Corps of Engineers, (304) 529-5127

caution is advised.

After the lower put-in, the rapids start slowly and begin to pick up speed. They quickly convert to obstructed, Class IV boulder drops, The Rapids, that continue without let-up in unbroken succession for four miles. The drops are often obstructed and frequently contain powerful holes at medium to high water levels. The banks are choked with rhododendrons and mountain laurels, so that most scouting must be done from eddies. This technique requires considerable experience, good boat control, and careful spacing between party members. A railroad on river right is convenient when walking out.

One place that should be scouted is Natural Weir, a seven-foot ledge drop plunging between giant boulders. Get off the river when you see the horizon line and take a good look, because all three chutes present problems. Of particular concern is the undercut rock found in the run on the right. Then, as suddenly as the hard rapids started, they end. The remaining three miles to the take-out is a fast run over easy Class II–III rapids.

To reach the put-in (A), take Route 41 to US 60 and head east. At Route 10 (the end of Corliss Road) take a left, then an immediate right onto a paved road. Bear right where the pavement ends, then follow the road through an old strip mine. Continue until you see the river on your left. In the summer, when the leaves are out, you will have to look hard to catch a glimpse of the river. You can also get to the river by following Snake Island Road north from East Rainelle and turning into the City Dump three miles downriver. This does not bypass the flatwater section, but the paddling passes quickly at high flows. Take out at the bridge on Quinwood-Nutterville Road (B), which intersects Route 41 a few miles upstream of Nallen.

Middle Meadow

The stretch between Russelville to Nallen is flat as it runs quietly along Route 41. A mile below Nallen, rapids

Section: Russelville to US 19 Bridge
Counties: Nicholas, Fayette
USGS Quads: Winona, Summersville Dam
Difficulty: Class III–III+
Gradient: 39 feet per mile
Average Width: 75 feet
Velocity: Fast
Rescue Index: Accessible to remote
Hazards: Some undercut rocks
Scouting: None
Portages: Possibly at very high water levels
Scenery: Beautiful
Highlights: Miracle Mile
Gauge: Mt. Lookout gauge

Runnable Water Levels	Minimum	Maximum
Mt. Lookout gauge	5.2 feet	6.6 feet

Additional Information: Summersville Dam, (304) 872-5809;
    Huntington District of U.S. Army Corps of Engineers,
    (304) 529-5127

appear. The river drops through boulder gardens between steep, forested banks, and then moves away from the road after passing a water treatment plant. Locals call this section the "Miracle Mile" because of its accessability and great play boating opportunities. The roadside section is a delightful place to hang out, even at low water levels. Interesting Class III–III+ rapids alternate with pools all the way to the take-out. As you travel, the gorge gets deeper and deeper. Soon spectacular, high, sandstone cliffs, fringed with hemlock, appear. Some of these drops develop a bad attitude at high water and must be approached cautiously. The biggest danger is the steep, uphill climb at the take-out (D), just below the Route 19 bridge on river left.

Lower Meadow

The Lower Meadow below the Route 19 bridge may be the most dangerous stretch of whitewater in West Virginia. While the gradient is not severe, the river has a drop pool character and many of its rapids flow around and under giant undercut boulders and dangerous rock sieves. Even the easier drops have run-outs that push you toward dangerous traps. There have been three fatal accidents on this section claiming the lives of expert paddlers in addition to several close calls. The last victim was a veteran guide with over 100 successful runs. But the unique challenge and spectacular beauty of the river draws a small group of paddlers to the run despite its risks. Those who follow them should be very, very careful.

The Lower Meadow was first run by Jack Wright, Tom Irwin, Frank and Bonnie Birdsong, Rick Rigg, and Donna Berglund in the fall of 1972. But while local experts run the river frequently and without incident these days, it is a very serious undertaking for first-timers. You and your party should be in top form and ready for anything. Fortunately, portaging the major rapids via an old railroad bed on the right is not difficult. The active railroad tracks on the left are much higher, but are ideal for walking out. Wear a good pair of shoes to facilitate your carries. It is always wise to go down with someone who knows the river, particularly at higher levels. The following descriptions are taken from notes provided by Donnie Hudspeth, a veteran guide for North American River Runners in Hico, West Virginia.

The first hard rapid, Rites of Passage (Class V), can be seen below the Route 19 bridge. A fast approach takes you over a four-foot ledge; the hole tries to shove you under a large rock on the left. The second drop, Hell's Gate (Class V+), trapped a veteran local guide underwater in a deep drain on the left side. Routes vary with water levels, and require you to catch small, guarded eddies to avoid dangerous rocks downstream.

A short distance later you'll encounter three steep, closely spaced drops. In the first, Brink of Disaster (Class V), a messy approach between gnarly pour-overs launches you over a 10-foot ledge. The run-out crashes angrily into the left bank and rushes toward an ugly Class VI rapid. The water in between, pushy and dangerous even at low water flows, carried an expert Southern paddler to his death at 2,500 cfs. Below is Coming Home, Sweet Jesus (Class V+), where after a tricky approach the river drops seven feet into a powerful ledge hole. The hole breaks right and pushes you into "the box," a huge drain under a giant boulder. A boater swam under the boulder in the 70s! And Sieve City (Class V+) is just below. At low flows there is a tight left line above horrible sieves. At levels over 650 cfs a "saner" right hand route opens up. Fortunately, all three drops can be easily portaged via an old railroad grade on river right.

You are now one mile into the run. The river opens up here for a half-mile stretch of good, Class IV rapids. There are multiple lines here and the water doesn't always push you into trouble. A short pool lies above Gateway to Heaven. After a tricky series of slots, the river narrows into a steep slide that should be scouted. There are some easier rapids between here and Let's Make a Deal (Class IV+). Here, the river tilts down a long, pushy, Class III+ approach into a strong hole. Below here are three doors;

Meadow River • West Virginia

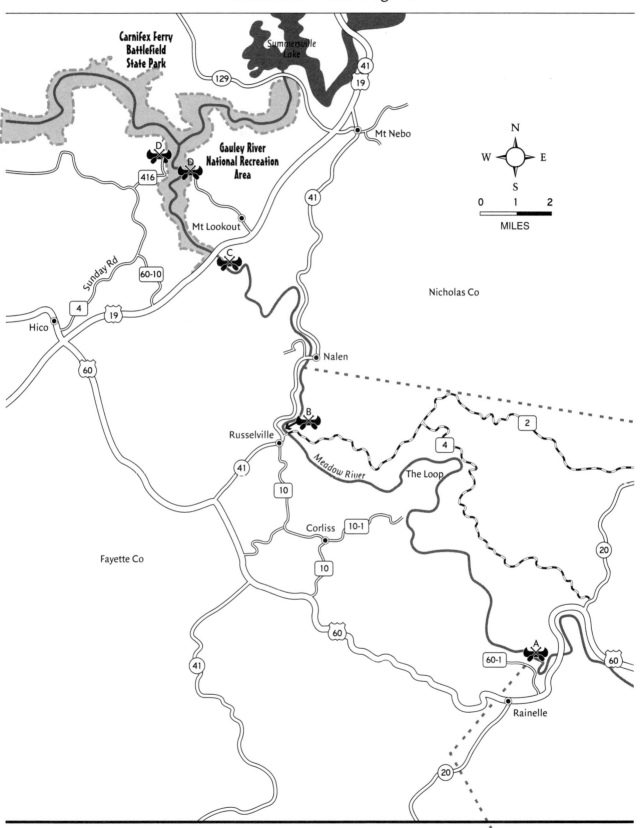

Section: US 19 Bridge to Carnifex Ferry
Counties: Nicholas, Fayette
USGS Quad: Summersville Dam
Difficulty: Class IV–VI
Gradient: 94 feet per mile (two miles at 125 feet per mile)
Average Width: 75 feet
Velocity: Fast
Rescue Index: Remote
Hazards: The entire section
Scouting: The entire section
Portages: Most big drops are often carried
Scenery: Beautiful
Highlights: Outstandingly beautiful canyon
Gauge: Mt. Lookout gauge

Runnable Water Levels	Minimum	Maximum
Mt. Lookout gauge	4.5 feet	6.0 feet

Additional Information: Summersville Dam, (304) 872-5809;
    Huntington District of U.S. Army Corps of Engineers,
    (304) 529-5127

the left looks tempting, but it's blocked by downstream rocks. The middle door is the best choice, a tight but runnable slot, and the far right is the safest. There's a nice pool below where you can relax and collect your wits before moving on.

Soon a huge bluff on the left marks the beginning of the Islands section. At the first island run right down a long stretch of Class III–IV. At the second island, the center line is blocked. A top expert from the Washington, DC area was vertically pinned and killed here, so finish on the left. Immediately downstream you'll encounter a big sliding ledge that tends to shove you left under a nasty undercut. There are a few Class IVs between here and the last big rapid, Double Undercut (Class V+), which can be easily scouted and carried on the left. It consists of a six- to seven-foot horseshoe-shaped ledge into a bad hole. The undercut right side is very hard to avoid. Below

here there's a nice stretch of Class III–IV water to the confluence with the Gauley.

To find the put-in (C), take the southbound lane of Route 19 and stop on the north side, about 200 yards above the bridge. On the other side of the guard rail is a steep dirt road down to the river. Most boaters take out at the base of Mt. Lookout Road (D), which turns into a very steep, rough dirt track as it approaches the river. You can also reach the river via Sunday Road (D'), but the approach to the river is even steeper. Both roads leave Route 19 on well-marked roads. Or you could run Lost Paddle Rapid and continue down the Upper Gauley.

The flow of the Meadow is measured at the Mt. Lookout gauge, just above the confluence with the Gauley. The upper and middle stretches are runnable at about 800 cfs, but most people will want 1,000–1,200 cfs for a good run. Anything over 2,000 cfs is considered high and makes the upper section rather pushy. The Lower Meadow is run between 450 and 1,500 cfs; most veterans consider 750 cfs ideal.

Mt. Lookout Gauge Conversions

4.2 feet	200 cfs
4.6 feet	500 cfs
5.0 feet	720 cfs
5.2 feet	840 cfs
5.4 feet	940 cfs
5.6 feet	1,140 cfs
5.8 feet	1,310 cfs
6.0 feet	1,500 cfs
6.2 feet	1,700 cfs
6.4 feet	1,900 cfs
6.6 feet	2,120 cfs
6.8 feet	2,360 cfs
7.0 feet	2,620 cfs
8.0 feet	4,100 cfs
9.0 feet	5,900 cfs
10.0 feet	8,000 cfs

Cranberry River

The headwaters of the Gauley River contain many outstanding whitewater streams. The best are collectively referred to as the "fruit basket" and the Cranberry is the sweetest of them all. Born along the state's high mountain backbone, it drains a remarkable wilderness area called the Cranberry Backcountry. The water is crystal clear and flows through an unspoiled Appalachian forest. The South Fork gathers in the Cranberry Glades, a unique, high-altitude swamp filled with rare plants. Part of it can be viewed from a boardwalk accessible via USFS Road 102. A dirt road (USFS Road 76) runs along the river from the Glades to Cranberry Campground, but it is gated and closed to motorized vehicles. Below this seldom-traveled wilderness run is an intense roadside section and a delightful intermediate wilderness stretch.

Section: Above Cranberry Recreation Area to Gauley River
Counties: Pocahontas, Webster, Nicholas,
USGS Quads: Lobelia, Webster Springs SE, Webster Springs SW, Canden on Gauley
Difficulty: Class II–V, depending on section
Gradient: 60 feet per mile
Average Width: 50 feet
Velocity: Fast
Rescue Index: Accessible to remote
Hazards: Steep technical rapids in upper section
Scouting: S Turn
Portages: None
Scenery: Beautiful
Highlights: Unspoiled wooded surroundings
Gauge: Richwood gauge; Summersville Dam, (304) 872-5809

Runnable Water Levels	Minimum	Maximum
Above Cranberry Rec. Area	4.6 feet	Flood stage
Below Cranberry Rec. Area	3.5 feet	5.0 feet

Additional Information: U.S. Army Corps of Engineers at Charleston, (304) 529-5127

Wilderness Section

This uppermost "wilderness" section is occasionally run at very high water, but it is difficult to catch up. You'll need high water—over 4.6 feet on the gauge at Richwood Bridge. Park near the locked gate at the end of the Cranberry Glades parking lot (A), shoulder your boat, and carry down the road until a small stream appears on the right. This is the South Fork. Initially the river meanders through a densely vegetated swamp, but it abruptly picks up speed and doesn't let up until the end. Most rapids are straightforward, open Class II–IIIs, but you should keep alert for small-stream tree hazards. Below the Dogway Fork you'll encounter the section known as The Roughs. The water reaches a Class IV rating here; then things calm back down until you reach the Cranberry Recreation Area downstream.

Upper Cranberry

The stretch from Cranberry Campground (B) to the Woodbine Bridge (C) is known as the Upper Cranberry. This is a small, steep, busy stream flowing swiftly around giant boulders. At low water flows the rapids are scrapy and very tight (Class IV), requiring intense maneuvering. At high water the drops open up and become more powerful; a lot like Maryland's Upper Yough. This section can be scouted from the road, where ample pullovers provide a variety of camping and access points.

After a mile of flatwater the river drops over a complex series of ledges; below here one steep drop follows another. Most can be scouted from your boat, but don't be afraid to stretch your legs if necessary. Toward the end of the run you'll encounter a nasty, blind, Class IV+ rapid called S Turn. A giant boulder marks the top of this drop. The left side entry looks pretty easy, but once you turn the corner there's no stopping! The water carries you into a second turn where you have to cut precisely between huge boulders. This is a tight and nasty move, so make

Cranberry River • West Virginia

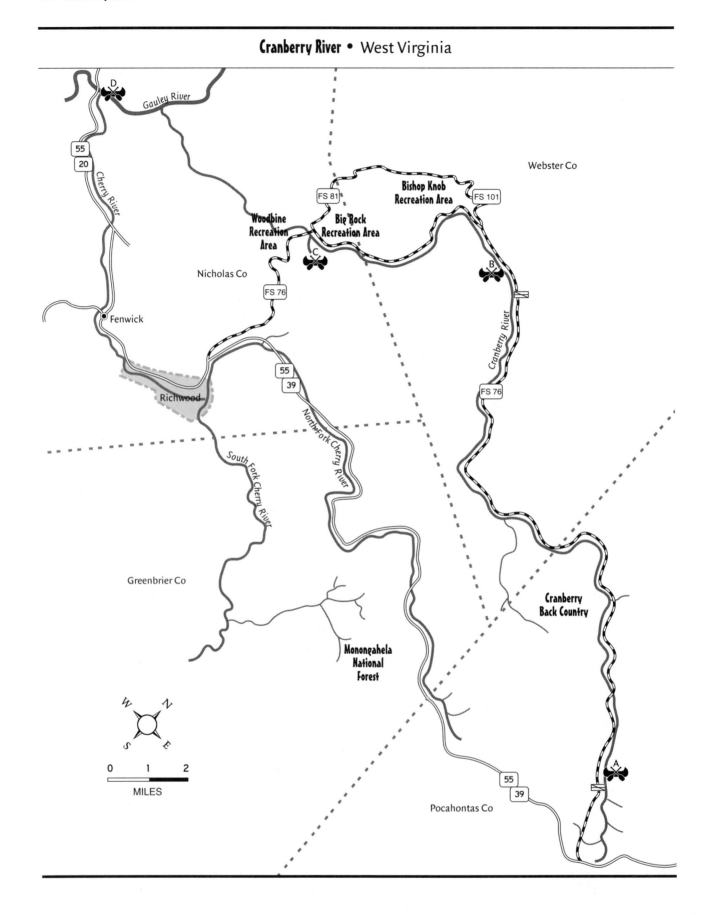

Gauley River

55
20

Cherry River

Webster Co

Bishop Knob
Recreation Area

FS 81

FS 101

Woodbine
Recreation
Area

Big Rock
Recreation Area

Nicholas Co

C

B

FS 76

Fenwick

Cranberry River

FS 76

55
39

Richwood

South Fork Cherry River

North Fork Cherry River

Greenbrier Co

Cranberry
Back Country

Monongahela
National
Forest

N
W   E
S

0   1   2
MILES

55
39

Pocahontas Co

A

sure you look it over first. The river starts to let up below here, but there are still a few more challenging drops before you float under the Woodbine Bridge.

Lower Cranberry

Below Woodbine the river changes character from a tough expert run to something suitable for intermediates. It starts out with two miles of practically continuous Class II–III rapids, then narrows down and picks up speed. The rapids culminate in what was once the Class V Cranberry Split. The infamous Split boulder was pushed aside by a flood, but although the rapid is probably no more than a Class III+, it's still a scramble to get by on the right. Here the river rushes to the right of a brushy island and necks down to about 10 yards wide. The tricky rapids downstream seem easy by comparison.

After five miles of paddling, the Cranberry flows into the Gauley. This is a big, powerful river with many wide-open Class II–III rapids, hidden boulders, and holes. Proceed downstream to the WV Route 20 Bridge at Curtin for an easy take-out. Because both the Cranberry and the Gauley flow in a westerly direction, the glare of the sun makes it hard to read the water and sunglasses are recommended for afternoon paddling.

Gauge information is obtained from the U.S. Army Corps of Engineers at the Summersville Dam (304-872-5809) or Charleston (304-529-5127). The latter gives you access to the USGS Richwood Gauge on the Cranberry at Woodbine; 3.5 feet (300 cfs) is the minimum flow; 5.0 feet (1500 cfs) would be considered high water. The Craigsville Gauge, which is listed on both recordings, measures the inflow to Summersville Lake. It should read at least 11.6 feet to justify a trip to the headwaters. The gauge itself is just downstream of Woodbine Bridge on river left.

The shuttle is easy. USFS Road 76 leaves WV 39 just outside Richwood, giving access to Woodbine and Big Rock. There's a nice restaurant at the turn-off. USFS Road 102 leaves WV 39 for the Cranberry Glades about 10 miles further uphill. The Curtin bridge (D) on the Gauley is reached via WV Routes 20 and 46

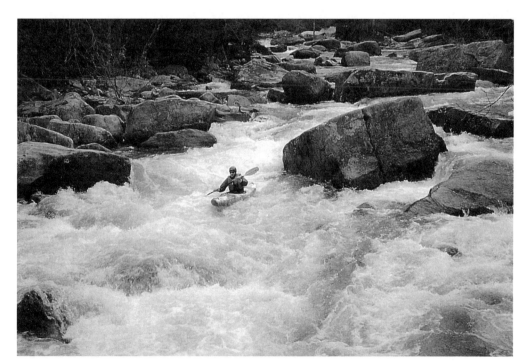

Chris Kerr paddling S Turn on the upper Cranberry. Photo by .

APPENDICES

Appendix A

Water Level Resources

National Weather Service

The National Weather Service accepts the main federal responsibility for disseminating current, forecast, and hydrological information to the public. The main office in Maryland operates a system of satellites that accepts gauge readings from USGS gauges. The regional river forecast centers collect information from local offices and distribute forecasts and warnings. Local offices are responsible for maintaining a river- and rainfall-reporting network within their hydrological service area and for local distribution of information. You may also access the NWS via the Web at http://www.nws.noaa.gov.

Main Office

National Weather Service
National Oceanic and Atmospheric Administration
Department of Commerce
1325 East West Highway
Silver Spring, MD 20910-3283
(301) 427-7622

River Forecast Centers

Lower Mississippi River Forecast Center
National Weather Service
62300 Airport Road
Slidel, LA 70460
(504) 641-4343

Middle Atlantic River Forecast Center
National Weather Service
227 West Beaver Avenue
Rider Bldg. No. 2, 4th Floor
State College, PA 16801
(814) 234-9701

Ohio River Forecast Center
National Weather Service
1901 South State Route 134
Wilmington, OH 45177
(513) 383-0527

Southeast River Forecast Center
National Weather Service
4 Falcon Drive
Peachtree, GA 30269
(404) 486-0028

National Water Information Center

The National Water Information Center is designed to be a hub for the dissemination of water resources information to all inquirers; call (800) 426-9000. This toll-free number will take your information requests and refer you to the appropriate source of hydrological information. E-mail requests can be sent to h2oinfo@usgs-gov.

National Water Data Exchange

The National Water Data Exchange (NAWDEX) is a group of water-oriented organizations working together to improve access to water data. Its primary objective is to assist users of water data and water information in the identification, location, and acquisition of water data.

National Water Data Exchange
US Geological Survey
421 National Center
Reston, VA 22092
(703) 648-6848

USGS Water Resource Division District Offices

The United States Geological Survey is the principal supplier of hydrological information in the United States. This agency maintains the system of automated gauges reporting river stages (often via satellite) to the National Weather Service and other agencies. The Water Resource

Division District Offices of the United States Geological Survey are NAWDEX assistance centers that can provide the public with water data and answer questions on the water resources of their specific regions.

Alabama

U.S. Geological Survey
2350 Fairlane Drive, Suite 120
Montgomery, AL 36116
(334) 213-2332

Connecticut

U.S. Geological Survey
Abraham A. Ribicoff Federal Building
450 Main Street, Rm 525
Hartford, CT 06103
(860) 240-3060

Delaware

U.S. Geological Survey
300 South New Street
Federal Bldg., Rm 1201
Dover, DE 19901-4907
(302) 573-6241

District of Columbia: See Maryland

Georgia

U.S. Geological Survey
Peachtree Business Center, Suite 130
3039 Amwiler Road
Atlanta, GA 30360-2824
(770) 903-9100

Kentucky

U.S. Geological Survey
9818 Bluegrass Parkway
Louisville, KY 40299
(502) 493-1900

Maine

U.S. Geological Survey
26 Ganneston Drive
Augusta, ME 04330
(207) 622-8208

Maryland

U.S. Geological Survey
8987 Yellow Brick Road
Baltimore, MD 21237
(410) 238-4200

Massachusetts

U.S. Geological Survey
28 Lord Road, Suite 280
Marlborough, MA 01752
(508) 490-5000

New Hampshire

U.S. Geological Survey
361 Commerce Way
Pembroke, NH 03275-3718
(603) 226-7800

New York

U.S. Geological Survey
425 Jordan Road
Troy, NY 12180
(518) 285-5600

North Carolina

U.S. Geological Survey
3916 Sunset Ridge Road
Raleigh, NC 27607
(919) 571-4000

Pennsylvania

U.S. Geological Survey
840 Market Street
Lemoyne, PA 17043-1586
(717) 730-6900

South Carolina

U.S. Geological Survey
720 Gracern Road
Stephenson Center, Suite 129
Columbia, SC 29210
(803) 750-6100

Tennessee

U.S. Geological Survey
810 Broadway, Suite 500
Nashville, TN 37203
(615) 736-5424 (x 3123)

Vermont

U.S. Geological Survey
361 Commerce Way
Pembroke, NH 03275
(603) 225-4681

Virginia

U.S. Geological Survey
3600 West Broad Street, Rm 606
Richmond, VA 23230
(804) 278-4750 (x 227)

West Virginia

U.S. Geological Survey
11 Dunbar Street
Charleston, WV 25301
(304) 347-5130

U.S. Army Corps of Engineers Offices

The Army Corps of Engineers builds and operates most public dams and water projects in the United States. Information on Corps projects, dam release schedules, and current releases can be obtained from district offices.

National

Public Affairs Office
U.S. Army Corps of Engineers
20 Massachusetts Avenue, NW
Washington, DC 20314
(202) 272-0010

Division and District

North Atlantic Division
U.S. Army Corps of Engineers
90 Church Street
New York, NY 10007-2979
(212) 264-7500

Baltimore District
U.S. Army Corps of Engineers
10 South Howard Street
Baltimore, MD 21201
(301) 962-2809

New York District
U.S. Army Corps of Engineers
26 Federal Plaza
New York, NY 10728-0090
(212) 264-2188

Norfolk District
U.S. Army Corps of Engineers
803 Front Street
Norfolk, VA 23510-1096
(804) 441-7606

Philadelphia District
U.S. Army Corps of Engineers
100 Penn Square East
Philadelphia, PA 19107-3390
(215) 656-6515

Ohio River Division
U.S. Army Corps of Engineers
P.O. Box 1159
Cincinnati, OH 45201-1159
(513) 684-3010

Huntington District
U.S. Army Corps of Engineers
502 Eighth Street
Huntington, WV 25701-2070
(304) 529-5452

Louisville District
U.S. Army Corps of Engineers
P.O. Box 59
Louisville, KY 40201-0059
(502) 582-6503

Nashville District
U.S. Army Corps of Engineers
P.O. Box 1070
Nashville, TN 37202-1070
(615) 736-7161

Pittsburgh District
U.S. Army Corps of Engineers
Federal Building
1000 Liberty Avenue, Rm 1801
Pittsburgh, PA 15222-4186
(412) 644-4130

South Atlantic Division
U.S. Army Corps of Engineers
77 Forsyth Street, SW, Rm 322
Atlanta, GA 30303-3490
(404) 331-7444

U.S. Army Corps of Engineers Support Center
P.O. Box 1600
Huntsville, AL 35807-4301
(205) 895-1691

Charleston District
U.S. Army Corps of Engineers
P.O. Box 919
334 Meeting Street
Charleston, SC 29402-0019
(803) 727-4201

Mobile District
U.S. Army Corps of Engineers
P.O. Box 2288
Mobile, AL 36628-0001
(205) 690-2505

Savannah District
U.S. Army Corps of Engineers
P.O. Box 889
Savannah, GA 31402-0889
(912) 652-5270

Wilmington District
U.S. Army Corps of Engineers
P.O. Box 1890
Wilmington, NC 28402-1890
(910) 251-4626

River Services, Inc.

A private company, River Services, Inc., offers a real-time, computer-based, hydrological information service.
River Services, Inc.
3414 Morningwood Drive, Suite 11
Olney, MD 20832
(301) 774-1616

Although the cost of this information service is probably out of the reach of individuals (currently a minimum of $100 per month, including one hour a month of connection time), clubs and outfitters might be interested. Using your personal computer with a modem, a toll-free number, and an access code provided by River Services, you can access a customized computer database of river forecasts and river levels (as well as a wide variety of other information). You should be able to get current readings for every USGS gauge that sends data to the National Weather Service satellite system.

Waterline National River Information Hotline

Waterline is the largest single telephone source of river information available to the public in the United States. Waterline is fully automated, operates continuously, and reports on over 1,100 river levels and flows. Most Waterline reports are updated six to twenty-four times per day via satellite directly from the gauges.

To use the service you need to know the six-digit code for the desired site. These codes are available by mail, fax, or Internet. For codes by mail or fax, call Waterline's customer service number at (800) 945-3376. To have codes and other information mailed to you, press 0 to speak to the operator or leave a message. Staff members are available 9 A.M. to 5 P.M. Eastern Standard Time. To get codes by fax at any time, follow the recorded instructions to fax yourself a state code list. Once you have the list, call back and get the information on the states you desire. The fax system responds within two minutes of your request. Site codes are also available on the Internet at http://h2oline.com.

Once you have the desired site code, you can call Waterline's 800 or 900 hotlines from a touch-tone phone. With the 800 line (800-297-4243), you can set up an account and access code to receive information. This line costs 68 cents per minute. A twelve- minute block of time is billed to your Visa or MasterCard. Unused time remains for future calls. You can recharge your account anytime by pressing 999 and following the prompts. Time spent setting up or recharging your account is free.

The 900 line (900-726-4243) does not require an account, but is available only if you call from home. The cost is $1.28 per minute and will be charged to your phone bill. Federal government rules require that you be eighteen years or older or have parental permission to call a 900 number.

After the initial messages, Waterline will ask for a six-digit site code. Enter the code whenever you want. You can interupt the message with a new site code whenever you want. You can also program Waterline to play a specified list of sites whenever you call. The average call time is two billable minutes. Once you are familiar with the system, a one-minute phone call will yield one to four readings for a single river or three to four different river readings.

Waterline also publishes the Waterline Guide to River Levels and Flow Information. This guide contains all the Waterline site codes as well as every known public source of current river level information in the United States including the Internet resources. Each copy includes a precharged access card with twelve minutes of time on Waterline's 800 number.

Appendix B

Map Sources

USGS Topographic Maps

Topographic maps are available at many outdoor shops and from other commercial vendors, but for the best prices and selection, you should order directly from the USGS of the Department of the Interior (but see TVA description below). They sell the topographic maps in the standard 7.5-minute (1:24,000) series of quadrangles and in a variety of other sizes as well. Write for the Index to Topographic and Other Map Coverage and the companion Catalog of Topographic and Other Published Maps for each state in which you are interested.

Mapping Distribution
U.S. Geological Survey
Box 25286 Federal Center
Building 41
Denver, CO 80225
(303) 236-7477

(Some of you will remember that the USGS used to have an Eastern and a Western Distribution Branch;that's no longer true.)

County Road Maps

Alabama

State of Alabama Highway Department
Bureau of State Planning
Attn: Map Room
Montgomery, AL 36130
(334) 832-5637
Carto-Craft Maps, Inc.
738 Shades Mountain Plaza
Birmingham, AL
(205) 822-2103

Georgia

Department of Transportation
Map Room, Room 10
Number 2, Capitol Square
Atlanta, GA 30334

Kentucky

Map Sales
Department of Commerce
Frankfort, KY 40601
(502) 564-6998

Maryland

Map Distribution Sales
Maryland State Highway Administration
Brooklandville, MD 21022

North Carolina

Head of Location and Survey Unit
N.C. Department of Transportation
Division of Highways
Attn: Map Sales
P.O. Box 25201
Raleigh, NC 27611

Tennessee

Map Sales Office
Tennessee Department of Transportation
505 Deaderick Street
Suite 1000, James K. Polk Building
Nashville, TN 37219
(615) 741-2195

Virginia

Department of Highways and Transportation
Attn: Map Sales
1221 East Broad Street
Richmond, VA 23219

West Virginia

West Virginia Department of Highways
Planning Division, Attn: Map Sales
1900 Kanawha Boulevard East
Bldg 5, Rm A848
Charleston, WV 25305-0430
(304) 559-3113

Other Map Sources

DeLorme Publishing Co.
P.O. Box 298
Freeport, ME 04032
(207) 865-4171 or (800) 227-1656
Marshall Penn York, Inc.
1538 Erie Boulevard
West Syracuse, NY 13204
(315) 422-2162

Appendix C

Whitewater Schools

The following list includes many of the nation's leading whitewater schools of instruction.

New England Outdoor Center
P.O. Box 669
Millinocket, ME 04462
(800) 766-7238

Zoar Outdoor Paddling School
Mohawk Trail
P.O. Box 245
Charlemont, MA 01339
(800) 532-7483.

Saco Bound's Northern Waters School
Box 119-C
Center Conway, NH 03813
(603) 447-2177

W.I.L.D./W.A.T.E.R.S.
Route 28 at the Glen
Warrensburg, NY 12885
(518) 494-4984 or (888) WILD H2O.

Endless River Adventures
P.O. Box 246
Bryson City, NC 28713
(704) 488-6199

Nantahala Outdoor Center
13077 Highway 19 W
Bryson City, NC 28713
(704)488-6737 or (800) 232-7238

Riversport School of Paddling
213 Yough Street
Confluence, PA 15424
(814) 395-5744 or (800) 216-6991

Whitewater Challangers Outdoor Adventure Center
P.O. Box 8
White Haven, PA 18661
(717) 443-9532

The Kayak Centre
9 Phillips Street
Wickford, RI 02852
(401) 295-4400

Adventure Quest
P.O. Box 184
Woodstock, VT 05091
(802) 484-3202

Bob Taylor's Appomattox River Company
614 North Main Street
Farmville, VA 23901
(804) 392-6645 or (800) 442-4837

Appendix D

Organizations

American Canoe Association
7432 Alban Station Boulevard, Suite B-226
Springfield, VA 22150
(703) 451-0141

America Outdoors
P.O. Box 10847
Knoxville, TN 37939
(423) 558-3595; (423) 558-3598 (fax)

American Rivers
1025 Vermont Avenue NW, Suite 720
Washington, DC 20005
(202) 347-7550

American Whitewater Affiliation
P.O. Box 85
Phoenicia, NY 12464

Friends of the Cheat
P.O. Box 182
Bruceton Mills, WV 26525
(304) 379-3141; (304) 379-3142 (fax)

Environmental Defense Fund
257 Park Avenue S
Ney York, NY 10010
(800) 684-3322

International Rivers Network
1847 Berkley Way
Berkley, CA 94703
(510) 848-1155

National Association for Search and Rescue
4500 Southgate Place, Suite 100
Chantilly, VA 20151-1714
(703) 222-6277

The Trade Association of Paddlesports
12455 North Wauwatosa Road
Mequon, WI 53097
(414) 242-5228

River Network
4000 Albermarle Street, NW, Suite 303
Washington, DC 20016
(202) 364-2550

River Watch
c/o American Rivers
1025 Vermont Avenue NW, Suite 720
Washington, DC 20005
(202) 547-6900 or (800) 296-6900

The Sierra Club
85 2nd Street, 2nd Floor
San Francisco, CA 94105-3441
(415) 977-5500

West Virginia Rivers Coalition
P.O. Box 578
Buckhannon, WV 26201
(304) 472-0025

Wilderness Society
900 17th Street, NW
Washington, DC 20016
(202) 833-2300

Appendix E

Web Resources

What follows are the World Wide Web sites and e-mail addresses available on the Internet. All Web addresses should have the http:// prefix. Keep in mind that the World Wide Web is a transient medium and changes often. If a Web address is unavailable, try looking for it through your favorite search engine.

American Canoe Association
Web: www.aca-paddler.org
E-mail: acadirect@aol.com

American Rivers
Web: www.amrivers.org/
E-mail: amrivers@amrivers.org

America Outdoors
Web: www.americaoutdoors.org
E-mail: infoacct@americaoutdoors.org

American Whitewater Affiliation
Web: www.awa.org

Blackwater Falls State Park, WV
Web: wvweb.com/www/blackwater_falls.html

Blue Ridge Outfitters, WV
Web: www.broraft.com
E-mail: broraft@intrepid.net

Environmental Defense Fund
Web: www.edf.org

Friends of the Cheat
Web: www.pitt.edu/~steckel/cheat/index.html

Great Outdoor Recreation Page (G.O.R.P.)
Web: www.gorp.com

Haw River Paddlers, NC
Web: www2.emji.net/haw

International Rivers Network
Web: www.irn.org
E-mail:irnweb@irn.org

Nantahala Outdoor Center, NC
Web: www.nocweb.com/
E-mail: programs@noc.com

National Association of Search and Rescue
Web: www.nasar.org
E-mail: info@nasar.org

National Organization of Whitewater Rodeos
Web: www.nowr.org

National Park Service
Web: www.nps.gov

National Weather Service
Web: www.nws.noaa.gov/

The Trade Association Paddlesports
Web: www.viewit.com/NAPSA/

The River Network
Web:www.teleport.com/~rivernet/
E-mail: rivernet2@aol.com

Sierra Club
Web: www.sierraclub.org

Tennessee Valley Authority (TVA)
Web: www.tva.gov

Tennessee Valley Canoe Club
Web: home.earthlink.net/~smgibbon/tvcc/

U.S. Army Corps of Engineers
Web: www.usace.army.mil

US Forest Service
Web: www.fs.fed.us/

USGS
Web: water.usgs.gov

West Virginia Tourism Whitewater Page
Web: www.state.wv.us/tourism/whitewat/default.htm

West Virginia Rivers Coalition
Web: www.msys.net/wvrc/
E-mail: wvrc@msys.net